THE WOMEN'S HEALTH BIBLE

AN ESSENTIAL GUIDE TO HEALTH AND
WELLBEING FOR EVERY WOMAN

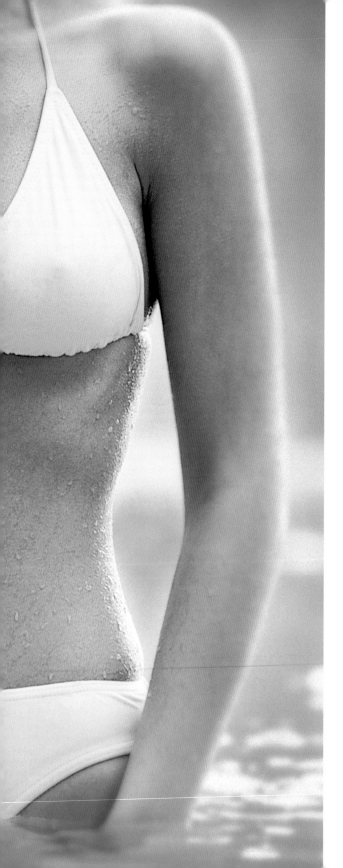

This edition first published in the UK in 2004 by
Rodale International Ltd
7–10 Chandos Street
London W1G 9AD
www.rodale.co.uk

Designed by Briony Chappell

Printed and bound in China

1 3 5 7 9 8 6 4 2

A CIP record for this book is available from the British Library
ISBN 1–4050–7330–1

This Edition Published for Index Books Ltd 2005

NOTICE

This book is intended as a reference volume only, not as a
medical manual. The information given here is designed to
help you make informed decisions about your health. It is not
intended as a substitute for any treatment that may have been
prescribed by your doctor. If you suspect that you have a
medical problem, we urge you to seek competent medical help.

   Mention of specific companies, organizations or authorities
in this book does not imply endorsement by the publisher, nor
does mention of specific companies, organizations or
authorities in the book imply that they endorse it.

   Internet addresses and telephone numbers given in this
book were accurate at the time it went to press.

Contents

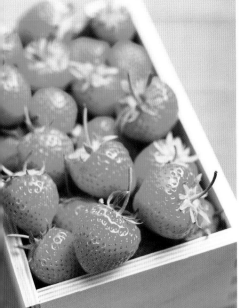

Introduction vi

PART 1: What's going on?
The wise woman's health planner

Chapter 1: The Female Body, Decade by Decade 2

PART 2: Your stay well, stay young 'to do' list

Chapter 2: Vitamins, Minerals and Nutrition:
the Complete Plan 28

Chapter 3: Using Herbs Wisely 49

Chapter 4: The Ultimate Ladder of Fitness 63

Chapter 5: *The Women's Health Bible*
Guide to Your Perfect Weight 80

Chapter 6: A Real-life Guide to Stress Relief 99

Chapter 7: A Stop-Smoking Programme
That Can't Fail 108

Chapter 8: Sun-proof (and Age-proof)
Your Skin 116

Chapter 9: Beauty Products That Rejuvenate . .122

Chapter 10: Balancing Your Emotions 130

Chapter 11: Healthy Sex at Any Age 142

PART 3: Hormonal wellness: the best-ever life-stage strategies

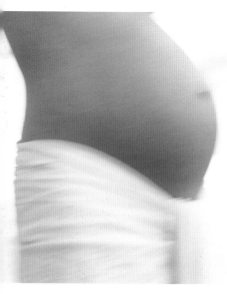

Chapter 12: PMS and Menstrual Discomforts 150

Chapter 13: Contraception 158

Chapter 14: Pregnancy 164

Chapter 15: Childbirth 169

Chapter 16: Infertility 172

Chapter 17: Polycystic Ovary Syndrome 177

Chapter 18: Fibroids 181

Chapter 19: Endometriosis 185

Chapter 20: Pelvic Inflammatory Disease 189

Chapter 21: Perimenopause 192

Chapter 22: Menopause 200

PART 4: Primary care: essential protection against major health threats

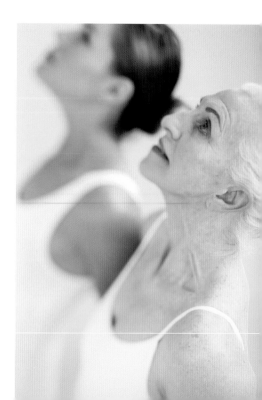

Chapter 23: Heart Disease 216

Chapter 24: High Blood Pressure and Stroke 225

Chapter 25: Diabetes 232

Chapter 26: Cancer 243

Chapter 27: Osteoporosis 259

Chapter 28: Alzheimer's Disease 270

PART 5: An A–Z of Women's Health

Abdominal Fat 276

Anaemia 278

Arthritis 280

Back Problems 284

Blemishes, Pimples and Spots 289

Breast Pain and Tenderness 291

Constipation 293

Depression 296

Fatigue 299

Fibromyalgia (Fibrositis) 302

Food Allergy 306

Haemorrhoids 310

Headaches 311

Irritable Bowel Syndrome 316

Kidney Infections 319

Memory Problems 321

Phobias and Panic Attacks 325

Thinning Hair 327

Urinary Incontinence 330

Urinary Tract Infections 333

Vaginal Dryness 336

Vaginal Infections 337

Varicose Veins 341

Get Fit Forever with Exercise 345

Guidelines for Safe Use of
Supplements 358

Index 364

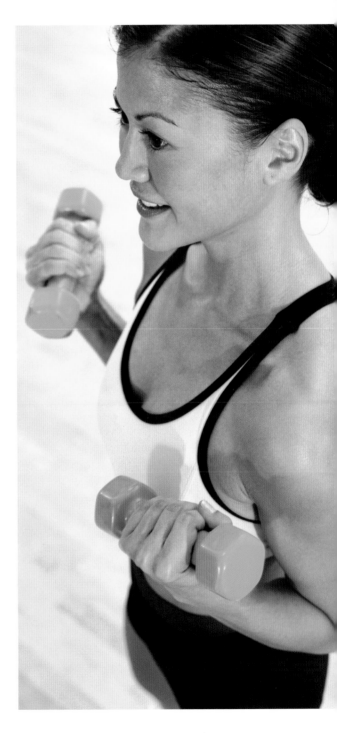

Introduction

Over the past century, remarkable advances in women's health care have almost doubled the average woman's life span, dramatically reduced maternal and infant mortality, and resulted in the development and delivery of medical services and treatments that previous generations could not have imagined. Women are not only living longer, they are also healthier than at any time in history. A new focus on women's health has provided women with greater knowledge and access to information about their health. Women's health issues have been integrated into medical research, health care professional training and clinical practice. Additionally, one of the most important accomplishments over the past decade has been the recognition that women and men have different health needs, and that gender matters in understanding health and disease.

Consider this: in the year 1900, a woman had beaten the odds if she saw her 49th birthday; the average female life expectancy was 48 years. The leading killers then were infectious diseases such as tuberculosis, smallpox, diphtheria and influenza, and the complications of childbirth. But thanks to the triumph of public health programmes including sanitation, vaccinations, health education, preventive health practices, safety and environmental regulations, increased access to health care, new medical diagnostic and treatment interventions, and the implementation of national public health policies, women are now living 30 years longer on average than they did a century ago. Consequently, the challenge is to keep women healthy over the course of their longer life spans.

Today, the major killers of women are chronic illnesses, including cancer, diabetes, heart and lung disease, and stroke, as well as injuries and violence. As much as 50 per cent of the causes of these conditions are linked to preventable behavioural, lifestyle and environmental factors, such as smoking (the single most important cause of premature death in the West), being overweight and lack of physical exercise.

That's why improving health today means focusing on prevention, and putting it to the forefront of our health care agenda. Knowledge is power when it comes to your health. Put prevention into practice and take an important step towards a healthier future for you and your family.

The Women's Health Bible, written by the Editors of *Prevention* – the world's largest circulation health magazine – draws on the wisdom and expertise of the magazine's large team of medical advisors and other healthcare experts, to provide an authoritative and useful reference book.

The Women's Health Bible is a unique health guide to every stage of a woman's life. With it to hand, you can find out about all your health options – medical treatments, natural alternatives, mind-body techniques, home remedies and preventive strategies.

The advice is targeted to a woman's biological needs and, where appropriate, to age and reproductive status. Use the book as a reference guide or symptom finder – or start with the simple, doctor-approved plans for acheiving optimum health.

The book is divided into five sections. **Part 1: What's going on?** is a health planner with preventive recommendations for every age group that can help you to stay healthy throughout your life.

Part 2: Your stay well, stay young 'to do' list shows how you can put these recommendations into practice, with advice on getting more exercise and re-energizing your body, reaching and maintaining your ideal weight, achieving emotional balance, enjoying a healthy sex life and reversing premature signs of ageing.

Part 3: Hormonal wellness discusses specific women's problems and life stages – from PMS to endometriosis, from childbirth to menopause. It looks at the changes that occur, how to get the most out of your doctor, and home and alternative treatments you can try.

Part 4: Primary care examines major health threats, such as heart disease, cancer and diabetes, and gives the latest advice on treating and managing these conditions. Again, the book looks not only at the conventional treatment for these illnesses, but also at home remedies, lifestyle strategies and alternative treatments that can help.

Finally, **Part 5: An A–Z of women's health** is a useful reference guide to dealing with many common complaints, including anaemia, fatigue, headaches and varicose veins.

With practical advice, recommendations and remedies from leading doctors, nutritionists, fitness instructors, psychologists and other health-care experts, *The Women's Health Bible* can help you to lead a healthier life and make the most of the health care options available.

Prevention.

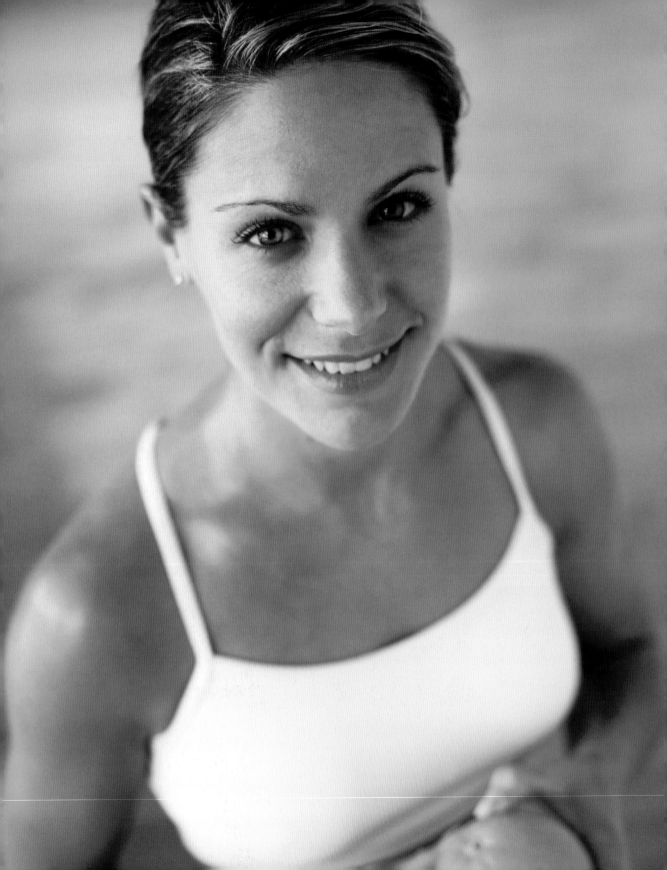

PART 1

What's going on? The wise woman's health planner

The Female Body, Decade by Decade

Centuries from now, anthropologists might look at today's 'over the hill' birthday cards as cultural indicators of women's attitudes towards getting older. Snide remarks about sagging breasts, expanding waistlines and disappearing sex lives may serve to help women shrug off changes as shared – and inevitable – declines.

Imagine, for a moment, an alternative Birthday Card Universe – an equally fertile market where the prevailing message is positive and congratulatory, applauding well-toned muscles, glowing skin, sparkling teeth, sharp eyesight and a reliable memory.

A fantasy, you say? Maybe; maybe not. Take the right steps and, with every birthday you celebrate, you can maintain the vibrancy and healthy glow you had at 20. And it's easier than you might think. Start with *The Women's Health Bible* 'Wellness Checklists' for every stage of a woman's life, from leaving school to career, marriage, kids, menopause, retirement and beyond.

At each life stage, you'll start with the building blocks of wellness: Self-care Checklists, which cover a healthy diet and nutritional solutions to problems that may pop up along the way – such as weight gain, high blood pressure or hot flushes – plus Professional Health Checklists, with special attention to conditions to watch for and medical screens and tests that can help you detect and manage small problems before they become unmanageable.

Once you get oriented, depending on your current age, turn to Part 2, Your Stay Well, Stay Young 'To Do' List, to learn more about getting the right exercise and the right vitamin and mineral supplements, and other preventive steps on your course to good health and well-being. You'll find step-by-step action plans for customizing medical advice for your personal needs.

Sceptical? If you don't think any of these strategies can really make a difference in 20 or 30 years, ask Dr Michael Lichtenstein at the University of Texas Health Science Center. 'People who have lifelong health maintenance habits like exercising and eating healthily will live long and healthy lives,' he says.

Whatever stage of life you're at, you can take the road to lifelong health and end up being a 70 year old who may never lay eyes on another 'over the hill' birthday card.

Ages 18 to 35

Imagine a group of runners at the start of a race. Their bodies are in superior shape, they're focused and they're primed to do their best.

As a young woman, you're at a similar starting line. You have every reason to expect a long and healthy life. Women's life expectancy has increased. Women aren't letting disease slow them down, either. In the past, a cancer diagnosis meant a slim chance of survival. But now, thanks to improved methods of prevention, detection and treatment, around half of the people living in the developed world who have cancer are outliving the disease.

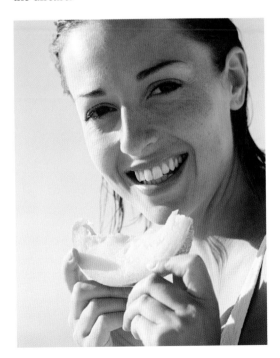

What's the best way to get to the finish line? Start with a base of healthy habits that continue throughout your journey.

The medical screens and tests you'll find here help detect cancer and other diseases early, when they're easier to treat or even cure. Even better, take steps to prevent illness. For instance, fruit and vegetables contain phytochemicals, substances that actually fight cancer. Whole grains provide fibre, which lowers risk for diabetes, heart disease and cancer. And omega-3 fatty acids, which are good for the heart, also help lift your mood.

And the sooner you take steps to keep your weight in check, the better. Putting this step off will make weight control harder, as your metabolism tends to slow once you approach the age of 40. Being obese – more than 30 per cent over your ideal body weight – puts you at greater risk for many conditions, including diabetes, high blood pressure, heart and artery disease, sleep disruptions, varicose veins, osteoarthritis, some cancers, respiratory problems, and complications during pregnancy and surgery. If you're overweight, the nutritional guidelines here will help you get started on eating a healthy diet. And for a more thorough programme to help you lose weight, see chapter 5.

Even if you don't have a weight problem, eating healthily throughout your lifetime is still important. Proper nutrition can increase your energy levels and improve your mood; eating healthily when pregnant could help you avoid birth defects in your baby.

The sooner you practise good health habits, the better off you'll be in the future.

'Most of us have eating patterns that were formed when we were very young,' says Dr Terri Brownlee, a nutritionist. 'Even at 20 years old, it's difficult to make changes. But it's certainly harder the longer you wait. If you wait until you're 50 or 60 years old, bad habits are much harder to break.'

Studies on people who have adopted a healthy diet and continued with it for years have shown that true lifestyle changes are the only way to do it.

Your Self-care Checklist

Multivitamins and mineral supplements
To be extra sure you're getting the vitamins and minerals you need, get in the habit of taking a multivitamin and mineral supplement that provides 100 per cent of the RNI (or recommended

daily allowance) for most nutrients, including vitamin A or beta-carotene, vitamin D, vitamin B_6, copper and zinc.

Consider taking separate supplements of 100 to 500 milligrams of vitamin C and 100 to 400 IU of vitamin E. They act as antioxidants, counteracting the natural effects of ageing and environmental damage at the cellular level.

Also make sure your multivitamin has a BP (British Pharmacopoeia) label on it. It means the manufacturer guarantees the supplement contains the amount of vitamins listed on the label.

For all women under 50, 500 milligrams of a calcium supplement is recommended. One type, calcium carbonate, should be taken with meals, while you may take calcium citrate on an empty stomach. Be sure not to overdo the vitamins. More is not necessarily better.

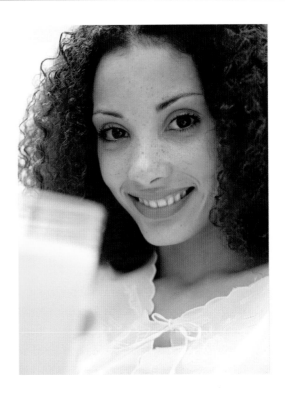

◯ **Folic acid/folate** The B vitamin folic acid (the supplement form of folate) prevents serious types of birth defects called neural tube defects. Women are advised to get 200 micrograms of folic acid. While pregnant, your doctor may advise you to increase your intake to 400 micrograms until at least 12 weeks.

Along with your supplements, eat two folic acid-rich foods a day, like spinach, kidney beans or orange juice.

◯ **Iron** One in five premenopausal women doesn't get the recommended daily allowance of 14.8 milligrams of iron. Without enough iron, you'll feel tired and have trouble concentrating. To battle that fatigue, eat iron-rich foods, such as pulses, dark green leafy vegetables and extra-lean meat. Consuming vitamin C products, such as orange juice, with iron-rich foods boosts absorption.

◯ **Good-mood foods** Women in their thirties who battle mood problems may be reacting to the food they eat, nutrients they're missing or drugs they take.

■ Premenstrual symptoms may be worse if you're not getting enough calcium, so make sure you're getting the RNI of 700 milligrams of calcium a day, from milk, yoghurt or calcium-fortified orange juice. This will help minimize mood swings from PMS.

■ Women who take birth control pills are usually low on vitamin B$_6$, which helps manufacture the mood-boosting chemical serotonin. Make sure you're getting enough by eating bananas and extra-lean meat.

Your Professional Health Checklist

◯ **Dental checkups** Go to the dentist every 6 months to help prevent cavities, gum disease and other oral problems.

◯ **Eye examinations** Ophthalmic opticians and optometrists (the names describe the same people: they are divided on what they should call themselves) are now fully equipped and trained to examine the eyes for many diseases, including the main problems of glaucoma, cataracts and macular degeneration. They can also detect early stages of other diseases such as high blood pressure and diabetes. So it is important to see your high-street eye professional for a first time and then regularly thereafter.

◯ **Serum ferritin test and transferrin saturation test** If you are tired or feel you don't have the energy you used to have, then your doctor will perform a 'full blood count' including your haemoglobin and red cell appearance and measurements. If from that test result there is a suspicion of an iron deficiency (a low haemoglobin and/or changes in the size and number of the red cells) then you will be offered further tests, including serum ferritin and transferrin saturation

'In people aged 35 and younger, **women have more skin cancers than men.** Evidence supports that sunbathing or tanning beds may contribute to this female predominance.'

DR SCOTT DINEHART, PROFESSOR OF DERMATOLOGY

levels. These are simple blood tests taken from a vein in your arm. Iron deficiency is the most common known form of nutritional deficiency, and it's highest among women of childbearing age. Almost one-third of British women and nearly half of adolescent girls are deficient in iron and 6 per cent of females have iron deficiency anaemia.

Iron overload, or haemochromatosis, is a relatively rare genetic disease. If you have liver disease, diabetes, arthritis or a family history of haemochromatosis, then the serum ferritin and transferrin saturation tests will find that, too.

◯ **Skin examination** Just one or two blistering sunburns in youth can set the stage for skin cancer later in life, though it might take decades for the signs to surface. Today around 200,000 cases of skin cancer are diagnosed each year in the UK and around 300,000 Australians visit their doctor to have skin cancers removed every year. Most skin cancers are curable if detected early enough.

Starting at the age of 18, examine your skin at least once a year for signs of skin cancer. 'Check your birthday suit every year on your birthday,' says Dr Ira Davis, an assistant professor of dermatology.

Use a mirror if you have to and look for:

- Pearly white bumps or spots that may bleed, may break down or don't heal, usually on the face or the arms (but they can appear anywhere on the body)

- Red and scaly bumps that resemble a scar and are shallow in the middle, usually on the face or the arms (but they can appear anywhere on the body)

- Dark spots that are asymmetrical, have irregular borders, have more than one colour and are bigger than the size of a pencil rubber, usually on the legs and trunk (but they can appear anywhere on the body); they may be flat or elevated

If you are worried about any spot or blemish on your skin, ask your doctor about it. If there is a doubt about it, you will be sent to a dermatologist. From then on, if it is judged that you are at extra risk, you will be called for a regular follow-up examination. Always attend these appointments. If you don't appear to have a skin problem, but have, or have had, a relative with melanoma (a potentially deadly form of skin cancer), and/or you are at risk for skin cancer (you've spent a lot of time in the sun, you have been sunburnt more than once, you have fair skin with freckles or have a lot of moles), then your doctor will assess your risk and arrange a follow up accordingly. Don't neglect the follow up.

○ **Tetanus jab** This may seem like stuff for primary school kids, but everyone needs a tetanus jab every 10 years to stay immune to the rare but fatal disease. Tetanus is caused when bacteria in an open wound attack the central nervous system.

○ **Blood pressure check** A blood pressure check is usually standard screening every time you see your family doctor or gynaecologist. If it has been found to be 140/90 or above, then there are standard guidelines for your doctor to follow it up – the rules change with rising figures. If you are on the contraceptive pill, your blood pressure will be measured each time you have a repeat prescription. If it is found to be raised, you will be put on a 'blood pressure register' and followed appropriately. You may need drugs to keep it in the normal range. Do take your drugs as advised, as you cannot tell from any particular symptom that your pressure is rising or too high. Modern drug treatment of high blood pressure has reduced early deaths from strokes and heart attacks by around half.

○ **Complete blood lipid profile** Today experts are seeing evidence of atherosclerosis (blood vessels with unhealthy deposits of cholesterol and other fats) in teenagers, which is why regular cholesterol checks are so important. With just one blood test, your doctor can measure your total cholesterol, HDL ('good') cholesterol, LDL ('bad') cholesterol, levels of triglycerides and total/HDL ratio. Blood will be taken to measure your lipid profile if your doctor considers you at risk (if you are obese, have high blood pressure, have diabetes, or have symptoms suggestive of circulation problems, such as chest pain, faintness or dizzy spells, or problems with your fingers and feet). If you have had relatives with early heart attacks or strokes, then you will also be offered the test. Smokers are at high risk, too, and will be asked to give blood for a lipid profile.

Healthy results are:

- Total cholesterol of 5 mmol/litre or below

- HDL 1.3 or above

- LDL 3 or below

- Total/HDL ratio of 4 or below

- Triglyceride levels under 1.5

○ **Electrocardiogram (ECG)** This important test identifies injury or damage to the heart, enlargement of the heart or abnormal rhythms. If you have risk factors for heart disease, such as hypertension or diabetes, and you've never had an ECG, get one no matter what your age, says Dr Elizabeth Ross, a cardiologist.

○ **Blood glucose tests (fasting and after food)** While the majority of women who develop type

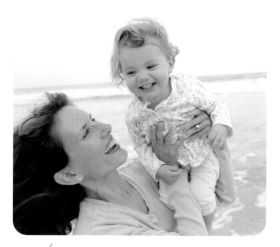

'Women should get in the habit at a very young age of not bending over at the waist to pick up anything, especially heavy children.

This helps prevent ruptured discs and back strain.

Bending at the knees and squatting down strengthens the muscles around the hip, which reduces your risk of hip fractures from osteoporosis later in life.'

DR MARJORIE LUCKEY, EXPERT ON OSTEOPOROSIS AND BONE DISEASE

2 diabetes don't do so until they are over 45, the incidence of the disease among younger women is rising. If you're at high risk, get tested now and at your doctor's recommendation.

Risk factors include:

- Being obese

- A family history

- Being from an at-risk ethnic group, such as African-Caribbean, South Asian or Pacific Islander

- Having high cholesterol

- Having a history of diabetes in pregnancy

- Having low HDL cholesterol and high triglycerides

○ **Pelvic examination and Pap (cervical smear) test** Since 1970, the incidence of and death rates from cervical cancer have gone down by 40 per cent, thanks in part to early detection with the test. Starting at the age of 18 – or younger if you are sexually active – visit your surgery for a pelvic examination and smear or Pap test.

During the pelvic examination, the doctor examines the genitals, vagina and cervix for infections, rashes or abnormal growths. The doctor also checks the size and position of the ovaries and uterus to make sure they're not enlarged.

She'll also take a sample of cells from your cervix for the test. This screens for cancer of the cervix, but it may also detect a sexually transmitted disease called human papillomavirus, which causes cervical cancer. This is essential

cancer protection since half of all women diagnosed with cervical cancer have never had a test. If you or your partner has multiple sexual partners, you should be tested for other sexually transmitted diseases as well.

○ **Breast examinations** Many women, or their partners, detect their own breast cancer. That's why you should give yourself regular breast self-examinations.

Symptoms to watch for: breast lumps, thickening, swelling, distortion, tenderness, skin irritation, dimpling, nipple pain, nipple inversion, discharge or scaliness.

Ages 35 to 40

Assuming you've established a healthy lifestyle, now is the time to deal with specific changes that typically occur as women approach midlife.

Some women experience perimenopausal symptoms as early as 35. During perimenopause, your levels of oestrogen and other female hormones drop as your body gets closer to menopause. You might experience irregular menstrual periods, hot flushes, night sweats, insomnia, mood swings and vaginal dryness.

Under the circumstances, it's harder to become pregnant at this time. In women, fertility gradually wanes after 35, and the risk of miscarriages increases to about 50 per cent by 45. Women in their forties also have a higher risk of pregnancy complications such as premature labour, stillbirth and the need for Caesarean section.

More than ever, exercise is essential to your

muscles and your bones. Beginning in their thirties, women lose 1 to 2 per cent of their muscle mass per year, but exercise can reverse the process and keep your metabolism up. Redouble your efforts not to put on weight now because once you reach 40, it won't be as easy to lose excess pounds at will.

And along with losing muscle, you could also lose bone if you're not careful. During childhood and puberty, your skeleton built more bone than it broke down. But by the time you reach 35, the process reverses and your body breaks down more bone than it builds. Weight-bearing exercise, such as walking and lifting weights, will strengthen your skeleton and help you avoid osteoporosis.

Your Self-care Checklist

◯ **A fertile weight** Obesity affects ovulation and could make it hard to get pregnant or carry a baby to term. In one study, a group of women who had a 75 per cent miscarriage rate lowered that rate to 18 per cent after eating a healthy diet, exercising and losing weight. If you're infertile and overweight, losing weight may help.

On the other hand, being underweight increases your risk for miscarriage, Caesarean deliveries or giving birth to a premature baby. A healthy weight is your best bet for fertility.

◯ **Folic acid/folate** Folic acid (the supplement form of folate) is recommended for all women of childbearing age. Once you get pregnant, your doctor may advise you to increase your intake to 400 micrograms until at least 12 weeks. But even if you're not pregnant, getting at least five servings of folic acid a day from food may decrease your risk of getting colon cancer later on. Folic acid, which is found in fruit and vegetables such as spinach and pulses, works on your DNA to keep it normal. Your suggested daily intake is 200 micrograms. If you're deficient in folic acid, you're more likely to develop the type of DNA damage that can lead to cancer.

◯ **Vegetables and calcium** You should already be exercising and getting enough calcium (recommended daily allowance is 700 milligrams) to keep your bones strong, but you also should be eating plenty of vegetables. Research shows that the nutrients in fruit and vegetables – zinc, magnesium, potassium, fibre and vitamin C – decrease the risk of having low bone mass.

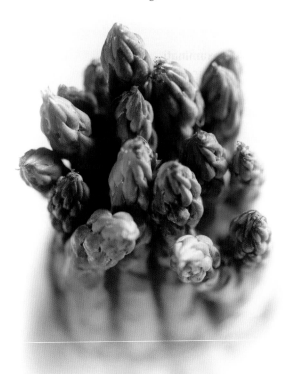

Your Professional Health Checklist

◯ **Dental checkups** Have them twice a year, or more often at your dentist's advice.

◯ **Eye examinations** If you have never had one, schedule an initial comprehensive eye examination. Then see an optometrist if you notice a change in your vision. Otherwise, you don't need regular eye tests until you reach 41.

◯ **Serum ferritin test and transferrin saturation test** If you're frequently fatigued or have liver disease, diabetes, arthritis or a family history of haemochromatosis, talk to your doctor about the most current recommendations regarding these iron tests.

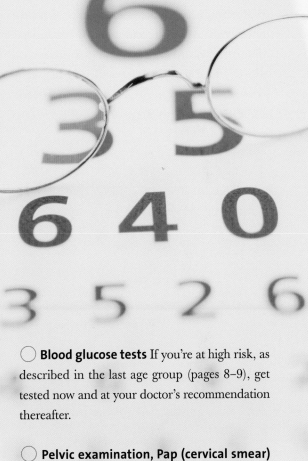

◯ **Skin examination** Continue examining your skin yearly if you're not at high risk for skin cancer, but check with your doctor if you're at high risk, as described on page 7.

◯ **Tetanus jab** If it's been 10 years, get another one.

◯ **Blood pressure check** Continue to have it checked at least every 2 years, or more frequently if it's been abnormal.

◯ **Complete blood lipid profile** As described for the last age group, on pages 7–8, your doctor will suggest a blood lipid profile if you are at risk.

◯ **Blood glucose tests** If you're at high risk, as described in the last age group (pages 8–9), get tested now and at your doctor's recommendation thereafter.

◯ **Pelvic examination, Pap (cervical smear) test and breast examination** Continue having them every year, and do regular breast self-examinations.

◯ **Mammogram** If two or more close relatives had breast cancer, particularly if they got it before the age of 40, start having annual mammograms in your thirties.

◯ **Bone-density test** If you're at high risk for osteoporosis because of another illness or a medication, talk to your doctor about getting a baseline bone-density scan prior to menopause. (For example, some medications to treat conditions such as rheumatoid arthritis, endocrine disorders, seizure disorders and gastrointestinal diseases may damage bone and lead to osteoporosis.) Otherwise, wait until the menopause for the test. You're at risk for osteoporosis if:

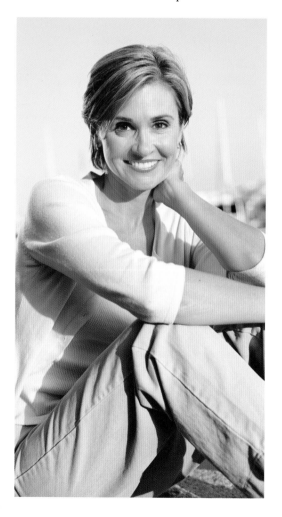

▪ You broke a bone after the age of 35 from low trauma (falling from a standing height or less)

▪ You have a family history of osteoporosis or hip fractures

▪ You weigh less than 57 kilograms (9 stone), even if you're short

▪ You smoke cigarettes or drink excessive amounts of alcohol

▪ You have taken steroids for 3 months or longer for conditions such as asthma

▪ You have a chronic disease that increases your risk for osteoporosis (both before and after menopause), such as seizure disorders, inflammatory bowel disease, chronic liver disease, kidney disease or coeliac disease

Ages 40 to 50

During this time, you might feel a few bumps in the road, particularly as you approach menopause, but paying attention to changes in your body, choosing foods that could lend relief to perimenopausal symptoms and getting the medical tests you need will help keep you healthy.

Almost all women – 85 to 90 per cent – experience symptoms of perimenopause, when the ovaries slow down their production of oestrogen and hormone levels fluctuate, the most common symptom being irregular periods.

'Anything is possible,' says Dr Margery Gass, a professor of obstetrics and gynaecology. Your periods could be completely normal and regular up until menopause, or they might move closer together or further apart, skip cycles or become heavier.

'Although more frequent periods are most common, it's important to stay in touch with your doctor to figure out what's normal for you during this time,' Dr Gass says. 'Heavy bleeding, irregular bleeding, periods every 2 to 3 weeks and breakthrough bleeding are always worrisome symptoms that should be checked by your doctor. They could be signs of cancer, polyps, fibroids, infections or miscarriages.'

Other symptoms include:

- Hot flushes, night sweats and extreme sweating (with or without chills)

- Vaginal dryness

- Changes in sexual desire

- PMS symptoms

- Mood changes

- Frequent urination

- Achy joints

- Difficulty in concentrating

- Headaches

- Insomnia

- Early wakening

Your emotional state also could affect the symptoms. Some life changes that are common during this time include an empty nest, divorce or widowhood, early retirement, anxiety about ageing or death, loss of friends and loved ones, loss of financial security, becoming a caregiver to an ageing parent and anxiety about your own health.

Together, the physical and life changes you face might leave you feeling as though you're going through puberty all over again. But there's plenty you can do to ease yourself through the 2 or 3 years it typically takes to make this transition.

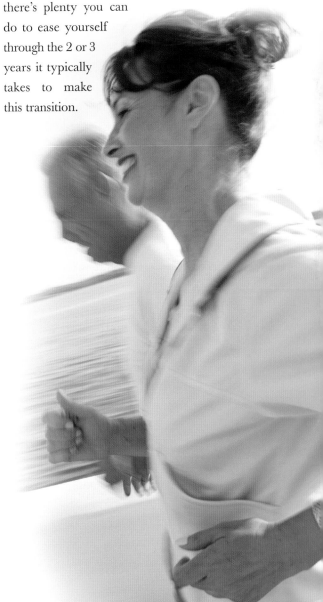

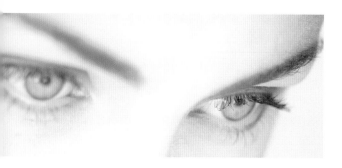

Your Self-care Checklist

◯ **Exercise, exercise, exercise** First and foremost, continue to rev up your metabolism with exercise. Researchers have found that women tend to put on about 0.5 kilograms (1 pound) a year in their forties, and it's easier to add fat to your abdomen, where it can do the most damage to blood sugar, cholesterol levels and blood pressure.

It's easy to blame weight gain on your changing hormones, but recent studies have found that added pounds have nothing to do with menopause or its treatments. Rather, lower physical activity is the culprit. Since women's risk for heart disease goes up after menopause and having more body fat could exacerbate the risk, work on keeping your weight down now by eating healthily and exercising.

◯ **Calorie control** With slower metabolism, you might find you're putting on weight even if you haven't changed your eating habits. But training the scales not to budge is as simple as eating one bite less at every meal. That adds up to about 100 fewer calories a day, the number of calories you should cut from your diet each decade.

◯ **Hunger signals** 'We each have our own unique metabolism, so you're the best judge of food that works best for you,' says Dr Jerianne Heimendinger, a scientist who has studied the antioxidant effects of fruit and vegetables. Listen to your hunger and satiety signals, and pay attention to how food makes you feel by pausing before you start your meal, eating slowly and chewing more carefully. You'll become more in touch with your body and less likely to overeat.

◯ **Fibre** A high-fibre diet of wholegrain bread and cereals and fruit and vegetables helps balance your oestrogen and could reduce symptoms of perimenopause. Fibre has also been shown to reduce the risk of heart disease, and may help lower your risk for some cancers.

◯ **Low-fat dairy** Another great way to stay slim and healthy: choose low-fat cheeses and yoghurt. They have all the calcium and other nutrients their high-fat counterparts carry – without the saturated fat.

'They're nutritional powerhouses without the guilt,' says Dr Leslie Bonci, a nutritionist.

◯ **Natural foods** Since women need fewer calories as they get older, avoiding processed foods – which are usually low in vitamins, minerals and fibre and high in fat and sugar – will give you the nutrients you need at a discount: fewer calories.

◯ **Vitamin E** Taking about 800 IU of a vitamin E supplement daily may not only cool hot flushes but also relieve mood swings and vaginal dryness

– three symptoms that result from fluctuating hormones during perimenopause.

Your Professional Health Checklist

○ **Dental checkup** Continue to go to the dentist every 6 months, unless your dentist advises more (or fewer) trips.

○ **Eye examinations** If you have never had one, schedule an initial comprehensive eye examination now. Then see an optometrist every 2 to 4 years, or sooner if you notice a change in your vision.

○ **Serum ferritin test and transferrin saturation test** If you're frequently fatigued or have liver disease, diabetes, arthritis or a family history of haemochromatosis and haven't had these tests, have them. Talk to your doctor about the most current recommendations regarding these iron tests.

○ **Skin examinations** Continue examining your skin yearly if you're not at high risk, but check with your doctor if you're at high risk of skin cancer, as described on page 7.

○ **Tetanus jab** Repeat every 10 years.

○ **Blood pressure check** The risk of developing hypertension tends to increase as we get older, so get checked at least every 2 years.

○ **Complete lipid profile** As described on pages 7–8, your doctor will suggest a blood lipid profile if you are at risk.

○ **Stress-echocardiogram test** If you're 40 or older and at high risk for heart disease (you have high blood pressure, have high cholesterol, have a history of bypass surgery or have had a heart attack or angioplasty) have a stress-echocardiogram test and an ECG. Also, if you're starting a vigorous exercise programme and you haven't been exercising, ask your doctor whether you should first have a stress-echocardiogram test.

○ **Flu jab** If you have any chronic condition (asthma, chronic obstructive lung disease, diabetes, heart disease, arthritis, kidney disease) or have had a transplant and/or are on immune suppressant drugs, get a flu jab annually. Even if you're in good health, the flu jab is 70 to 90 per cent effective at preventing the fever, cough, sore throat, runny or stuffy nose, headaches, muscle aches and fatigue the infection is likely to cause.

◯ **Blood glucose tests** All women 45 and older should have their blood sugar tested every 3 years to screen for diabetes. If results are abnormal or if you're at high risk for diabetes, get tested more often.

The signs of diabetes are unexplained weight loss, unusual thirst, frequent desire to urinate, extreme fatigue, extreme hunger, irritability, frequent infections, blurred vision, slow-healing cuts and bruises, tingling or numbness in the hands or feet, or recurring skin, gum or bladder infections.

◯ **Bone-density test** If you're at high risk for osteoporosis, as described in the last life stage (page 12) – or at the first signs of menopause – get a bone-density scan.

◯ **Pelvic examination and Pap (cervical smear) test** It's a fact. Many deaths from cervical cancer could have been prevented through safe sex practices and routine tests. Do yourself a favour and go to your doctor when you are called for this important test. If you think you may be due for a test but have heard nothing, contact your surgery and ask about it.

Also, talk to your doctor if you have questions about signs of perimenopause you might be experiencing.

Symptoms to watch for: heavy bleeding, bleeding longer than 7 days (or 2 or more days longer than usual), having fewer than 21 days between periods, spotting between periods and bleeding after intercourse. They could indicate a hormone imbalance, misuse of the Pill, pregnancy, fibroids, thyroid dysfunction, abnormalities in the uterine lining, cancer or bleeding outside the uterus (such as in the vagina or cervix).

◯ **Pelvic ultrasound** Women at high risk for ovarian cancer (several family members had breast or ovarian cancer) should have a pelvic ultrasound and a CA-125 test, a blood test that looks for cancer markers in the blood.

Women with BRCA1 and BRCA2 mutations are also at higher risk for ovarian, breast and some other cancers. If you know you have a gene that could give you cancer, talk to your doctor about getting tested every 6 months.

A new blood test is being studied that could provide more reliable results than the CA-125. It will measure lysophosphatidic acid (LPA), a lipid in the blood. Women with ovarian cancer have high quantities of this acid. This new test could detect the cancer early, when it's most treatable. Some controversy surrounds the testing, as in certain cases it may yield false-negative or false-positive results.

Symptoms to watch for: enlargement of the abdomen is the most common sign of ovarian cancer, but it's not always present. A large tumour could make you look 5 months pregnant. Another sign is persistent digestive problems, such as unexplained stomach discomfort, flatulence and abdominal swelling. In rare cases, abnormal vaginal bleeding will occur.

◯ **Breast examination** Continue your regular breast self-examinations. Symptoms to watch for: breast lumps, thickening, swelling, distortion, tenderness, skin irritation, nipple pain, nipple inversion, scaliness or dimpling.

Ages 50 to 60

From here on in, you can look forward to relief from perimenopausal symptoms. Fluctuating oestrogen levels, which have been causing hot flushes, insomnia, headaches, night sweats, vaginal dryness and mood swings, finally drop off completely. The ovaries no longer produce eggs. Menstruation ceases.

After 12 months without a period, you've reached menopause. It could happen anywhere between the ages of 40 and 58, but the average age is 51. Women who smoke usually go through menopause about a year and a half earlier than women who don't, and women with a higher body mass index (discussed on page 83) or who have had more than one pregnancy usually experience later-than-average menopause. You'll probably reach menopause at the same age your mother did.

For some, menopause may be a day to mourn the loss of fertility. For others, it's a day to celebrate having no more periods, premenstrual symptoms and fear of pregnancy. In fact, postmenopausal women are the *least* likely of all women to be depressed – due to a sense of well-being.

In the past doctors thought a decline in health after menopause was a normal part of ageing. Now we know that a healthy lifestyle can keep women vibrant. Good thing, too, since many women lead at least one-third of their lives after menopause.

Menopause does bring new health challenges, however. Without some form of hormone replacement therapy, women can lose between 2

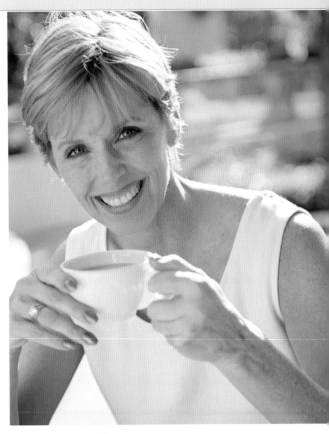

and 5 per cent of bone mass on average per year in the first 3 to 5 years after menopause.

Your risk of dying from breast cancer, too, rises with age (although it's still a distant third behind heart disease and lung cancer for women in general). When you were 35, your chance of getting breast cancer was only one in 622. By the age of 60, the relative risk is one in 24 (although the risk varies greatly from woman to woman).

And while oestrogen protected you in younger years from heart disease, losing it in menopause raises LDL ('bad') cholesterol levels and, by the time you're 60, your risk will have increased to equal a man's. Oestrogen also kept your blood vessels naturally elastic. Without it, the risk of heart disease and stroke increases.

Again, these risks are relative and within your control. That's why a healthy diet and screening are extra important at this age. Calcium and vitamin D help fight bone loss, but if a bone-density scan finds that you have low bone mass, your doctor can put you on protective therapy early to fight it. If a breast tumour is found with a mammogram or breast examination, the earlier it's detected, the easier it is to treat and cure. In the meantime, you can eat food associated with low breast cancer risk. And eating a low-fat diet, getting exercise and not smoking can lower your odds of getting heart disease.

The scales present another challenge. It's getting harder and harder to keep your weight down. Increasing your muscle mass with exercise will help you burn calories.

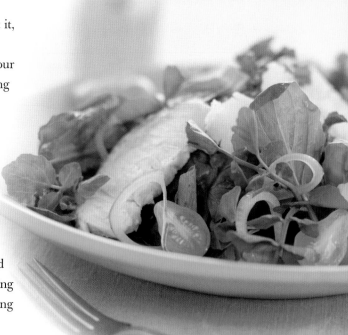

Your Self-care Checklist

◯ **Calorie reduction** To compensate for slower metabolism, cut another 100 calories from your daily diet. Cut down on the size of your meals instead of completely eliminating a food group, such as carbohydrates like bread. To fill your plate without overeating, use a salad plate for dinner and you won't feel deprived.

◯ **Mini-meals** To keep your metabolism up, ditch the usual three big meals and eat six smaller ones of about 250 calories each throughout the day. Researchers have found that women who eat larger meals may burn 60 fewer calories per day than women who eat mini-meals – the equivalent of 2.5 kilograms (6 pounds) a year.

◯ **Portion control** To make sure you're not eating double or triple portions of snacks, biscuits and other packaged foods, check the serving size on food labels, and limit yourself to single servings, not the whole amount provided.

◯ **Low-fat, high-fibre diet** A diet low in fat and high in fibre has been associated with a lower risk of both heart disease and colon cancer. Reach for fruit, vegetables, wholegrain breads and cereals, pulses, soya foods, and fat-free or low-fat dairy foods.

◯ **Calcium** Postmenopausal women get only half the calcium they need, yet they need more calcium than ever. The loss of oestrogen from menopause gives you less protection from bone loss, so increase your daily calcium consumption to 1,000 milligrams.

You don't have to drink three glasses of milk a day if you don't want to. Instead, you may take calcium supplements equal to 700 milligrams towards that recommended daily allowance. Experts recommend that for better absorption you spread the dose out over the day, and take no more than 500 milligrams at one time. Though you need to take one type, calcium carbonate, with meals, you may take calcium citrate on an empty stomach. Look for a calcium supplement formula with vitamin D. You may need more D than the amount your daily multi provides.

◯ **Vitamin B$_{12}$** Women need only 1.5 micrograms per day of vitamin B$_{12}$ to fight heart disease, but after the age of 50 it's harder for us to absorb the vitamin when we get it from food. Take it in a multi supplement – it's well-absorbed.

◯ **Spinach** Lutein and zeaxanthin, antioxidants found in spinach, may protect the retina from age-related macular degeneration. Eat spinach once a day, with olive oil, since fat promotes lutein absorption.

◯ **Fall prevention** As you approach 60, step up your efforts to prevent falls, to guard against wrist and hip fractures. Keep electrical cords away from through traffic areas of your home, use night-lights, arrange for handrails (and non-slip tape) to be installed in the shower, clean up spills in the kitchen right away, wear sturdy, rubber-soled shoes and put rubber mats under rugs to keep them from sliding under your feet.

Your Professional Health Checklist

◯ **Height measurement** You should be getting your height measured every time you're at the doctor's surgery, or at least once a year. Over

WHEN CALCIUM ISN'T GOOD

Calcium supplements can help preserve bone density, protecting you from fractures. But did you know that taking calcium just before a bone scan might blur your bone-density test results?

The very best test for measuring bone density in the spine and hip – dual energy X-ray absorptiometry, or DEXA – works by reading how much calcium is present, not only in the bone but also within a cross section of the body. Poorly absorbed calcium can linger in the intestines and mimic dense bone on a spine scan, obscuring telltale signs of thinning bone.

This rarely happens, but it could at least cause inconvenience: if your doctor notices an odd reading, she may suggest a second scan. Don't stop taking supplements or cancel your DEXA. And don't take any calcium supplement within an hour of a DEXA.

your lifetime, a gradual loss of about 4 centimetres (1.5 inches) is normal. But if you've lost more height than that – or you've lost 4 centimetres (1.5 inches) in 10 years or less – it could indicate vertebral compression fractures as a result of osteoporosis.

◯ **Bone-density test** Get a bone-density measurement if you're menopausal or past menopause and you've never had a test. One in three women in the UK over 50 have osteoporosis: an estimated 3 million people.

The best measurement for women is a DEXA scan of the spine and the hip, the two places that usually have the most serious fractures. The spine is also where the first bone loss most often occurs after menopause.

◯ **25-hydroxy vitamin D serum level check** If you're older than 49, especially if you're at risk of osteoporosis, have your level of vitamin D checked. Vitamin D helps calcium get absorbed in the body. Your levels should be over 20 nanograms per litre.

◯ **Dental checkup** Go to the dentist every 6 months, or more often if you experience pain or other problems.

◯ **Eye examinations** Go for a comprehensive eye examination, if you have not already done so. You should be having an eye test every 2 to 4 years, or sooner if you notice a change in your vision.

◯ **Serum ferritin test and transferrin saturation test** Talk to your doctor about the most current recommendations regarding these tests.

◯ **Skin examinations** Don't let up on checking your skin for changes, as described on page 7.

◯ **Blood pressure check** Get your blood pressure checked at least every 2 years, more often if it's abnormal.

◯ **Complete lipid profile** As described on pages 7–8, your doctor will suggest a lipid profile if you are at risk. Note, though, that women typically get cardiovascular disease 10 to 15 years later than men, when they experience the postmenopausal loss of oestrogen. Also, cholesterol levels change after menopause. 'Bad' LDL cholesterol levels go up, while 'good' HDL cholesterol levels go down, putting postmenopausal women at greater risk of cardiovascular disease.

◯ **Pelvic examination and Pap (cervical smear) test** As with your previous decade, make sure you attend whenever your doctor writes to you for your repeat test. If you feel that you have been forgotten (that you haven't had one for some time), contact the surgery and ask about it.

◯ **Mammogram** Once you reach 50, it's time to start having a regular mammogram. A mammogram is a low-intensity X-ray that can confirm whether lumps you or your doctor found are in fact tumours. It can also detect tumours when they're too small to feel with your hand. When tumours are found early, they're easier to treat and the cancer could be cured because it hasn't spread to other parts of the body.

◯ **Colorectal screening** Colorectal cancer is the second most-common cancer among women in the UK, but it's almost always curable if found early enough. If everyone started having regular screenings for colon cancer at 50, many lives a year could be spared from the disease.

If you have close relatives who have had colorectal cancer (with or without 'polyps') then you should have been screened for it early. The screening involves colorectal endoscopy and biopsy of any suspicious area of bowel. If there is no history of colorectal cancer in your family, and you have no symptoms, then a rectal examination at 50, which will be done at your well-woman clinic appointment, is probably enough. If you start to have symptoms (see below), you should see your doctor immediately.

Risk factors for colon cancer include:

- A family history
- A genetic predisposition
- Chronic inflammatory bowel disease
- A previous history of colon polyps or colon cancer

Watch out for rectal bleeding, blood in stool, persistent pain in the lower abdomen or back, unexplained tiredness or anaemia, unplanned loss of weight or a change in bowel habits.

◯ **Flu jab** Everyone over 50 should have a flu jab annually. If you're healthy, the jab can prevent illness, and if you have a chronic medical condition, such as asthma, it can reduce the flu's severity and risk of serious complications.

◯ **Tetanus jab** The majority of people over 60 haven't had a tetanus shot in the previous 10 years, which means they're not immune to tetanus. If you're one of those people, make sure you get the jab.

'Studies show that **aspirin reduces the growth of polyps** that lead to colon cancer. The dose and frequency are not clear, but talk to your doctor about taking either regular or baby aspirin at least every other day. It's probably a good idea if you're not bothered by aspirin's side effects, which can include stomach upsets and gastrointestinal bleeding.'

– DR HAROLD FRUCHT, EXPERT IN GASTROENTEROLOGY

Ages 60 and Older

There's no doubt about it: we're living longer than ever before – and these years bring unique health concerns.

Screening for colon cancer and mammograms are absolutely necessary now. Almost every time, colon cancer can be cured if screening detects the cancer early. And while women over 60 who have had several negative Pap or smear tests don't have to get them any more, it's important to see your doctor for pelvic examinations and clinical breast examinations.

Getting exercise should also be high on your list of priorities. Go for walks, garden, dance. Spend 30 minutes three times a week doing this type of weight-bearing aerobic exercise. On the other days, lift weights for 15 or 20 minutes. You'll burn extra calories and strengthen your bones and muscles.

Even if you have low bone mass or osteoporosis, lifting weights is safe if you start with a light weight of no more than 2 kilograms (5 pounds) and go slowly. You'll build muscle, bone mass and balance. To avoid injury, give yourself a day to rest between strength-training sessions. Besides keeping you strong, exercise could let you lose weight, which will help you avoid pain in your hips, knees, ankles and feet.

But your muscles and skeleton shouldn't be the only thing you're exercising, say health experts. Filling up your social calendar, connecting emotionally with friends and family and staying stimulated also keep you happy and healthy.

'There's no question that people who remain intellectually active and socially engaged in older years do better,' says Dr Eugenia Siegler, an associate professor of clinical medicine. Use this time to travel, learn new things, take classes at a local college, volunteer and connect to friends and family. Most retired people are already active. Nearly 10 per cent of women of retirement age are still in employment. Women are challenging themselves by going back to college or work,

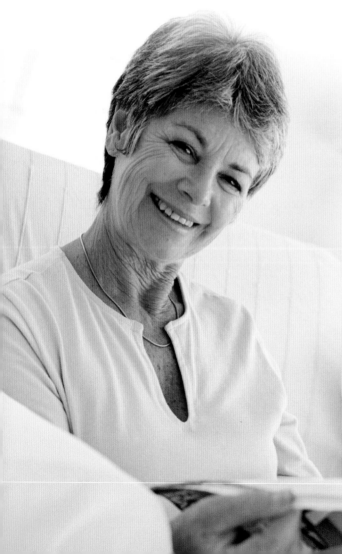

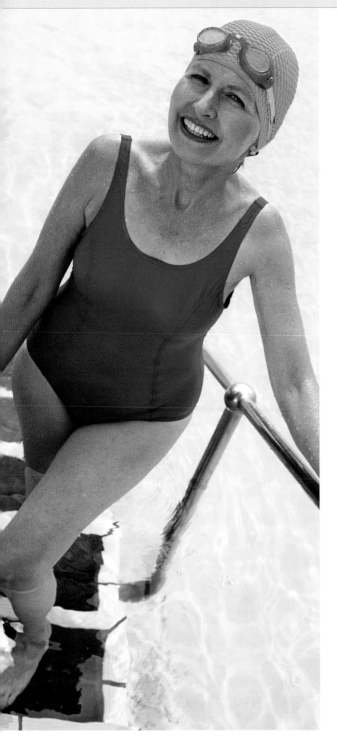

volunteering and making use of the Internet. In one survey, 37 per cent of older adults said continuing their education was important in retirement. Numerous University of the Third Age (U3A) groups around the UK, Australia and New Zealand organize themselves, for the purpose of learning, after retirement.

Attitudes towards these years have changed, too. Compared with a generation ago, today fewer Westerners over 65 say poor health, loneliness, few job opportunities and too little money are problems for people in their age group.

Your Self-care Checklist

◯ **Nutrient-dense food** Because your calorie needs are still dropping while your nutritional needs are rising, make every calorie count by eating whole grains, beans, low-fat dairy foods, fruit and vegetables and small amounts of extra-lean meats. Take a multi supplement just to make sure you're getting all your nutrients.

◯ **Antioxidant-rich food** Antioxidants found in fruit, vegetables and whole grains stimulate your immune system and help you avoid infections like flu or pneumonia. So finish off your vegetable stir-fry with a bowl of berries.

◯ **Restaurant choices** When ordering fast food, choose salads with fat-free dressing, a plain hamburger or a grilled chicken sandwich. At sit-down restaurants, you could ask your waiter to wrap half your meal in a doggy bag before even setting it down in front of you.

Your Professional Health Checklist

◯ **Flu jab** Continue having a flu jab every year. If you have a chronic medical condition, the jab might not prevent the flu, but it could make your illness less severe if you do get it and lower your risk of complications. The flu jab is offered free to all over-60s, regardless of their health status. You will get notice of the date from your doctor.

◯ **Pneumococcal vaccine** Get this vaccine for pneumococcal pneumonia at least once after the age of 60. You'll want to avoid the trip to the hospital or the infections that could result from pneumonia.

◯ **Dental checkups** Continue going to the dentist every 6 months, and don't ignore gum pain, swelling or bleeding.

◯ **Eye examinations** After you reach 65, start going to the optometrist every 1 to 2 years if you haven't been already. If you have diabetes, go every year to make sure you don't get diabetic retinopathy, a disease in which tiny blood vessels in the eye weaken and leak, causing blurred vision or even blindness.

◯ **Skin examinations** This is no time to slack off on skin care, especially if leaving the workforce affords you more time in the outdoors.

◯ **Tetanus jab** Two out of three people over the age of 60 aren't immune to tetanus, a disease in

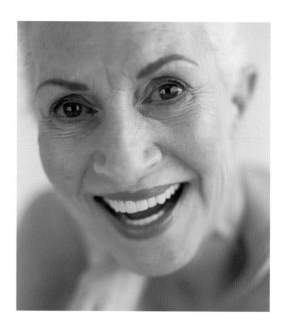

which bacteria enter an open wound and attack the nervous system, causing muscle spasms, lockjaw, difficulty swallowing, rigid muscles, fever and a raised heart rate. Get vaccinated every 10 years.

◯ **Bone-density test** You should be having a DEXA scan regularly by now. Nine out of 10 women have osteoporosis by the age of 75, so being screened regularly is essential.

If your test results are normal, go back for another scan every 3 to 5 years. If you have low bone mass and you're on therapy to treat it, go back in 2 years to track your progress. After that, your doctor will put you on your own screening schedule to see if you're progressing from the therapy.

The following checks are a guide for women over 60. It is not a rigid plan of action. How often you really need to have these checks depends on your own physical state and risks, which, of course, are different from those of other women. So discuss them with your doctor, and you will be able to work out between you what is correct for you. Here is one such plan, which probably is about right for most women of your age.

◯ **Blood pressure check** Continue getting your blood pressure checked at least every 2 years, or more often if your readings are abnormal.

◯ **Complete lipid profile** Consider having this test every 2 years if results are normal, and every 4 months if abnormal.

◯ **Blood glucose test** Screening for diabetes is important, so consider having a blood glucose test every 3 years.

◯ **Colon cancer screening** Have a digital rectal examination every year and a colonoscopy every 10 years, along with a yearly faecal occult blood test. If you don't have risk factors for colon cancer, you can have a flexible sigmoidoscopy every 3 to 5 years instead of a colonoscopy.

◯ **Thyroid-stimulating hormone test** You should consider getting screened every 5 years for thyroid disease.

◯ **Pelvic examination, Pap (cervical smear) test and breast examination** Smear or Pap tests are not offered to women who have had normal results when they reach 60. That's because there is very little new disease in the cervix after that time. However, it is correct to have a pelvic examination if any new symptoms arise after this time, such as new bleeding, itching, discharge, painful intercourse, general pelvic pain and incontinence.

◯ **Mammograms** Mammograms are not offered after the age of 60, unless you feel you need one, or have a strong family history of late breast cancer. Most new cancers after the age of 60 are self-diagnosed: they are slower to grow and have a lower mortality rate than cancers arising in women before the menopause. Again, the risk of repeated X-rays may outweigh the risks of missing a new fatal breast cancer.

WHEN SHOULD I GO DOWN TO CASUALTY?

Most illnesses and conditions can wait until you're able to see a doctor – but some symptoms require emergency attention. They include:

- Chest pain that lasts longer than 2 minutes
- Difficulty breathing or shortness of breath
- Any sudden or severe pain that lasts longer than half an hour.
- Uncontrolled bleeding
- Coughing or vomiting blood
- Sudden dizziness, weakness or a change in vision
- Severe or persistent vomiting or diarrhoea to the point of fainting due to dehydration
- Marked changes in mental function, such as confusion.

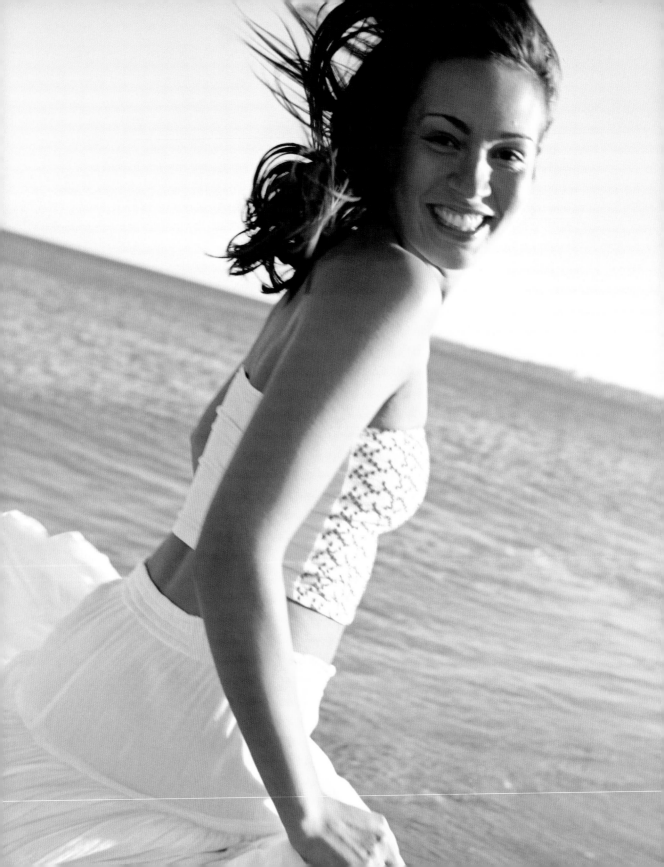

PART 2

Your stay well, stay young 'to do' list

Vitamins, Minerals and Nutrition: the Complete Plan

Just a few years ago, most health experts felt that women could get all of the vitamins and minerals that they needed from a healthy diet and that supplements were unnecessary. Today, many have changed their minds.

Even women who are conscientious about eating a healthy diet will occasionally fall short of essential nutrients. And let's face it: on any given night, most women are more likely to eat pizza and ice cream than baked wild salmon and a green salad.

'Most women don't meet even conservative recommendations for fruit and vegetable intakes,' says Dr Michael Fossel, a clinical professor of medicine. 'Even I probably don't eat enough fruit and vegetables, and I know better.'

Surveys have shown that well below half of adults in the West – women included – eat five servings of fruit and vegetables daily. Even if they do, that's probably not enough: many experts advise that for optimal health protection, women should eat nine daily servings of fruit and vegetables.

Our dietary shortcomings aren't the only reasons that nutritionists advise women to use nutritional supplements. Recent studies have shown that some key nutrients provide the most benefits when they're consumed in amounts greater than it's possible to get from foods alone.

Consider folate. This nutrient has been shown to reduce the risk of heart disease as well as certain birth defects. Unless you eat fortified breakfast cereals, you'd have to eat more than 5 large servings of romaine lettuce daily to meet the daily requirement. Taking a 200-microgram folic acid (the synthetic form of folate) supplement makes good sense.

The same is true of vitamin E. Only nuts and vegetable oils have appreciable amounts, which is why women only get about 13 IU of vitamin E daily. Studies have shown that getting at least 100 IU daily is associated with a reduced risk of heart disease. 'There's no way that anyone could get that amount without taking a supplement,' says Dr Jane Higdon, a scientist who researches the role of vitamins, minerals and micronutrients.

Even though every woman should do everything possible to eat a healthy, balanced diet, adding a multivitamin and a few key nutritional supplements is a reasonable approach for preventing deficiencies and safeguarding your long-term health.

Nutrition: Where to Start

Calories. Calorie needs vary from woman to woman depending on height, weight, age and body composition. A very muscular woman might need 2,500 calories per day, and a woman with less muscle might only need 1,800 calories.

Carbohydrates. Carbohydrates are the foundation of a healthy diet. Try to get 60 to 65 per cent of your calories from carbohydrates, and make three to six of those servings whole grain, such as wholemeal bread and bran cereal.

Whole grains provide all the nutrients from the grain, like fibre, that are taken out of refined products. They're also satisfying. You feel like you're really eating something and you feel fuller when you're finished.

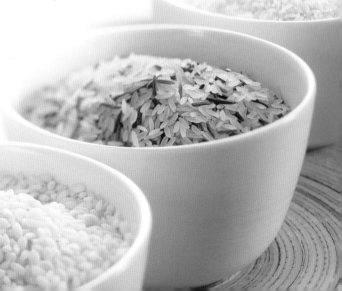

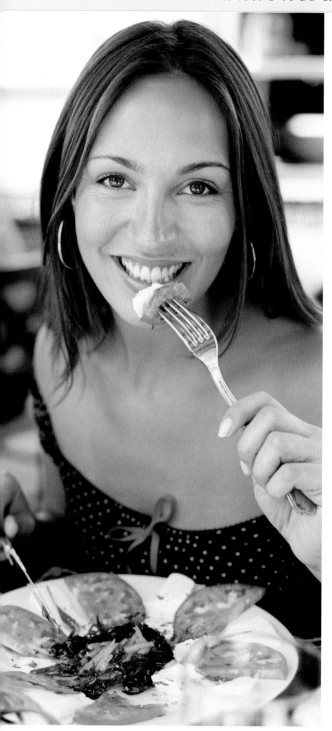

To make sure you're eating whole grains, check the label. 'Whole wheat' should be listed in the ingredients of bread and biscuits, and '100 per cent whole grain' should be included on your box of cereal.

Fruit and vegetables. Aim for five servings of vegetables and four servings of fruit a day, and you'll get a good helping of antioxidants, substances that protect your DNA, the genetic information in every cell of your body, from cancer. (For more on antioxidants, see page 36.)

If you're not accustomed to eating so many fruits and vegetables, increase the number gradually. Start out by tossing a handful of chopped onions or mushrooms into your pasta sauce. Substitute grilled aubergine parmigiana made with low-fat cheese for chicken parmigiana with cheese high in fat. Bake an apple with cinnamon for dessert. Add in two extra servings of vegetables while you make dinner by snacking on hummus or another bean dip and baby carrots.

You'll be glad you did. Not only are fruit and vegetables good for you, but they also bring crunchiness, sweetness or a savoury taste to your meals.

To get the best health protection, choose from a variety of botanical families. For instance, kiwi fruit, strawberries, bananas, apples, oranges and grapes come from different families. As for vegetables, mushrooms, spinach, watercress, sweet potatoes, broccoli, courgettes, sweetcorn, lentils, garlic, tomatoes and carrots come from different families, too. Or look for different colours. There are some exceptions, but fruit and vegetables of different colours usually come from different botanical families. Try to buy two or three fruits and two or three vegetables a week, and try to make them slightly different every time you visit the supermarket, says Dr Terri Brownlee, a nutritionist.

You'll also benefit from eating the fruit and vegetables themselves rather than taking a supplement, says Dr Jerianne Heimendinger, a scientist who has studied the antioxidant effects of fruit and vegetables. 'Many of the components of food work synergistically, so it's much better to have the food than it is to isolate one component and give it to people in larger amounts.'

Lean protein. Now, and in the years to come, you should be getting 10 to 15 per cent of your calories from lean protein, such as beans and peas, nuts, fish, skinless chicken and turkey and lean red meat (if you eat meat), and low-fat milk and eggs (if you eat dairy products).

Don't be fooled by meat labelled 'lean', though. Check the fine print, and take note of how many grams of fat the meat really contains. Don't buy it if it has more than 10 grams of fat per serving.

Dairy. Eat two or three servings of low-fat dairy products a day – or 1,000 milligrams of calcium. Low-fat and fat-free milk, yoghurt and cheese are excellent sources of calcium, which helps keep your bones strong.

By the time you reach your early thirties, your body begins to lose more bone than it builds. Calcium will help you put bone in the bank, so to speak. The recommended 1,000 milligrams of calcium

is the equivalent of about three servings of dairy food: 240 millilitres (8 fluid ounces) of skimmed milk, 230 grams (8 ounces) of yoghurt, and 60 grams (2 ounces) of low-fat mozzarella cheese. If you have trouble getting calcium from dairy food, try calcium-fortified food, such as orange juice or cereal.

Fat. You probably already know that you're supposed to eat fat and sweets 'sparingly'. That means no more than 25 per cent of your total calories should come from fats. Reach for the healthiest fats and you'll start a habit that will benefit you for the rest of your life. The best choices are monounsaturated: olive oil, rapeseed oil, peanut oil (as long as allergy is not a problem for you) and avocado. Monounsaturated fats bring down total cholesterol without affecting HDL ('good') cholesterol levels – a strong asset, given that researchers have detected high cholesterol levels even in teenagers.

Polyunsaturated fats – such as safflower,

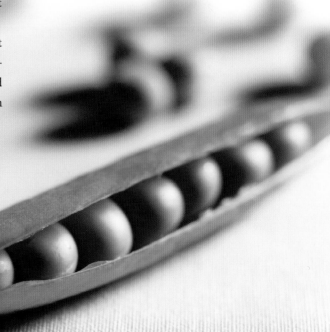

sesame and sunflower seeds, corn and soya beans, and other nuts and seeds and their oils – are also good choices. These fats bring down all cholesterol levels.

Foods high in saturated fat and trans fatty acids (processed fats that resemble saturated fat) should be eaten sparingly, if at all. Both raise cholesterol levels and contribute to heart disease. Saturated fat is found in animal products, such as beef, whole milk and ice cream, as well as in so-called tropical oils: cocoa butter, coconut oil, palm oil and palm kernel oil. Trans fats are manufactured by adding hydrogen to polyunsaturated fats to make them more solid. Also called hydrogenated oils, they're the primary fat in most vegetable fats, biscuits, desserts, snacks, crisps and some margarines.

A good rule of thumb is to choose items with hydrogenated oils listed as far down the ingredients list as possible. Also, look for 'trans fatty acid–free' margarine (the label will say something like 'contains no trans fats').

Making good choices now could affect your cholesterol all the way through menopause and beyond, when women's risk of heart disease increases. A study found that when women had low cholesterol levels during premenopause, they significantly lowered their risk of heart disease after menopause.

Fish. Eat two servings of wild salmon, mackerel, herring or sardines each week, and you'll get 3.5 grams of fish oil omega-3 fatty acids. This type of fat isn't made by the body, but it's necessary for growth and development. It also helps

EXTRA HELP FOR SMOKERS

The smoke from cigarettes does more than damage the lungs. It also triggers the formation of free radicals, which 'use up' vitamin C in the body. That's why smokers are advised to take 80 milligrams of vitamin C daily, compared with 40 milligrams for non-smokers.

There's another reason smokers may need greater amounts of vitamin C and other nutrients. If you smoke, your diet may not be as good as it should be – in part because

nicotine suppresses appetite, and also because smokers are more likely to light up than to enjoy nutritious snacks, says Dr Michael Fossel, a clinical professor of medicine.

The best thing, of course, is to quit smoking. But in the meantime, be sure to take a vitamin C supplement daily. You also may want to get extra amounts of vitamin E and selenium, which will lower levels of free radicals in the body.

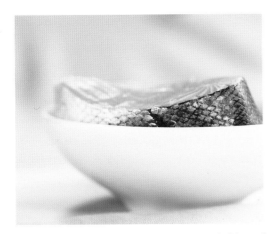

prevent heart disease, hypertension, arthritis and cancer, and reduces inflammation.

Flaxseed/linseed. Flaxseed or linseed is the vegetable source of omega-3 fatty acids and helps prevent heart disease and possibly cancer.

Add a tablespoon of ground flaxseed to your diet every day in addition to your two servings of fish a week. (Both foods are exceptionally high in omega-3s.) Because the seeds come in hard shells, you'll be able to digest flaxseed better if you grind it in a blender or food processor and store it in the fridge or freezer. Then sprinkle the ground seeds on salad, porridge or muffins. Another option: buy flaxseed oil and use it in place of other oils in your cold dishes. But don't cook with flaxseed oil because heat changes its structure. Store the oil in the refrigerator as soon as you bring it home.

Fibre. Try to get 25 to 35 grams of fibre a day. Eating high-fibre foods such as beans and pulses, whole grain cereal and bread, vegetables, fruit and nuts also lowers cholesterol and the risk for heart disease.

Garlic. Eating nine to ten cloves of garlic a week may protect women against stomach and colorectal cancers. In fact, garlic has killed cancer cells in the test tube. Brush a mixture of olive oil and crushed garlic on to fish, or make your own garlic bread with a spray of olive oil and fresh crushed garlic. After you peel and chop garlic, let it sit for 15 minutes before cooking to allow time for the cancer-fighting compounds to develop.

Low sodium. Eating food naturally low in sodium, such as fresh fruit and vegetables, and avoiding excessively salty food – such as smoked, cured or processed meat; soy sauce; garlic salt; tinned soup; some frozen meals; and salty crackers, crisps, popcorn and nuts – will help lower your blood pressure. Try to consume fewer than 800 milligrams of sodium per meal, or 2,400 milligrams a day – the equivalent contained in 1 teaspoon of table salt.

Cinnamon. Cinnamon increases glucose metabolism and lowers your risk of diabetes, which is becoming increasingly prevalent. Doctors who have studied cinnamon's effects recommend stirring a quarter to a full teaspoon of cinnamon into orange juice, coffee or porridge every day.

Carotenoids. Although giving up smoking is the best way to reduce your risk of lung cancer,

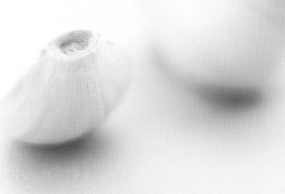

studies have found that a diet high in phyto-chemicals called carotenoids is associated with a significantly lower risk of lung cancer for both smokers and non-smokers.

Carotenoids are found in fruit and vegetables such as sweet potatoes, tomatoes, carrots, spinach, broccoli, cantaloupe melon, pumpkin and apricots. Carrots in particular, which are a major source of a carotenoid called alpha-carotene, have been shown to benefit non-smokers. Tomatoes, which contain a carotenoid called lycopene, have been shown to benefit smokers.

Vanadium. Certain foods containing this trace mineral help keep blood sugar levels normal.

Foods with vanadium include skimmed milk, gelatine, lentils, kidney beans, lobster, vegetable oils, radishes, potatoes, squash, lettuce, hazelnuts, buckwheat, rye seed, grains and cereal.

Potassium. Potassium in fruit and vegetables can help reduce your blood pressure. It is a

A VEGETARIAN'S GUIDE TO SUPPLEMENTS

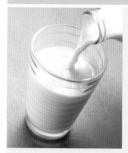

Doctors agree that following a vegetarian diet is among the healthiest lifestyle choices a woman can make. But even if you're careful to eat well – ideally a vegetarian diet will include fruit, vegetables, pulses and whole grains with almost every meal – it may be a challenge to get all the essential nutrients that you need.

If you're a vegan – one who avoids eggs and dairy as well as meats – you'll have to work harder to get adequate amounts of all vitamins and minerals. Doctors usually advise vegetarians to take a few key supplements, including:

■ **Iron.** Menstruating women who eat meat are advised to get 14.8 milligrams of iron daily. Women who are vegetarians may need more, because the iron in plant foods is less easily absorbed. Advice is to take less than 17 milligrams per day as a supplement,

unless under a doctor's supervision. If you're postmenopausal, you may not need supplemental iron unless you are anaemic or have a very low dietary intake.

■ **Vitamin D.** It's found mainly in fish and dairy foods. If you're a strict vegetarian, the only way to get enough vitamin D is to use a supplement that contains it.

■ **Vitamin B_{12}.** Vitamin B_{12} is found in animal products and milk but is not generally found in plant foods. Vegetarian women should make sure they get at least 2.4 micrograms daily by taking a multivitamin.

■ **Calcium.** Even though plant foods contain some calcium, they can't compete with the amounts found in milk, yoghurt or other dairy foods. If you're premenopausal, aim for 1,000 milligrams a day; after menopause try to get 1,200 milligrams per day. Take a supplement, if necessary.

mineral similar to sodium, but it has the opposite effect on the body. Foods high in potassium include acorn squash, green beans, tomato juice, potatoes, spinach, bananas, watermelon, pulses and avocados.

Blueberries. The dark blue colour of blueberries holds antioxidants, which keep free radicals from harming your DNA and causing cancer. With just 115 grams (4 ounces) of blueberries, you'll get the antioxidant power of nearly 700 grams (1½ pounds) of chopped spinach. You also might slow down the short-term memory loss that comes with age, according to studies done on rats. Blueberries can even help prevent urinary tract infections and improve your night vision and adjustment to bright lights.

Sprinkle the berries on your morning cereal, on a bed of mixed lettuce and feta cheese, or in frozen yoghurt, or pour skimmed milk over them with a little sugar or honey.

Recycled nutrients. Make your nutrients work harder. After you cook vegetables such as broccoli, carrots or spinach, use the water as a soup stock. You'll get the vitamins, minerals and nutrients the vegetables had.

Moderate alcohol consumption. For women, having up to three drinks of wine, beer or spirits a week raises HDL ('good') cholesterol levels, prevents blood clots and interferes with cell growth in the blood vessels, all factors that lower risk of heart disease. Even better news: the effects are most apparent in people over 50 or people with risk factors for heart disease. It's best to limit yourself to no more than one drink a day, however. Drinking more than that appears to be a risk factor for cancer and, in susceptible women, could lead to alcohol dependency.

Tea. In animal and some human studies, tea shows antioxidant effects, which lower risk of cardiovascular disease and cancer.

Tea also has protective compounds called isoflavonoids that keep our bones strong, particularly if you add milk to your cup. Researchers think the isoflavonoids' oestrogenic effect maintains bone density in women after they go through the menopause.

Foods that fight breast cancer. Although research hasn't proven it, several studies suggest that eating some foods could lower the risk of breast cancer. Protection may come from the beta-carotene in carrot juice, lycopene in V8 vegetable juice, linoleic acid in skimmed milk, omega-3 fatty acids in wild salmon and antioxidants in grape juice.

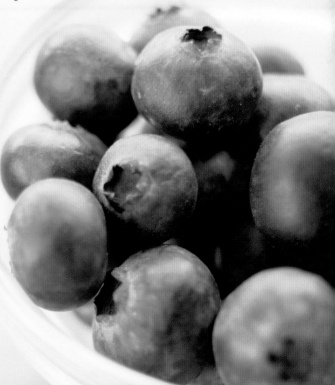

The Antioxidant Edge

Vitamins C and E are among the best-known (and best-studied) antioxidants, but many other vitamins and minerals have similar effects. Because antioxidants are so important to your overall health, it's worth taking a moment to explain what these nutrients are and how they protect against dozens (if not hundreds) of illnesses and conditions, including many common among women.

As your cells work, they use oxygen to create energy. But during normal metabolic processes, some oxygen molecules lose an electron and become unstable. These molecules, called free radicals, career around your body, trying to stabilize themselves by stripping electrons from other molecules. When they succeed, they create still more free radicals – and damage healthy tissues in the process.

Every day, your body faces thousands of assaults from free radicals. Free radical damage is what causes low-density lipoprotein (LDL, the 'bad' cholesterol) to stick to artery walls and impede or block the flow of blood. When free radicals damage the DNA in cells, the result can be cell mutations that lead to cancer. Free radicals can damage tissues in the eyes and cause cataracts or macular degeneration, the leading causes of vision loss in the elderly. Many scientists believe that free radicals are the prime force behind ageing itself.

There's no way to completely eliminate free radicals. As we've seen, they're a normal by-product of the body's metabolism. They're also formed by exposure to such things as sunshine, pollution, tobacco smoke, and simple everyday wear and tear.

Nature anticipated the harmful effects of free radicals, and created a number of countermeasures. Just as your body produces free radicals, it also produces antioxidants, enzymes that 'voluntarily' give up their own electrons to the marauding molecules. In other words, they essentially come between free radicals and your body's cells, preventing potential damage. These

MENUS WITH THE MOST

There's nothing wrong with using supplements as extra insurance against nutritional deficiencies, but you shouldn't depend on them. Experts agree that you'll get the best nutritional value for money when you get most of your nutrients in their natural form – from deliciously wholesome foods.

'Supplements are like seat belts,' says Dr Jeffrey Blumberg, a professor of nutrition. 'You don't buckle your seat belt and drive through red lights. You wear one for added security.'

Even though supplements can make up for shortfalls in your diet, foods always provide a greater range of health benefits, as they provide protein and fibre, along with a host of protective plant chemicals called phytonutrients.

Unfortunately, even women who try to eat a nutritious diet don't always succeed. The average Western diet is often deficient in such nutrients as calcium, iron and vitamins A and C, says Dr Leslie Bonci, a nutritionist.

antioxidant enzymes can do only so much, however. In fact, they can easily get overwhelmed by the sheer volume of free radicals.

That's when women need to call in the reserves – the antioxidant nutrients found in foods and many supplements. There are hundreds of natural food compounds with antioxidant properties. The main advantage of these compounds, unlike your body's natural enzymes, is that they're available in inexhaustible quantities. As long as you eat healthy foods and take supplements as necessary, you'll constantly replenish the supply.

In any discussion of antioxidants, you'll come across a lot of references to vitamins C and E, simply because they're the ones that scientists have studied most. But it's worth keeping in mind that they're only a small part of a massive army of protective compounds.

For example, the minerals zinc and selenium, which are included in most multi supplements, act as potent antioxidants. So do many of the B

To get the optimal amount of vitamins and minerals from your diet, here's what she advises.

Think plant-based. As long as your diet consists primarily of plant-based foods, such as fruit, vegetables and whole grains, you'll almost automatically get enough nutrients and fibre.

Colour your plate. Foods that are colourful are often the ones that are most nutritious. The colours in plant foods come from phytochemicals, plant-based chemical compounds that are among the most healthy things you can eat. When you have a whole grain cereal, for example, top it with red strawberries or dewy blueberries. Add mange-tout to rice dishes, or watercress to meat dishes. The more colours you get, the healthier your diet will be.

Give desserts a nutritional kick. There's nothing wrong with enjoying rich desserts on occasion. But why not make them healthier? Topping a slice of chocolate cake with delicious berries, or adding fruit slices to a bowl of ice cream, will provide important nutrients along with the sweet tastes you crave.

vitamins, as well as minerals such as magnesium. Even though the individual antioxidants are effective on their own, they perform best when they're working together. Vitamin E, for example, is one of the most powerful antioxidants ever discovered, but it's quickly exhausted in the body. When you get vitamin C at the same time, it 'recharges' vitamin E and allows it to protect your body longer. This is one reason that health experts encourage people to eat many different healthy foods or to take multivitamins instead of individual nutrients. The greater the variety of antioxidants that you consume, the more protection you'll get.

Vitamins and minerals do much more than fight free radicals, of course. In the following pages, we'll look at the many ways in which the essential nutrients in supplements and foods can prevent some of the most serious health threats that women face today.

Supplements Every Woman Should Take

You may already take vitamin or mineral supplements. It is estimated that around 10 million people in the UK take supplements every day. Do doctors disapprove? Not at all. When researchers conducted a survey of 4,500 female doctors, they found that half used vitamin and mineral supplements. Which supplements do you, as an individual, really need? It's not an easy question to answer because every vitamin and mineral does something different in the body. Many women do the easiest thing and take a multi supplement that contains a variety of vitamins and

THREE THINGS I TELL EVERY FEMALE PATIENT

Dr JANE HIGDON, a leading vitamin researcher, appreciates the benefits that come from taking supplements. But to be effective, supplements have to be used wisely. Here's what she advises.

1

EAT A NUTRITIOUS DIET – AND USE SUPPLEMENTS AS A BACKUP. There's no substitute for eating nutritious foods every day. For most women, increasing their intake of fruit and vegetables is the best way to stay healthy. But when you need a little push in the right direction – for example, getting extra calcium because you don't eat dairy foods – taking a supplement is a good way to go.

2

SHOP WISELY. Women often spend far too much on multivitamin and mineral supplements. You don't need to buy fancy brands at health food shops. Look for a multivitamin and mineral supplement that contains 100 per cent of the RNI (or recommended daily allowance) for most nutrients. Don't worry about phosphorus, pantothenic acid or potassium, because you easily get adequate amounts from food.

3

DON'T IGNORE OTHER ASPECTS OF GOOD HEALTH. People who take supplements sometimes feel as though it's acceptable to slack off in other ways. But supplements can't protect you if you don't take care of all aspects of your health – by not smoking, for example, or by getting regular exercise and a good night's sleep.

minerals. But this isn't always the solution, either. Some multi supplements contain laughably small amounts of some key nutrients, and unnecessarily high levels of others.

For example, some multis provide large amounts of vitamin A. If you're pregnant or have a history of liver problems, that can be a problem because doses higher than 10,000 IU of vitamin A in the form of retinol can increase the risk of birth defects or liver damage. Zinc is another mineral that may cause problems in doses of 25 milligrams or more daily because it interferes with the body's ability to absorb copper.

In addition, supplement manufacturers sometimes try to wow consumers by providing every conceivable nutrient – even those that researchers aren't even sure that people need. When you read supplement labels and see nutrients such as nickel, tin or silicon, you may be paying good money for substances that may not be necessary for health.

Spend a few moments surveying the shelves at the supermarket, pharmacy or health food shop, and you'll see enough different supplements to make your head spin. Many of them are helpful in certain situations, but for most women, the goal should be to get extra amounts of just a few key nutrients. Here are the supplements that we recommend.

A multi that contains 100 per cent of the RNI (or recommended daily allowance) of all nutrients – but not iron. Except for women who have been diagnosed with low iron levels or iron deficiency anaemia, supplementary amounts of this mineral aren't needed and may be harmful.

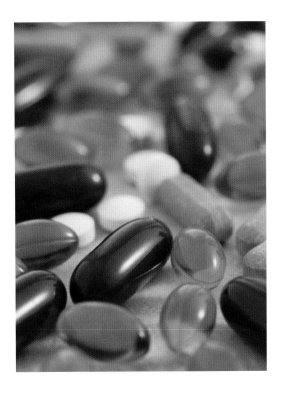

Vitamin C. We recommend a daily dose of 100 to 500 milligrams. A powerful antioxidant, vitamin C may prevent cholesterol buildup in the arteries. It also increases levels of high-density lipoprotein (HDL, the 'good' cholesterol), improves blood pressure and enhances the body's absorption of iron.

A study of more than 11,000 people found that all causes of death were lower among those who took up to 300 milligrams of vitamin C daily.

Supplemental vitamin C even appears to help people with mild to moderate hypertension lower their blood pressure. A study of 39 people with high blood pressure found that those who took vitamin C were able to lower their systolic blood pressure from an average of 155 to 142, and their diastolic blood pressure from 87 to 79. These findings have not yet been replicated in larger studies, however.

People with high blood pressure who are thinking about taking vitamin C should continue their current therapy (medication, lifestyle changes etc) and follow up with their doctor.

It's worth mentioning a potential downside to vitamin C. A study presented at an American Heart Association meeting reported that people who took 500 milligrams of vitamin C daily were more likely to develop atherosclerosis, hardening of the arteries, which increases heart disease risk.

The study got a lot of attention by the media and from scientists, but it's important to remember that it's only one study.

'Many more studies have found positive results from vitamin C supplementation, so it's important to look at the totality of the studies,' Dr Higdon says.

Vitamin C is easy to get in the diet. If you eat five servings of fruit and vegetables daily, for example, you could get at least 200 milligrams of vitamin C. If you do decide to take supplements, follow the advice from experts and take 100 to 500 milligrams daily.

Vitamin E. Look for a separate supplement that provides 100 to 400 IU. It's especially important for women who have reached the menopause, when the risk of heart disease climbs dramatically. As we mentioned earlier, vitamin E helps prevent free radicals from oxidizing, or damaging, cholesterol in the arteries, the process that makes it more likely to cling to artery walls and increase the risk of heart disease or stroke.

Natural forms of vitamin E are easy for the body to absorb, but they tend to be more expensive than synthetic forms. If you use synthetic vitamin E, plan on taking about 50 per cent more. For example, to get the equivalent of 400 IU of natural vitamin E, you'll need to take about 600 IU of the synthetic form.

If you're taking blood-thinning medications such as warfarin or regularly taking aspirin, talk to your doctor before supplementing your diet with vitamin E. It inhibits the ability of blood to clot, which can be dangerous in those who are also using clot-inhibiting medications.

Calcium with vitamin D. If you're under 50, you should be taking a daily calcium supplement that contains 500 milligrams; if you're over 50, take 1,000 milligrams. You may want to choose a calcium supplement that also contains vitamin D, which will help the body absorb calcium and keep the immune system strong. Fortified milk also has vitamin D.

Calcium supplements made with calcium carbonate are the least expensive, but for best absorption you'll want to take them with meals. Calcium citrate costs a little more but can be taken on an empty stomach.

You can absorb only about 500 milligrams of calcium at a time. If you're taking 1,000 milligrams daily, be sure to divide it into two doses.

B vitamins. These help your body turn food into the energy that you need to stay active. Doctors often advise women to take a B-complex supplement that contains vitamins B_6 and B_{12}, folic acid, thiamin, riboflavin, niacin, biotin and pantothenic acid.

Magnesium. It allows the arteries to relax, which helps control blood pressure. It also plays a role in transmitting electrical signals that keep the heart beating. Most women get about 230 milligrams of magnesium daily – a lot less than the recommended 320 milligrams for women over 30 and 310 milligrams for women under 30.

Those are just a few of the main nutrients that you need every day, but they're among the most important. When they're combined with trace minerals and essential nutrients, such as calcium and vitamins C and E, they'll go a long way towards protecting your long-term health.

Different Women, Different Supplements

The complete nutrition action plan that follows will make it easy for you to eat well at every decade of life. A woman in her twenties who's thinking of getting pregnant, for example, requires different nutrients to a woman who's entering her menopause. The vitamins and minerals you need to watch for in your thirties and forties aren't necessarily the same ones that you need to focus on in your fifties and sixties.

In Your Twenties

Get relief from PMS. For most women, the bloating, breast tenderness and other symptoms of premenstrual syndrome tend to get better as the decades pass.

But for women in their twenties, PMS can be a real problem. There's some evidence that taking extra amounts of magnesium and vitamin B_6 can ease anxiety, premenstrual bloating and other monthly discomforts.

One study found that women who took 200 milligrams of magnesium daily for 2 months had significantly less fluid retention than women who took a placebo.

'Magnesium is very important, and it's often short in women's diets,' says Dr Ann Walker, senior lecturer in human nutrition at the University of Reading. Her studies have shown that women who take 200 milligrams of magnesium and 50 milligrams of vitamin B_6 will suffer less from premenstrual tension, mood swings, irritability and anxiety.

Calcium is also helpful for women who experience PMS. One study found that women who supplemented their diets with 1,200 milligrams of calcium daily for 3 months were able to reduce their symptoms by 45 per cent.

WHAT YOU NEED DURING PREGNANCY

A woman's body changes dramatically during pregnancy. Everything gets larger and more active: the uterus and its supporting muscles enlarge, the joints get more flexible in anticipation of childbirth and blood volume increases by as much as 60 to 80 per cent.

Even if you eat a nutritious diet, it's not always possible to get enough vitamins and minerals to supply your needs as well as those of the baby-to-be. That's why doctors usually advise women to take prenatal supplements during pregnancy.

Every woman needs different kinds of supplements, depending on her diet. A woman who's a vegetarian, for example, may need a supplement with higher-than-usual amounts of iron or vitamin B_{12}. On the other hand, a woman who eats a lot of meat or seafood will want to avoid high-iron supplements because she'll probably get more than enough of this mineral in her diet.

If you're pregnant now or are planning to get pregnant, here are a few nutrients you'll need to pay attention to.

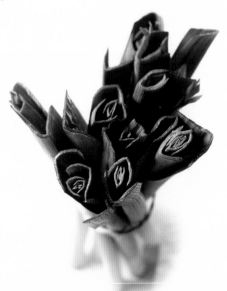

- **B vitamins**. You don't have to worry about getting too much of the B vitamins during pregnancy because these nutrients do not accumulate in the body. Two B vitamins to focus on are folic acid or folate and vitamin B_{12}. Folic acid prevents birth defects called neural tube defects, and vitamin B_{12} aids in foetal metabolism and maintains healthy levels of red blood cells. Foods high in folic acid include fortified cereals, bread and pulses. Foods high in vitamin B_{12} are meats and fish. If you've had a baby with neural tube defects and you're planning another pregnancy, your doctor may prescribe taking 400 micrograms of folic acid.
- **Vitamins A and D.** Unlike the B vitamins, your body accumulates vitamins A and D over time. The amount of these nutrients you should get in your prenatal supplement will depend on the amounts you get in your diet. Foods high in vitamin A include squash and carrots; vitamin D-rich foods include fatty fish and fortified milk.
- **Calcium.** Women who are pregnant often have low levels of calcium, which is essential for strengthening foetal bones.
- **Iron.** Women who are pregnant are sharing their blood supply with the growing foetus, and they require a large amount of iron in order to keep up with the increased demand for red blood cells. Even if you have a healthy diet, you have a high risk of becoming anaemic during pregnancy.

Before your doctor gives you a prescription for prenatal nutrients, be sure to mention whether you're eating a lot of iron-rich foods, such as red meat, liver or green leafy vegetables. This will help your doctor determine how much additional iron you'll need.

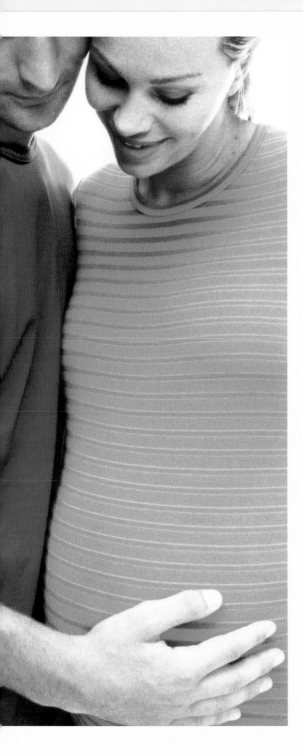

Dodge diabetes. There's a good reason to take action against diabetes right away. Women in their teens and twenties are increasingly being diagnosed with type 2 diabetes, which is often triggered by weight gain. In the past, this condition usually affected women after the age of 45.

Vitamin and mineral supplements are unlikely to prevent diabetes, but they may reduce its severity and potential side effects if you do get it.

After reviewing data collected on almost 10,000 men and women over 20 years, researchers found that people who had the highest levels of vitamin E were the ones who were least likely to develop diabetes. Vitamin E also protects against heart disease, which is important because people with diabetes have a very high risk of getting it. In fact, heart attack and stroke are leading causes of death among those with diabetes.

In addition to vitamin E, you may want to be sure that your multi supplement contains chromium and magnesium. Both minerals have been shown to make cells in the body more sensitive to insulin's effects, thereby reducing the risk of developing full-fledged diabetes.

Keep your gums healthy. Young women who don't get enough vitamin C and calcium in their diet are more likely to develop periodontal disease, an infection of the gums and other tissues that support the teeth. Take a multi supplement that contains at least 60 milligrams of vitamin C. For calcium, women in their twenties should take a supplement that provides 500 milligrams daily.

Build strong bones. When women reach menopause, they have a high risk of developing osteoporosis, a bone-thinning condition that's the leading cause of fractures in elderly people. This doesn't mean you can put off thinking about it, however. Keeping your bones strong when you're young will help prevent problems decades down the road. One of the simplest things that you can do is make sure you get enough calcium and vitamin D.

In one study, women who took 500 milligrams of calcium and 700 IU of vitamin D daily for 3 years were able to reduce the loss of supportive bone throughout their bodies. This was impressive enough – but the most important lesson occurred after the study ended. About a third of the participants stopped taking the supplements, and within 1 year they lost all of the bone density gains.

If you're in your twenties, plan on taking 500 milligrams of calcium daily. The body can absorb only so much calcium at a time, so it's best to take these supplements between meals, or with meals that don't contain a lot of calcium.

Vitamin C is also important for strong bones. It helps stimulate the body's production of bone and of collagen, a connective tissue. When researchers tested the bone mineral density of 994 postmenopausal women, they found that those who took an average of 745 milligrams of vitamin C daily had bone densities that were about 3 per cent higher than those who didn't supplement.

Your regular multivitamin will help, too, as long as it contains the RNI (or recommended daily allowance) of 400 IU of vitamin D. In northern latitudes, such as the UK, there is insufficient ultraviolet light available for the body to produce vitamin D. Taking a supplement year-round will ensure a woman has adequate vitamin D stores throughout the year.

Some multis also contain vitamin K, which helps with bone formation and reduces bone breakdown. The minerals magnesium and potassium have been shown to help prevent fractures. Magnesium keeps blood calcium at healthy levels, and potassium keeps acid in the blood from pulling calcium from the bones. Look for multis that provide 100 per cent of the RNI (or recommended daily allowance) of these nutrients.

In Your Thirties

Kick the common cold. Women in their thirties are often juggling careers and family responsibilities. The non-stop stress makes the body vulnerable to upper respiratory infections – especially when children are always coming home from school with sneezes and runny noses.

On average, Westerners get two to six colds a year. Although there is little evidence that vitamin C prevents colds, a number of studies have found that taking at least 1,000 milligrams of vitamin C daily at the first symptoms of a cold reduced the duration of colds by an average of 1 day. This may be due to vitamin C's ability to block the effects of histamines, chemicals in the body that at high levels cause cold symptoms.

The vitamin C in multi supplements can also be helpful if you're suffering from low energy. Studies have shown that 20 to 30 per cent of Western adults get less than the RNI (or recommended daily allowance) of 40 milligrams of vitamin C. This can be a problem because one of the jobs of vitamin C is to move fatty acids into heart and skeletal muscles to provide energy.

Protect your heart. One in three women currently under 40 will eventually develop heart disease. An effective way to protect the heart, as well as getting regular exercise, refraining from smoking and avoiding saturated fats in the diet, is to get enough antioxidant nutrients in the diet.

We've already discussed how vitamin E prevents free radicals from damaging cholesterol and making it more likely to stick to arteries. Unfortunately, most women don't get anywhere near enough of this important vitamin.

Vitamin E is important even if you already have blood vessel disease. It relaxes blood vessels and helps prevent the formation of blood-blocking clots. Studies have shown that when people with heart disease take vitamin E supplements, their risk of dying from the disease declines by 40 to 60 per cent.

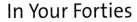

Many doctors advise women to take 100 to 400 IU of vitamin E daily. At the same time, it's helpful to take a multi that contains vitamin C. It 'recharges' vitamin E in the body, which increases its effectiveness.

The nutrients in your multivitamin and mineral supplement can also protect the heart. For example, selenium, a mineral found in most multis, reduces the amount of cholesterol that's damaged by free radicals. Multis also contain folic acid, vitamin B_6 and vitamin B_{12}. These B vitamins lower blood levels of homocysteine. High homocysteine levels have been linked to heart disease.

In Your Forties

Fight cancer with supplements. Studies have clearly shown that women who consume an abundance of fruit and vegetables have a lower risk of cancer. Some of the credit for this goes to folic acid (or folate), which is present in fruit,

---

WHAT WORKS FOR ME

DR CHRISTINE K. CASSEL, chair of the department of geriatrics and adult development at a leading medical school, doesn't take a lot of supplements – but there are a few that she makes sure to take every day.

I take a multivitamin, along with vitamins C and E for their antioxidant protection. I've

started taking additional B vitamins, including folic acid, now that there's some evidence that folic acid may protect against heart disease by lowering homocysteine levels in the blood. I also take a calcium supplement as insurance against bone loss.

vegetables and other plant foods. Studies suggest that women who don't get enough folic acid in their diet have a higher risk of developing cancers of the cervix, colon and rectum, lung, oesophagus, brain, pancreas and breast. The body uses folic acid to synthesize DNA. If you don't get enough, the DNA becomes more vulnerable to damage, which increases cancer risk. Doctors advise women to get 200 micrograms of folic acid daily. In addition, be sure your multi supplement contains vitamin B_{12}. This nutrient is necessary for folic acid to function in the body.

Another cancer-preventing nutrient is calcium. One study found that people who took 1,200 milligrams of calcium daily were less likely to develop recurring polyps, growths in the colon that often precede the development of cancer.

Vitamin D, too, may help. American scientists have noticed that deaths from colon cancer are more common in parts of the United States that have the lowest amounts of sunshine. Sunshine, you'll recall, triggers the production of vitamin D in the body. This is important because vitamin D has been shown to suppress tumour growth. One study found that women with lower-than-normal levels of vitamin D had an increased risk for colorectal adenoma, damaged areas in the colon that may occur 10 years or more before cancer actually develops.

Selenium is another nutrient that protects against cancer. One study found that people who took 200 micrograms of selenium daily were significantly less likely to die from cancer. The mineral also reduced the incidence of cancers of the lung, colon and rectum.

Reduce joint pain. By the time women reach their forties, their joints start to rebel against a lifetime of flexing. Osteoarthritis, also known as 'wear and tear' arthritis, occurs when tissues in the joints begin to break down over time. One way to prevent this is to take vitamin E, which inhibits the effects of inflammation-causing molecules in the joints. In fact, vitamin E has been shown to relieve arthritis pain better than ibuprofen or other over-the-counter anti-inflammatory drugs. The recommended dosage for easing arthritis is 400 IU of vitamin E daily.

Another way to reduce joint damage from arthritis is to take a supplement that provides 400 IU, or 100 per cent of the RNI (or recommended daily allowance) for vitamin D.

Vitamin C and calcium also appear to protect the joints. In a study of almost 200 participants, those given a powder supplement that contained vitamin C and calcium reported less pain and stiffness and an improvement in joint function.

Sharpen your eyesight. Studies suggest that people who take supplemental vitamin C when they're young are less likely in their later years to develop cataracts, a common cause of vision loss.

Cataracts occur when proteins in the lenses of the eyes are oxidized, or damaged, by free radicals. When you take vitamin C, the nutrient saturates the tissues of the eye and prevents the oxidation. One study of more than 5,000 women found that those who took vitamin C for 10 years reduced their risk for cataracts by 45 per cent. So far, evidence suggests that taking 150 milligrams of vitamin C daily is enough to provide long-term protection against cataracts.

In Your Fifties

Protect against breast cancer. A woman's risk for breast cancer rises dramatically once she reaches her 50th birthday. It's hardly news that a high-fat diet increases the risk for breast cancer, probably because it increases levels of tumour-promoting lipids in the breast. Eating more fruit and vegetables and reducing fat in the diet are your first lines of defence, but it's also helpful to supplement your diet with calcium and vitamin D. Researchers aren't sure why, but these nutrients appear to inhibit breast changes that can lead to cancer.

If you drink alcohol, be sure to use a multi that contains folic acid. A study of more than 88,000 nurses found that those who had one measure of alcohol (one 120-millilitre glass of wine, one 350-millilitre glass of lager or one 45-millilitre measure of spirits) a day had a 24 per cent greater risk for breast cancer than those who drank less.

Those who supplemented their diet with folic acid were able to cut their risk in half.

Doctors advise taking a multi supplement that contains 200 micrograms of folic acid. The folic acid you get from foods such as pulses, fortified fruit juice, spinach and asparagus will easily take care of the rest.

Maximize your immunity. The immune system becomes less effective over time, which is why older women may be more susceptible to infections as well as cancer. Once again, vitamin E can make a difference. Studies have shown that when older adults take as little as 222 IU of vitamin E daily, their immune systems become more active and are better able to fend off infections.

Strengthen your memory. Nearly everyone experiences declines in short-term memory in the latter half of life. Doctors theorize that this may be due in part to the harmful effects of free radicals in the brain. Taking 100 to 400 IU of a vitamin E supplement, which 'neutralizes' free radicals, may be one of the best approaches to keeping your memory strong. In fact, a study of almost 5,000 people found that those who had high levels of vitamin E consistently performed better on memory tests than those with lower levels.

Vitamin B_{12}, too, plays a role in memory. It's not uncommon, in fact, for people to go to their doctors because they're experiencing memory loss or other mental declines, only to discover that they aren't getting enough vitamin B_{12} in their diet.

Deficiencies of vitamin B_{12} are common because, as people age, their digestive tracts become less efficient at absorbing this nutrient.

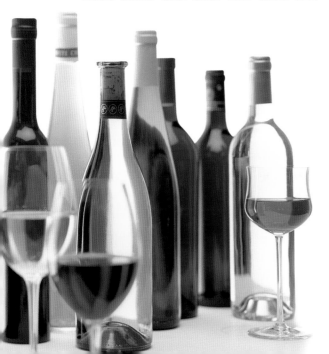

That's why doctors often advise adults aged 50 and over to take a multi supplement that provides 100 per cent of the RNI (or recommended daily allowance) of vitamin B_{12}, which is 1.5 micrograms.

Say goodbye to kidney stones. If you don't get enough vitamin B_6 in your diet, you may be putting yourself at risk of the agonizing pain of kidney stones. A study of more than 85,000 women found that those with the highest levels of vitamin B_6 in the blood were least likely to develop kidney stones. For protection against stones, doctors advise getting 10 milligrams of vitamin B_6 daily.

In Your Sixties and Beyond

Enhance your hearing and protect your mind. Are you always asking your friends to speak up? It's possible that getting too little vitamin B_{12} and folic acid is interfering with your hearing. About 24 per cent of those aged 65 to 74 have some degree of hearing loss; that number rises to 40 per cent after the age of 75. Your best protection may be to take supplements that contain the RNI (or recommended daily allowance), or 1.5 micrograms, of vitamin B_{12} and 200 micrograms of folic acid.

The same nutrients also appear to play a role in preventing Alzheimer's disease. In one study, researchers looked at 370 people 75 years and older and found that those with low levels of vitamin B_{12} or folic acid were twice as likely to get Alzheimer's disease as those who had normal levels.

Control ageing with copper. Women need only 2 milligrams of copper daily. Unfortunately, most women get half that amount. Over time, low levels of copper can speed up an ageing process called protein glycation, which breaks down tissues in the heart, blood vessels and kidneys. When shopping for a multi supplement, choose one that provides it as an amino acid chelate. Some multis contain a related compound called cupric oxide, which can't be absorbed by the body.

Improve your mood. A minority of those aged 65 years and older experience depression – and studies have shown that about 30 per cent of older people hospitalized for depression have low levels of vitamin B_{12}. In fact one study found that women over 65 who were deficient in vitamin B_{12} were twice as likely to suffer from severe depression than those who got enough of this nutrient.

In addition, up to 79 per cent of depressed adults are deficient in vitamin B_6. On average, women get only about half as much vitamin B_6 as they should. In addition, birth control pills and other supplemental hormones can interfere with the vitamin's action.

As long as you take a supplement that contains the RNI (or recommended daily allowance) of 2 milligrams of vitamin B_6 and 6 micrograms of B_{12}, you'll have sufficient levels of these nutrients to help protect your long-term mental health.

3

Using Herbs Wisely

From echinacea for colds to black cohosh
for menopausal changes and ginkgo for memory
problems, women often turn to herbal remedies
to solve everyday health problems. And indeed,
throughout this book, doctors who practise
complementary or alternative medicine offer herbal
solutions to everyday problems. Women have used
herbs as medicine for generations. Long before the
development of prescription and over-the-counter
drugs, herbs were commonly employed to fight
infection, reduce pain, soothe anxiety and relieve
menopausal discomfort.

The ancients knew what they were doing. Scientists have learned that herbs contain dozens or even hundreds of chemically active compounds. In fact, the active ingredients in many prescription drugs are very similar (or even identical) to the chemicals in herbs.

Unfortunately, shopping for medicinal herbs can be a challenge. Herb manufacturers are prohibited from making health claims on the labels; nor are they allowed to give advice on how to use herbs to treat medical problems. Without medical guidance, it can be difficult to know which herbs are most effective for treating different conditions, or how to use them to get the best results. And because the herb industry isn't strictly regulated, some unscrupulous manufacturers use ingredients that aren't effective or tout herbal combinations that don't work, says Douglas Schar, a leading herbalist.

Used as directed, the herbs suggested in this book can be very effective. When taken correctly, they're often less likely than drugs to cause side effects. They're often milder than drugs, yet still have beneficial effects. But because herbal medicines are sold over the counter, you become the doctor and pharmacist. It's important to have the same respect for herbs as you do for prescription drugs.

In the following pages, you'll find a comprehensive guide to dozens of important medicinal herbs used for women's wellness.

We explain which herbs are best for different conditions, tell you how to take the herbs and offer information on possible side effects or interactions. Schar provides dosage recommendations; the practitioner or experts that you consult for specific conditions may recommend slightly different amounts.

THREE THINGS I TELL EVERY FEMALE PATIENT

DOUGLAS SCHAR is a leading herbalist who specializes in preventing disease with herbal treatments. He offers this advice to women who use herbs.

1 **DON'T ASK THE ASSISTANTS IN HEALTH FOOD STORES FOR ADVICE.** They're not medically trained, and they rarely have expertise in the actions (and interactions) of herbal medicines. Instead, consult a professional herbalist, or a doctor who incorporates medicinal herbs in his or her practice.

2 **READ LABELS CAREFULLY.** The best products contain a single herb. Those that contain multiple herbs are less likely to be effective.

3 **TRUST YOUR INSTINCTS.** When manufacturers make claims that seem too good to be true, they probably are. Does the label 'guarantee' you'll lose 10 kilograms a month? Save your money. The manufacturer is more interested in marketing the product than in protecting your health.

How Herbs Heal

We have dozens of healing herbs at our disposal, but their active ingredients can all be grouped in a few chemical families. These chemicals, which occur in herbs in varying proportions, are what give herbs their healing powers. They include:

Bitters. As the name suggests, these are bitter-tasting chemical compounds. They stimulate bile flow and digestive juices.

Flavonoids. They're among the most important antioxidants. They protect cells from oxidation, strengthen blood vessel walls, and reduce water retention, inflammation and muscle spasms.

Volatile oils. They give herbs their unique scents, and they also have a mild antiseptic action. When inhaled, volatile oils relieve stress. They may also enhance appetite, stimulate circulation and reduce water retention associated with the menstrual cycle.

Alkaloids. They've been shown to fight bacterial and fungal infections.

Gums and resins. They bind to lipids (fats) in the blood. Herbs that contain gums and resins are often used to lower cholesterol.

Mucilage. It's a slippery substance in herbs that helps relieve constipation. Mucilage also soothes irritated mucous membranes in the throat, intestine and other parts of the body.

Saponins. These have anti-tussive (cough-relieving) properties. They also regulate women's hormones, reduce stress and strengthen blood vessels.

Tannins. These promote skin healing. They

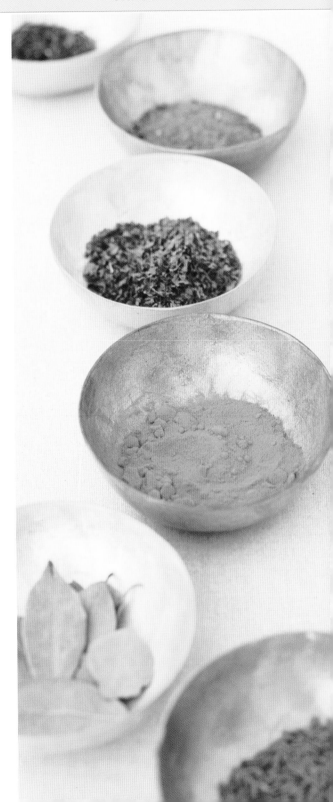

also help speed the healing of mucous membranes (as with sore throats).

Anthraquinones. They're good for digestion because they stimulate bile production. They're also helpful for strengthening and restoring proper liver function.

Cautions and Caveats

Men and women alike often assume that because herbs are natural, they're inherently safer than synthetic drugs. Nothing could be further from the truth. The chemical compounds in herbs can have powerful effects in the body – including powerful side effects. For the most part, herbs are safe as well as effective, but only when you use them properly. Here's what doctors advise.

Avoid herbs during pregnancy. Very little research has looked at the effects of medicinal herbs taken during pregnancy. Your doctor may recommend certain herbs if you're pregnant – but all of the information in the following pages is designed for women who aren't pregnant and aren't breast-feeding.

Don't double dip. Some herbs have similar actions to prescription or over-the-counter drugs. If you elect to take herbs suggested for various ailments discussed in this book, don't combine them with medication. The antidepressant Prozac, for example, shouldn't be combined with St John's wort, a herb commonly taken for depression. We'll talk more about herb–drug interactions in the chart opposite.

Stick to one herb. Just as it may be harmful to combine herbs and drugs that have similar actions, it can be risky to take two similar herbs.

Know which plant parts you need. The medicinal part of echinacea is the root, but that doesn't stop unscrupulous manufacturers from selling the leaves. In the chart below, we've included information on the parts of herbs that are most effective.

Avoid creative but misleading product names. Products with intentionally misspelled names, such as 'Clenze', 'Nutra-mune' or 'Staminex', are marketing gimmicks; they're unlikely to be effective herbal medicines. Also, avoid products that say 'pro', 'max', 'turbo' or 'plus' on the label. Instead, stick to the herbs recommended in this book.

Know when to stop. Herbs act more slowly than drugs, but you should still notice an improvement in your condition within a few weeks to a month. If a herb doesn't seem to be helping, stop taking it and get professional advice, Schar advises.

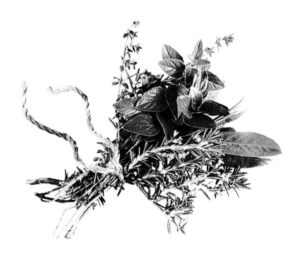

Your Personal Herb Guide

Allergies

Herb and Standard Doses	What It Does	General Cautions	Drug Interactions
NETTLE (*Urtica dioica*) Three times daily: 20 drops 1:1 tincture or 1 tsp 1:5 tincture. Use only the plant, not the root.	Relieves allergies, allergic skin rashes, hay fever and seasonal rhinitis.	None.	None known.

Anxiety

Herb and Standard Doses	What It Does	General Cautions	Drug Interactions
AMERICAN GINSENG (*Panax quinquefolium*) Four 500-mg root tablets once daily (use the root only).	Reduces stress.	Don't take if you have high blood pressure. May cause irritability if taken with caffeine or other stimulants.	Insufficient data.
PASSIONFLOWER (*Passiflora incarnata*) Two 500-mg tablets before bed. Use only the flower, leaves and vine.	Treats insomnia due to anxiety.	None.	Don't take with sedatives, sleeping pills or anti-anxiety medication.
SKULLCAP (*Scutellaria laterifolia*) 3 cups of tea daily. Use only leaves and flowers.	Treats anxiety, restlessness and nervousness. Also, reduces premenstrual symptoms and kidney problems.	None.	None known.
VALERIAN (*Valeriana officinalis*) Two 500-mg root tablets 30 minutes before bed. Use only valerian root.	Reduces nervousness and insomnia. Reduces digestive discomfort.	None.	Don't take with sleep-enhancing or mood-regulating medication.

continued

Cancer Protection

Herb and Standard Doses	What It Does	General Cautions	Drug Interactions
GREEN AND BLACK TEAS (*Camellia sinensis*) 1 cup green or black tea three times daily.	Green and black tea act as antioxidants, reducing cell damage that may lead to cancer. Also reduce joint inflammation in those with arthritis.	The caffeine in green and black tea may result in anxiety or insomnia.	None known.
MAITAKE MUSHROOM (*Grifola frondosa*) For prevention, two 350-mg tablets, three times daily. For those with cancer, the recommended dose is six 350-mg tablets three times daily during alternating months. Use only dried maitake supplements.	Improves immune system's ability to recognize or destroy damaged cells. Stimulates production of white blood cells.	None.	None known.

Cardiovascular Disease and High Blood Pressure

Herb and Standard Doses	What It Does	General Cautions	Drug Interactions
ELDERBERRY (*Sambucus nigra*) Three times daily: 1 tsp syrup or 1 tsp 1:5 tincture. Use only the ripe berry and flower.	Acts as a powerful antiviral agent that minimizes coughs, colds and flu.	None.	None.
GARLIC (*Allium sativum*) One 500-mg tablet three times daily. Use supplements with standardized amounts of alliin or allicin. (Avoid garlic oil gel caps.)	Acts as an antioxidant. Lowers blood pressure, cholesterol and the risk of cardiovascular disease.	A blood thinner, it should be discontinued 2 to 3 weeks prior to surgery, and for 2 weeks after surgery. Increases stomach acid production in some people.	Do not use if you're on blood-thinning medication.
GUGGUL (*Commiphora mukul*) 500 mg standardized guggul extract twice daily.	Reduces cholesterol levels and eases joint inflammation.	In rare cases, may cause diarrhoea, restlessness, apprehension or hiccups. Avoid this herb if you have hyperthyroidism.	None known.

Cardiovascular Disease and High Blood Pressure (continued)

Herb and Standard Doses	What It Does	General Cautions	Drug Interactions
HAWTHORN (*Crataegus oxycantha, C. laevigata, C. monogyna*) Two or three times a day: 20 drops 1:1 tincture; or 1 tsp 1:5 tincture. Use only the berries, flowers and leaves.	Reduces the risk of cardiovascular disease.	If you already have a cardiovascular condition, don't take without medical supervision. Use with caution if you have low blood pressure – it can lower the pressure even further.	May necessitate lower doses of blood pressure and other medication.

Constipation

Herb and Standard Doses	What It Does	General Cautions	Drug Interactions
FLAXSEED (LINSEED) (*Linum usitatissimum*) 2 tbsp ground flaxseed daily.	Contains soluble fibre to keep you regular.	Take with at least 240 ml (8 fl oz) water. Don't take flaxseed if you have a bowel obstruction or diverticular disease.	May interfere with the absorption of drugs.

Depression

Herb and Standard Doses	What It Does	General Cautions	Drug Interactions
ST JOHN'S WORT (*Hypericum perforatum*) Two 500-mg tablets three times daily. Use only the leaves, stems and flowers.	Improves mood and symptoms of depression. Eases muscle aches; prevents wound infection when applied topically.	May cause sensitivity to light. May cause gastrointestinal symptoms, allergic reactions and fatigue.	Don't use with antidepressants such as Prozac or Seroxat, or other prescription medicines. May lower amount of some prescription drugs in your blood.

Endometriosis

Herb and Standard Doses	What It Does	General Cautions	Drug Interactions
EVENING PRIMROSE (*Oenothera biennis*) Two 500-mg tablets once daily. Use oil made from the seeds.	Reduces inflammation and eases pain from endometriosis.	None.	None known.

continued

Fever

Herb and Standard Doses	What It Does	General Cautions	Drug Interactions
CINNAMON (*Cinnamomum zeylanicum*) Pour 1 cup boiling water over 1 tsp powder; steep covered for 20 minutes. Use only the bark. Drink 3 cups daily.	Reduces inflammation and pain and fever.	None.	None.
GINGER (*Zingiber officinale*) Three times daily: two 500-mg tablets; or 1 tsp 1:5 tincture; or, for tea, grate 1 tsp ginger, cover with 1 cup boiling water, and steep for 10 minutes. (Fresh root is most effective.)	Reduces fever.	Avoid therapeutic amounts of ginger if you have gallstones.	None known.
WILLOW BARK (*Salix alba*) Steep 2 tsp dried bark in 1 cup boiling water for 20 minutes.	Reduces fever.	Can cause stomach irritation. Do not give to children under 16 who have fever or any viral infection, including chickenpox or flu. May contribute to Reye's syndrome, which affects the brain and liver.	Do not take if you need to avoid aspirin, especially if you are taking blood-thinning medication because its active ingredient is related to aspirin. May interact with barbiturates or sedatives.

Headaches

Herb and Standard Doses	What It Does	General Cautions	Drug Interactions
FEVERFEW (*Tanacetum parthenium*) One 50-mg tablet every morning. Use only fresh or freeze-dried feverfew leaves. Or take 20 drops 1:5 tincture, or 10 drops 1:1 tincture.	Prevents migraine and cluster headaches.	Chewing fresh leaves can cause mouth sores in some people.	None known.
GINGER (*Zingiber officinale*) Three times daily: two 500-mg tablets; or 1 tsp 1:5 tincture; or, for tea, grate 1 tsp ginger, cover with 1 cup boiling water and steep for 10 minutes. (Fresh root is most effective.)	Improves circulation and prevents migraines.	Avoid therapeutic amounts of ginger if you have gall-stones.	None known.

Headaches (continued)

Herb and Standard Doses	What It Does	General Cautions	Drug Interactions
ROSEMARY (*Rosmarinus officinalis*) Steep 1 tsp dried rosemary in 1 cup boiling water for 10 minutes (use only the leaves). Take 2 cups per day.	Dilates blood vessels and prevents stress-related headaches; acts as digestive aid; may protect against diabetes and artery disease.	None.	None known.

Hepatitis

Herb and Standard Doses	What It Does	General Cautions	Drug Interactions
MAITAKE MUSHROOM (*Grifola frondosa*) 4 to 6 g powder tablets.	Stimulates immune system and may reduce symptoms of hepatitis.	Safe.	None known.

Hives (nettle rash, urticaria)

Herb and Standard Doses	What It Does	General Cautions	Drug Interactions
NETTLE (*Urtica dioica*) One or two capsules freeze-dried nettle leaf extract every 2 to 4 hours until symptoms disappear.	Reduces hives, nettle rash, urticaria.	None.	None known.

Inflammatory Bowel Disease

Herb and Standard Doses	What It Does	General Cautions	Drug Interactions
CHAMOMILE (*Matricaria recutita*) Pour 1 cup boiling water over 1 to 2 tsp dried herb, cover, and let steep for 10 to 15 minutes. Use only the flowers.	Relaxes muscles in the stomach. Eases indigestion, irritable bowel problems and colitis.	Causes allergic reactions in rare cases. Those who are allergic to related plants, such as ragwort, asters and chrysanthemums, should drink the tea with caution.	None known.
PEPPERMINT (*Mentha piperita*) Pour 1 cup boiling water over 1 to 2 tsp dried herb, cover, and let steep for 10 to 15 minutes. Use only the leaves.	Helps ease indigestion, flatulence and nausea.	None.	None known.

continued

Irritable Bowel Disease

Herb and Standard Doses	What It Does	General Cautions	Drug Interactions
CHAMOMILE (*Matricaria recutita*) Three times daily: 20 drops 1:1 tincture, or 1 tsp 1:5 tincture. Use only the flowers.	Eases irritable bowel problems and colitis.	Causes allergic reactions in rare cases. Those who are allergic to related plants, such as ragwort, asters and chrysanthemums, should drink the tea with caution.	None known.
CRAMP BARK (*Viburnum opulus*) Three times daily: 1 g dried-bark capsules, or 20 drops 1:1 tincture, or 1 tsp 1:5 tincture.	Relaxes intestines.	Safe.	None.
PEPPERMINT (*Mentha piperita*) Enteric-coated peppermint oil capsules, 0.2–0.4 ml, twice daily between meals.	May lessen bloating and diarrhoea.	None.	None known.

Laryngitis

Herb and Standard Doses	What It Does	General Cautions	Drug Interactions
CINNAMON (*Cinnamomum zeylanicum*) To make tea, pour 1 cup boiling water over 1 tsp powdered; steep covered for 20 minutes. Drink 1 to 3 cups daily.	Reduces inflammation and pain.	None.	None.

Low Energy

Herb and Standard Doses	What It Does	General Cautions	Drug Interactions
ASIAN GINSENG (*Panax ginseng*) Four 500-mg tablets once daily (only tablets that contain the root).	Acts as a mild stimulant and mood enhancer. Also acts as an antioxidant.	Don't take if you have high blood pressure, with caffeine or other stimulants, or when under acute stress. May cause menstrual irregularities or intensify menopause symptoms. May cause headaches, nervousness and insomnia in women under 45.	Insufficient data.
SCHISANDRA (*Schisandra chinensis*) Two 500-mg tablets twice daily. Use only tablets that contain the fruit.	Supplies energy by increasing circulation and improving heart function. Protects the liver, improves respiration, speeds reflexes and reduces symptoms of nervous exhaustion, such as headaches, insomnia, dizziness and palpitation.	None.	None known.
SIBERIAN GINSENG (*Eleutherococcus senticosus*) Two 500-mg tablets three times daily. Use only the root bark.	Similar properties to Asian ginseng.	None.	None known.

Low Sexual Desire

Herb and Standard Doses	What It Does	General Cautions	Drug Interactions
SAW PALMETTO (*Serenoa repens*) Two 500-mg berry tablets three times daily. (The berries are the most effective part.)	Increases sex drive in women. Also blocks the effects of androgens, male hormones that can cause excessive hair growth.	May cause stomach problems in rare cases.	None known.

continued

Macular Degeneration

Herb and Standard Doses	What It Does	General Cautions	Drug Interactions
BILBERRY (*Vaccinium myrtillus*) Pour 1 cup hot water over 1 or 2 tbsp dried whole berries (or 2 or 3 tsp crushed berries). Let tea steep, covered, for 10 minutes, then strain. Drink 1 cup daily. Commercial tea bags are also available.	Improves night vision.	None.	None.
GINKGO (*Ginkgo biloba*) 15 drops extract dropped into a sip of water, once or twice daily for 1 month.	Improves circulation in the eyes.	In very rare cases ginkgo can cause headaches, digestive upset and skin reactions. Thins blood, so don't take it 2 to 3 weeks before or after surgery. Can cause skin inflammation, diarrhoea and vomiting in doses larger than 240 mg.	Don't take with monoamine-oxidase inhibitors (MAOIs), such as phenelzine (Nardil) or tranylcypromine; aspirin or other non-steroidal anti-inflammatory drugs; or blood-thinning drugs, such as warfarin.

Memory

Herb and Standard Doses	What It Does	General Cautions	Drug Interactions
GINKGO (*Ginkgo biloba*) One tablet standardized to 24 per cent ginkgo flavone glycosides, three times daily.	Improves memory, concentration and alertness.	In very rare cases ginkgo can cause headaches, digestive upset and skin reactions. Thins blood, so don't take it 2 to 3 weeks before or after surgery. Can cause skin inflammation, diarrhoea and vomiting in doses larger than 240 mg.	Don't take with antidepressant monoamine-oxidase inhibitors (MAOIs), such as phenelzine (Nardil) or tranylcypromine; aspirin or other non-steroidal anti-inflammatory drugs; or blood-thinning drugs, such as warfarin.

Menstruation and Menopause Problems

Herb and Standard Doses	What It Does	General Cautions	Drug Interactions
ANGELICA (*Angelica sinensis*) Take three times daily: two 500-mg tablets or 20 drops 1:1 tincture or 1 tsp 1:5 tincture. The root is the most effective part.	Relieves hot flushes, increases sex drive and improves skin. Also stimulates digestion and production and action of immune cells. Binds to free radicals, making them harmless.	Use for short periods of time. Don't take it if you have oestrogen-dependent cancer or a bleeding disorder. Increases sun sensitivity.	Don't take if you're on blood-thinning medication or undergoing cancer treatment.

Menstruation and Menopause Problems (continued)

Herb and Standard Doses	What It Does	General Cautions	Drug Interactions
BLACK COHOSH (*Cimicifuga racemosa*) Three times daily: two 500-mg dried root tablets or 20 drops 1:1 tincture. The root is the most effective part.	Relieves menopausal symptoms, such as thin vaginal tissue, vaginal dryness, memory loss, depression, mood swings and hot flushes.	Don't use for longer than 6 months. Avoid this herb if you have oestrogen-dependent cancer. May cause occasional gastric discomfort.	Don't use if you're on hormone replacement therapy.
EVENING PRIMROSE (*Oenothera biennis*) 1,000 mg daily. Use oil made from the seeds.	Reduces inflammation and eases pain triggered by surges in prostaglandins during the menstrual cycle.	None.	None known.
FLAXSEED (LINSEED) (*Linum usitatissimum*) 1 tbsp ground flaxseed daily.	Helps balance shifting hormones at perimenopause. Contains omega-3 fatty acids, which lower the risk for heart disease. Contains soluble fibre to keep you regular. Also lowers cholesterol and fights breast cancer and depression.	Take with at least 240 ml (8 fl oz) of water. Don't take flaxseed if you have a bowel obstruction or diverticular disease.	May interfere with the absorption of drugs.
SAGE (*Salvia officinalis*) 4 heaped tbsp dried leaves steeped 4 hours in 1 cup boiling water. The leaves are the most effective part.	Helps reduce and even eliminate night sweats. May slow progression of Alzheimer's disease; may reduce indigestion and, when gargled, may soothe throat irritation. Acts as an antioxidant.	None.	Can increase sedative side effects of drugs.
VITEX (ALSO CALLED CHASTEBERRY) (*Vitex agnus-castus*) Twice daily: two 500-mg tablets or 60 drops 1:5 tincture or tablets containing 250 mg 4:1 extract. The seeds (also called the berries) are the most effective part.	Relieves premenstrual symptoms. Helps treat irregular, painful and heavy periods.	See your gynaecologist if you experience bleeding between periods.	May lower the effectiveness of contraceptive pills.

continued

Pneumonia

Herb and Standard Doses	What It Does	General Cautions	Drug Interactions
THYME (*Thymus vulgaris*) Steep 2 tsp herb in 1 cup water for 10 minutes. (Use the leaves and flowers.) Drink three times daily.	Reduces bronchial spasms and eases coughs.	None.	None known.

Skin Problems

Herb and Standard Doses	What It Does	General Cautions	Drug Interactions
ALOE (*Aloe barbadensis*) Apply three times daily to injured area. Buy pure (clear) aloe gel.	Heals sunburn and minor burns and wounds. Also treats chronic skin disorders such as psoriasis, eczema and acne.	Don't use on surgical incisions; don't take internally.	None known.
GOTU KOLA (*Centella asiatica*) Apply externally as needed.	Aids wound healing. Eases pain of insect bites and sunburn. Improves acne, acne rosacea, eczema and psoriasis.	None.	None known.

Urinary Tract Problems

Herb and Standard Doses	What It Does	General Cautions	Drug Interactions
GOLDENROD (*Solidago virgaurea*) Steep 1 tsp dried herb in 1 cup boiling water; drink 1 cup daily. Use only the flowering tops.	Promotes healthy urinary function.	Don't use if you have a chronic kidney disorder.	None known.

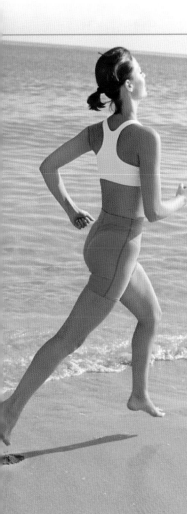

The Ultimate Ladder of Fitness

Women weren't officially allowed to run marathons until 1970, largely because of the outdated (and unspoken) perception that we were the weaker sex. But in 1984 Joan Benoit changed that thinking for ever. Benoit (now Samuelson) ran in the first women's Olympic marathon – and her time was faster than 11 of the 20 male winners who had run before her.

Is Joan unique? Of course. Élite athletes are in a class by themselves. But every woman, regardless of her current level of fitness, can be athletic – and then notch it up a few levels.

Like many women, perhaps you enjoy walking. You can easily increase the time you walk and the distance you go. Pretty soon, you might be ready to participate in a 5-K walk.

Do you lift weights? It just takes seconds to add more weight or to lift the weights more often. It doesn't matter what physical activities you engage in. Running, hiking, swimming, aerobics, weight training – they're all great workouts, and the more you do, the fitter you're going to be.

More is involved than just fitness. Studies have shown that regular exercise lowers anxiety, reduces the risk of heart disease, and even improves the frequency and quality of sex.

Exercise is more important today than it ever was. Researchers have found that the labour-saving inventions of the past 25 years – everything from computers to remote controls – have shaved an average of 800 calories of daily activity from our lives.

That's why we created the Ultimate Ladder of

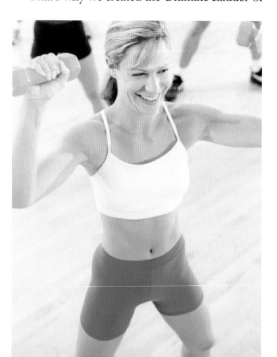

Fitness – a six-step plan for improving mobility, burning calories and trimming inches off your waistline. You'll also discover ways to make exercise a lot more fun, which is the real key to making it part of your life.

Exercise: You Can't Live without It

When it comes to your health, exercise isn't an option – it's a necessity.

We all know that being sedentary increases the risk of heart disease and of other serious health threats. Yet surveys have shown that as many as three-quarters of women in the UK don't get regular physical activity. In 2001 the Australian Bureau of Statistics reported the proportion of sedentary adults as 31 per cent, while in New Zealand the 2000/1 Physical Activity Survey found that 32 per cent of adults were 'inactive'.

What, exactly, can you gain from exercise? Here are some examples.

- It reduces your risk of heart attack and stroke. Exercise lowers blood pressure, slows resting heart rate, lowers cholesterol and burns abdominal fat.

- A number of studies have shown that exercise protects against colon cancer. It may lower the risk of breast and ovarian cancers as well.

- It helps the body secrete insulin, which can reduce the risk of diabetes.

- It boosts immunity and can prevent colds and other infectious diseases.

WHAT WORKS FOR ME

With work, family and constant travel vying for their time, exercise experts are every bit as swamped as the rest of us, yet they still manage to work out most days of the week. Here are their secrets for practising what they preach!

Use your weekends. 'I confess, when I'm seeing patients from 7 a.m. to 7 p.m., I don't exercise. But at weekends (including most Fridays), it's priority number one. I take an hour these days just for me and have a quality run or workout. Then I find a smaller chunk of time 2 more days of the week. The trick is preparation: I always have my gym bag with me. So if I suddenly have 30 minutes free, I'm out of the door for a walk or jog!' says Dr Mary Jane Minkin, clinical professor of obstetrics and gynaecology at Yale University School of Medicine and co-author of *What Every Woman Needs to Know about Menopause.*

Have a plan B. 'I start the day with an exercise plan. But as a doctor, my plans are routinely disrupted. So I have a plan B and plan C. For instance, I always carry exercise bands. If I can't make it to the gym, I can do resistance training at home, in my surgery or in my hotel room. I also carry my trainers. If I have lots of meetings, I take short walks in between to clear my head. Every 5 seconds counts!' says Dr Pamela Peeke, assistant clinical professor of medicine at the University of Maryland School of Medicine and author of *Fight Fat after 40.*

Make it a family affair. 'I have three school-age kids, so my life is out of control. I still exercise at least 4 days a week, but I don't lock myself into a routine. I take advantage of my children's desire to play outside. I run while they bike, I play tennis with my son or we all play soccer. It's so much better than watching TV,' says Dr Miriam Nelson, associate chief in the physiology laboratory at Tufts University and author of *Strong Women, Strong Bones.*

Focus on the benefits. 'I practise what I preach: I exercise every day or almost every day. One way I keep myself on track is by focusing on the rewards of my efforts: that time spent exercising will help reduce my risk for heart disease, control my weight and handle stress more effectively – and I can eat dessert now and then without worrying or feeling guilty!' says Dr James Blumenthal, professor in the department of psychiatry at Duke University.

Give it top priority. 'It would be easy to put off working out until the house is clean, more writing is done or I've gone through the mail. But I still put on my shorts and get going. The endless household and work duties will always be there. And if my exercise actually helps me live longer – I'm gaining time,' says Dr Christiane Northrup, co-founder of the Women to Women Health-Care Center, and author of *Women's Bodies, Women's Wisdom* and *The Wisdom of Menopause.*

- It strengthens bones. Older women who are active suffer fewer bone fractures than women who don't exercise.

- It burns fat, builds muscle and may lower levels of leptin, a hormone that seems to contribute to weight gain.

- It helps you live longer. A study of 14,000 women and men showed that moderate levels of physical fitness increased life span. In fact, walking as little as 2 miles daily could potentially add years to your life.

It's clear that exercise can improve the long-term quality (and quantity) of your life. But what will it do for you right now? Research has shown that women who exercise may have less menstrual discomfort. They're less anxious or depressed. They have less back pain and more self-confidence. They even sleep better.

Convinced? *So let's get started.*

Step 1:
Make the Change

If you haven't exercised regularly in the past, getting started can be a challenge. Your muscles won't be primed for action, and you won't have the force of habit to help you along. But once you get out of the door and get moving, it won't be long before exercise feels natural and comfortable. In fact, you may find yourself craving it. Before you do anything, have a checkup and let your doctor know about your plans to start exercising. Women who have been sedentary can easily injure themselves if they start too quickly.

Look for exercise opportunities. Women often think that physical fitness requires running, biking, swimming or other vigorous forms of exercise. But anything that gets your body moving counts. It could be walking the dog. Working in the garden. Raking leaves. Even cleaning the house can give you a decent workout if you move quickly and your total daily exercise is at least 30 minutes. There are many ways to sneak in exercise. We all have to go to places, so park a couple of streets away and walk the rest. Take the stairs instead of the lift. Or walk about while you talk on the phone.

Make it more like play. The problem with formal exercise is that it can easily feel like one more responsibility in an already hectic day. But it shouldn't be like that. Exercise is any physical activity that you enjoy. Why not indulge in some of the activities that you enjoyed when you were young – but with a twist?

Used to climb trees? Try rock climbing – in the wild or on the 'rock wall' at a local health club. Are you a dancer? Aerobics might be the ticket. For that matter, swing, salsa or line dancing can give you quite a workout.

Set reasonable goals. One reason so many women start an exercise programme and then give it up is that they don't feel they're making progress. Don't set impossible goals for yourself; keep things simple. Try to walk 10 more minutes than you usually do. Swim one extra length. Lift the weights two more times. Studies have shown that people who believe they can achieve a goal – any goal – are much more likely to stick with the programme.

Learn to
stretch
your muscles

Stretching is most effective when it's done before and after every workout. If that sounds like too much work, it's fine to do your stretches after exercising. Don't stretch when your muscles are cold; you're more likely to get injured.

These stretches hit every major muscle group in the body. For each one, hold the stretch for 10 to 30 seconds, breathing deeply all the time.

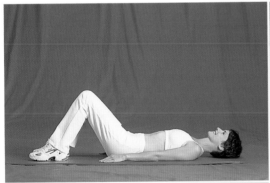

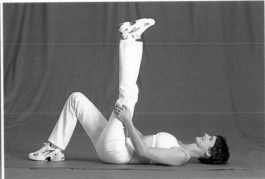

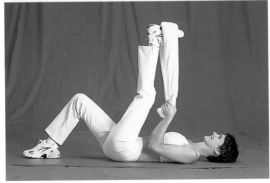

Hamstrings

Lie on your back with your legs bent and both feet on the floor (top left). Straighten and raise your left leg. Gently pull your thigh towards your body and hold (above). If you can't reach your leg, loop a towel under your foot and, with a slight bend at the knee, gently pull your leg towards your chest (bottom left). Repeat with the right leg.

continued

Learn to
stretch
your muscles

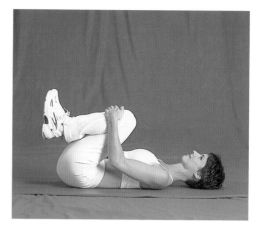

Lower Back

Lie on your back and pull both knees to your chest. Keep your upper body relaxed on the floor.

Calves

Stand facing a wall, with your right foot about 45 centimetres (18 inches) from the wall, and your left foot about 60 centimetres (2 feet) behind it (below). Place your hands against the wall for support and lean forwards while pressing your left heel to the floor. Switch legs.

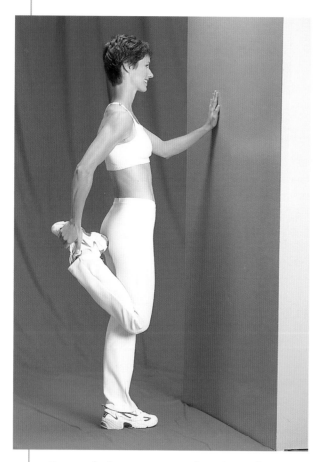

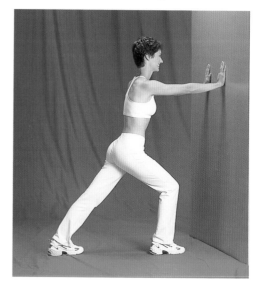

Quadriceps and Hip Flexors

Put your left hand on a wall (above). Bending your right knee, bring your right foot towards your buttocks; hold it in place with your right hand. Keep your knees together and do not arch your back. Repeat with the left leg, putting your right hand on the wall.

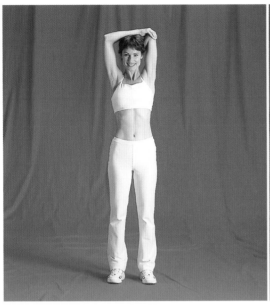
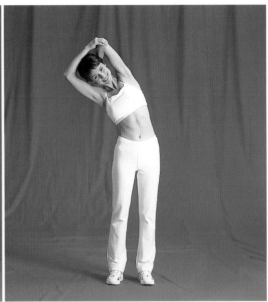

Triceps and Sides

Stand straight and raise your left arm over your head; bend the elbow, and drop the hand towards the middle of your back (left). With your right hand, gently pull your left elbow to the right. Tilt your body to the right (right) to stretch the muscles in your side. Keep your stomach tight. Repeat with your right arm.

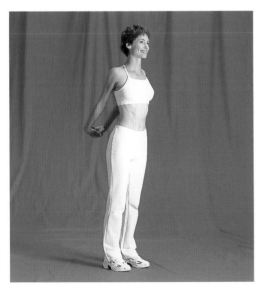

Chest

Stand with your feet shoulder-width apart and knees slightly bent. Clasp your hands behind your back with your palms facing in towards your body. Slowly push your chest forwards, keeping your back and abdomen stable. (If this movement is uncomfortable, do the stretch without your hands touching.) You can lean forwards slightly, but don't allow yourself to become pitched forwards.

continued

Learn to
stretch
your muscles

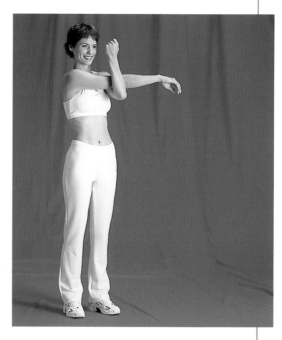

Upper Back
and Shoulders

Cross your right arm in front of your
chest (right). With the opposite arm,
gently pull your right arm towards your
body and hold. Repeat with left arm.

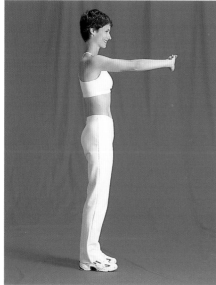

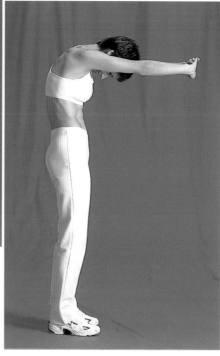

Upper Back

Clasp your hands in front of you with your
palms facing away (above). Round your
back, drop chin to chest, relax your
shoulders and press hands forwards (right).

Step 2: Learn to Stretch Your Muscles

Stretching is an integral part of any fitness plan. It improves your range of motion, helps you stay flexible, improves coordination, and helps prevent muscle strains and other injuries. Start with the stretches that begin on page 67, recommended by Carol Espel, an exercise physiologist.

Step 3: Work In Regular Aerobic Exercise Four or Five Times a Week

Nearly every health club offers an astonishing variety of aerobic dance classes, and women often confuse 'aerobics' with 'aerobic dance'. They're not the same thing.

Dancing is one form of aerobic exercise, but it's not the only one. Aerobic exercise simply means that you're moving fast enough to increase your heart and respiratory rates. When you exercise aerobically, the heart pumps more blood and the lungs fill the blood with more oxygen. Aerobic exercise makes the heart work harder, which makes it stronger: it pumps more blood with each beat, which means that it beats less often. In other words, aerobic exercise lowers your resting heart rate. Aerobic exercise can also result in drops in blood pressure because the blood moves more easily through arteries and veins.

You don't have to be an exercise fanatic to get impressive gains from aerobic exercise. Experts recommend that you accumulate 30 minutes of moderate activity most days to stay healthy and fit.

One more point about aerobic exercise: don't waste time doing something you don't enjoy very much. For years, women felt that they had to run in order to be aerobically fit. But a lot of them hated running, and naturally they didn't do it for very long. You have to do something that you like doing. It could be tennis. Bicycling. Climbing the stairclimber. Or even country dancing.

Step 4: Add Strength Training

The next time you go to the health club, take a look at the people lifting weights. Chances are, most of them are men. That's unfortunate because weight lifting, also called strength training or weight training, is among the best workouts for women.

For starters, strength training makes the bones stronger, which is critically important for women.

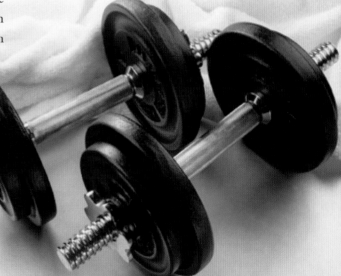

strength
training

Plan on repeating each of the following exercises 8 to 12 times. For those that involve weights, choose weights that are heavy enough so that you can barely complete the set of 12.

To get the most benefits from each exercise, do two or three sets of 12, resting for a few minutes in between. Repeat the exercises two or three times a week, but not on consecutive days. Remember to do your stretches when you've finished.

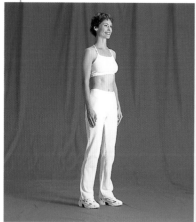

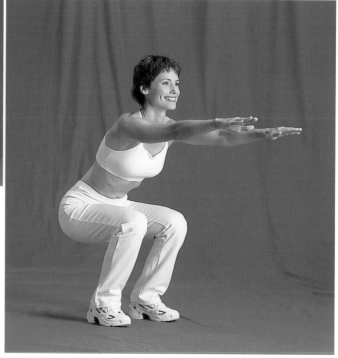

Squat

Stand with your feet shoulder-width apart (above). Bend your knees and squat as though you're sitting; hold your arms in front for balance (right). Make sure that your knees don't extend beyond your toes. Then return to the starting position.

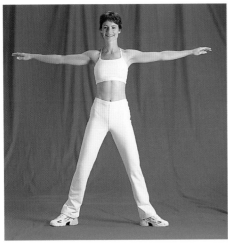

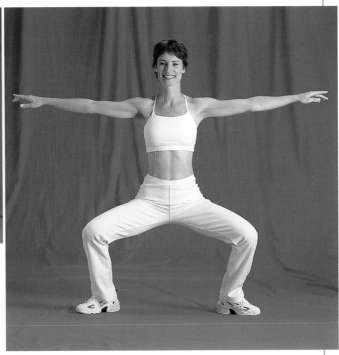

Plié

Stand with your feet about 60 centimetres (2 feet) apart; your legs should be turned out (above). With your back straight, lower your body (right). Then, as you straighten your legs, squeeze your inner thighs. Your knees should be in line with your ankles. Return to the starting position.

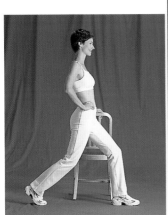

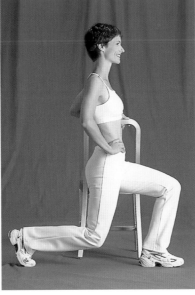

Lunge

Lightly place your left hand on the back of a chair for balance. Step forwards with your left foot (far left). Your knee should be above your left foot, not sticking out past your toes. Lower your body by bending your knees and dropping your hips straight towards the floor (near left). Return to the starting position, then repeat with the other leg.

continued

strength
training

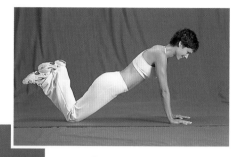

Pushup

Start on hands and knees, hands in line with shoulders. Your hips should be extended so that your body forms a straight line from head to knees. Cross your ankles in the air (left). Push yourself up (above), then return to the starting position. Repeat.

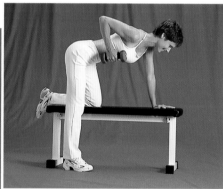

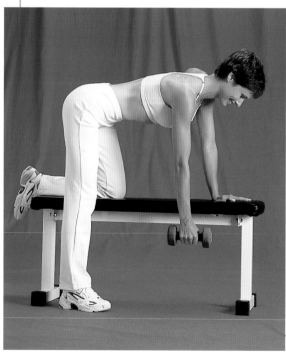

One-Arm Row

Put your left knee and left hand on a bench or a chair, keeping your back flat. Hold a weight in your right hand with your right arm straight and the weight hanging towards the floor, parallel to the bench (left). Raise the weight, keeping it close to your body, until it's even with your waist; your elbow should be pointed towards the ceiling (above).

Military Press

While sitting, hold a weight in each hand. Start with the weights at shoulder height; your palms should be facing forwards (near right). Raise the weights above your head without bringing them together or locking your elbows (far right), then bring them back down to your shoulders.

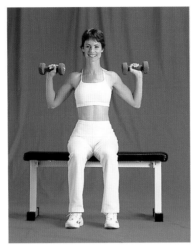

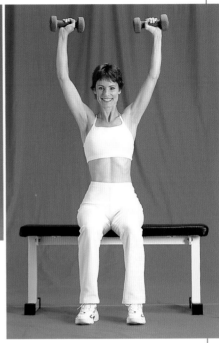

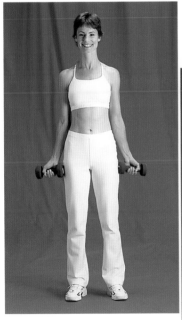

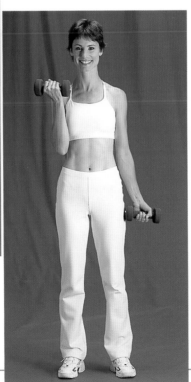

Biceps Curl

Stand straight and hold a weight in each hand, palms facing forwards (far left). Keeping your elbow close to your body, bend your right arm and lift the weight towards your shoulder (near left). Return to the starting position, then repeat with the other arm.

continued

strength
training

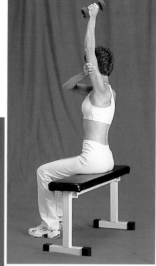

Triceps Extension

Sit on a bench or a chair while holding a weight in your left hand with your palm facing in. Bend your arm and raise it over your shoulder; your elbow will be pointing towards the ceiling, and the weight will be behind your head (near right). Hold your left elbow steady with your right hand, and raise the weight until your arm is straight (far right); return to the starting position.

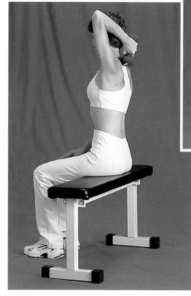

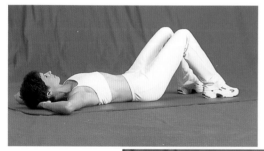

Abdominal

Lie on a mat with your knees bent, your feet flat on the floor and hip-width apart, your hands behind your head, elbows out to the sides (left). Contract your abdominal muscles and raise your shoulder blades off the ground about 30 degrees (below). Return to the starting position.

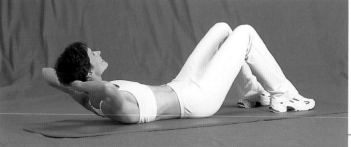

After a woman reaches the menopause, she can lose up to 20 per cent of her bone strength. Strength training literally adds mass to the bones, which makes them stronger and helps prevent fractures.

Strength training is also among the best ways to keep your figure trim. Muscle tissue is much more active metabolically than fat. When you lift weights and build muscle, you'll automatically burn more calories, even when you aren't exercising.

After the age of 40, women can lose 250 grams (about 1/2 pound) of muscle and gain 500 grams (about 1 pound) of fat every year. By the time a woman reaches her 65th birthday, she could have lost half of her muscle tissue – and her slower metabolism means she burns 200 to 300 fewer calories daily than when she was younger.

Strength training boosts the metabolism and reverses muscle loss. In fact, women who lift weights or do other forms of strength training twice a week for a few months can replace between 5 and 10 years of 'lost' muscle tissue. To make things easy, we've created a customized strength-training plan (see page 72) for women.

Step 5: Increase the Intensity

When you've being doing the same exercises for a while, you'll find that they get easier. This is because your body has adapted to the workload and is no longer feeling the strain. This is satisfying, in a way, because it means that you've made progress. But it also means that you won't progress further until you push your body a little harder. To keep your workouts at maximum pitch, increase the intensity. In other words, lift more weights, run faster and generally exercise harder two or three times a week. The boost in intensity can have substantial health and fitness benefits. One study found that people who regularly pushed their workouts to the limit had higher levels of high-density lipoprotein (HDL, the 'good' cholesterol) than those who exercised at lower intensities.

There are a number of ways to boost the intensity of your workouts. They include:

Exercise longer. Suppose you're currently exercising for 30 minutes. To increase the intensity, kick it up to 35 minutes. Keep it at that level for a few weeks, then add another 5 minutes – and then another. Exercising hard for 45 minutes will quickly add up to impressive fitness gains.

Try interval training. Instead of going all-out all the time – or, conversely, coasting along at a comfortable pace – shake things up with interval training. For example, exercise at a moderate pace for 4 minutes, then switch to high intensity for 4 minutes. Interval training will keep your body challenged without exhausting your muscles and lungs, says fitness expert Wayne Westcott, author of 15 books on strength training.

Add new exercises to your workout. Remember the strain you felt when you first started exercising? It's good to repeat the experience periodically because it puts a beneficial load on your whole body. As you challenge different muscles, your heart and lungs will work harder, and that's the key to boosting overall fitness.

Step Up To Fitness

If you haven't been active in the past but are getting ready to start, you may be wondering what types of activities you'll enjoy most – and what the fitness benefits will be.

Our Ladder of Fitness makes it easy. You'll find dozens of exercises – from 'formal' workouts to recreational activities and hobbies – along with the number of calories that they burn (based on a 64-kilogram (10-stone) woman who exercises for 15 minutes). You're sure to find some that will satisfy your interests as well as your fitness goals.

The activities at the bottom of the ladder are low intensity. As you go up the rungs, the exercises become more intense.

140 CALORIES

Mountain biking, hiking a moderate-to-difficult gradient, running a 10-minute mile, running up stairs, karate or tae kwon do, kickboxing, skipping with a rope, swimming vigorously, using a stairclimber or a ski machine

120 to 139 CALORIES

Running a 12-minute mile, singles tennis, volleyball, downhill skiing, rock climbing, swimming lengths, water jogging, having a snowball fight

95 to 119 CALORIES

Backpacking, doubles tennis, power-walking, briskly walking uphill, jazz and modern dance, basketball, soccer, high-impact aerobics, using a stationary rower, cycling at a moderate pace, ice-skating, sledding, digging flowerbeds

70 to 94 CALORIES

Golf (carrying your clubs), downhill skiing on beginners' slopes, gardening, calisthenics, step aerobics, walking at a brisk pace, dancing (country, jive or disco), playing tag, washing the car, canoeing, mowing the lawn with a push mower

40 to 69 CALORIES

Lawn and ten-pin bowling, badminton, croquet, dancing (cha-cha or swing), tai chi, golf (using a buggy), raking leaves, playing catch or Frisbee, walking the dog

Exercise to music. It's a good way to make the time go quickly, but music – as long as it has a fast tempo – also promotes impressive fitness gains. In one study, 24 men and women cycled to music. The intensity of their cycling increased when they listened to music with a fast beat.

Step 6: Keep Yourself Motivated

We've talked about how hard it can be to launch into an exercise programme when you haven't been active recently. What's even harder is sticking to it: many people who take up strength or aerobic training will slack off within a few months. People offer all sorts of reasons for giving up their workouts. Not enough time. Too much work. Family responsibilities. They're all valid reasons, but what it usually boils down to is this: women give up exercising because they aren't sufficiently motivated. It's a common

problem, which is why creating motivation is an essential part of any training plan. Here are some things you may want to try.

Test yourself often. Try keeping an exercise log, in which you record how long you exercised, the distance covered the amount of weight lifted. With every workout, you should try to push yourself just a little bit harder.

Show your competitive side. Some women do their best work – and their best workouts – when they're in competition with someone else. You may want to ask a like-minded friend to exercise with you – and keep a friendly competition going to see who improves the most in a certain period of time.

Push past the doldrums. When you find your motivation flagging, mentally force yourself to be active, even if it's only to go for a quick walk. Once you get off the sofa and start moving, you'll find that you enjoy the way you feel – and you'll probably keep going.

WHAT TO DO IF YOU HAVE ONLY **5 MINUTES**

You don't have to do 'formal' exercise to get a great workout: all you have to do is move.

Skip with a rope, walk up stairs, dance or play tag with the kids. Just keeping moving – while you wait for a pan of water to boil, for example, or when you're waiting for the laundry to dry.

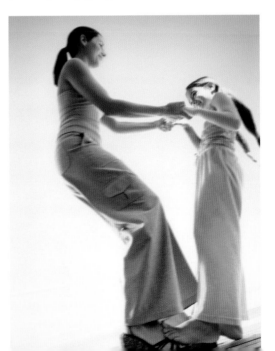

The Women's Health Bible Guide to Your Perfect Weight

A hundred years ago, only about 10 per cent of adults were overweight. Today an estimated one in five adults is obese. Yet we have the same genes as our ancestors. What's changed isn't our genes but our lifestyle.

It took Great-Grandmother hours to make dinner from scratch. She scrubbed clothes clean with her own hands. And without a car, she walked everywhere.

Today we can buy everything ready-prepared to feed the family. We load the washing machine to clean clothes. And a short car ride takes us to work, the shops or a friend's house.

In the 19th century, machines did 70 per cent of the work on farms and factories. Men and women did the rest. Now machines do 99 per cent of the work, and many of us earn a living sitting at a desk or computer. Cars have taken the place of walking or cycling. We burn rubber instead of calories. And computers, mobile phones and fax machines only make our society more fast-paced and stressful, which can send extra weight straight to our middles.

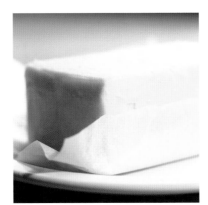

Superimpose stress and inactivity on a world where it's practically impossible not to come face-to-face daily with food that makes us fat, and it's easy to see why so many more women (and men) have a weight problem today than did our ancestors.

That said, a few people genuinely have a genetic disposition towards being overweight. Children of obese parents have an 80 per cent chance of being obese themselves, while children of normal-weight parents have less than a 10 per cent chance. Even adopted children tend to follow their biological parents' weight patterns. The culprits: metabolism and the hormone leptin.

Some people simply have lower metabolisms than others. That means their bodies burn off fewer calories in the course of eating, breathing, sleeping and performing other life functions. Metabolic rates seem to vary somewhat from family to family, or ethnic group to ethnic group. A study has found that women of African origin, for example, have lower resting metabolic rates than white women. And when scientists gave sets of twins an extra 1,000 calories a day, some sets of twins put on 13 kilograms (2 stone) – while others put on only 4.5 kilograms (10 pounds). (For conversion from calories to kilojoules see page 361.)

We all know women who can eat whatever they want and stay thin, while others seem to put on weight just looking at food. Experts believe that overweight people may be insensitive to leptin, a hormone that turns off appetite once you've had enough to eat. The more fat on the body, the more leptin is produced to keep us from overeating and to increase the amount of energy we expend. Scientists have found that obese people have high levels of the hormone leptin, which suggests that heavy individuals don't respond to leptin. Some compare this to insensitivity to insulin among people with type 2 diabetes.

Does this mean you were born to be fat?

'No, there is no "fat gene",' says obesity expert Dr John P. Foreyt. You may have been predisposed to put on weight in a culture of high-fat foods and sedentary jobs. And being overweight may run in your family. But ultimately, your behaviour determines the number on the scales.

'The only way to gain weight is to eat more than you burn,' Dr Foreyt says. Even if you have a tougher time losing weight, that doesn't mean you're doomed to be overweight.

Your Healthy Weight

Reaching or maintaining a healthy weight pays off in many ways. It lowers your risk of heart disease by lowering your blood pressure, cholesterol levels and triglyceride levels. In fact, weight loss works better than drugs at lowering blood pressure in women with and without hypertension. Losing weight also helps you become more sensitive to insulin, which will help you avoid type 2 diabetes. These effects are especially beneficial to women after the menopause, when they're more vulnerable to heart disease.

Because obesity contributes to five of the leading causes of death in the West – heart disease, stroke, high blood pressure, cancer and diabetes – losing weight can even help us live longer.

Regardless of the major health benefits, slimming down also improves quality of life. Think about it, losing extra weight will help you:

■ Breathe more easily

■ Sit more comfortably in cinema and aeroplane seats

■ Get into and out of your car with ease

■ Wear belted skirts and trousers

OVERWEIGHT? GET YOUR THYROID CHECKED

About 3 per cent of the population suffer from hypothyroidism, or an underactive thyroid. More than half of all women experienced three or more symptoms of hypothyroidism in the past year. If you're one of them, it could be why you're overweight.

The butterfly-shaped thyroid gland wraps around the front of the windpipe just below the Adam's apple and produces a hormone that regulates metabolism and organ function. It influences every organ, tissue and cell in the body.

When the thyroid doesn't produce enough of the hormone – often because the immune system creates antibodies that damage or destroy it – you could experience:

■ A weight gain of 4.5 kilograms (10 pounds) or less of fluid
■ Fatigue
■ Mood swings
■ Dry, coarse skin or hair
■ Hoarseness
■ Forgetfulness
■ Difficulty swallowing
■ Intolerance of cold

Women are at higher risk than men of an underactive thyroid. But just because you are overweight and feeling tired it doesn't mean you have thyroid dysfunction.

'I think a lot of us hope that when we gain weight, it's because of our thyroid,' says Dr Gay Canaris, an assistant professor of internal medicine.

So how do you know if you should get tested?

Talk to your doctor about your symptoms. Fatigue could be caused by other disorders, such as anaemia, cancer, depression or sleep disorders. It could also result from too much work.

- Tie up your shoes effortlessly

- Wear a swimsuit and enjoy going to the beach without feeling self-conscious

- Give you the confidence to try new things, like rock climbing

- Live to see your grandchildren and great-grandchildren

- Improve your sex life and overall energy level

As you slim down, you'll probably discover other, personal benefits of your own.

Here's everything you need to know to lose weight and keep it off, once and for all.

Step 1: Calculate Your Body Mass Index

Successful weight loss begins with setting the right goals. 'So many of the women I work with feel defeated if they don't meet the goal they set for themselves, even if they're within 2 kilograms (4½ pounds) of their ideal weight,' says Dr Stephen P. Gullo, president of the Institute for Health and Weight Sciences in New York. 'Some only get so far, then throw in the towel.' Others hope to reach whatever weight they were at college or on their wedding day. But that might not be realistic. A better strategy is to set a goal based on your body mass index (BMI), a ratio of weight to height.

Along with waist circumference (discussed in Step 2), body mass index is a more accurate indication of total body fat than body weight alone.

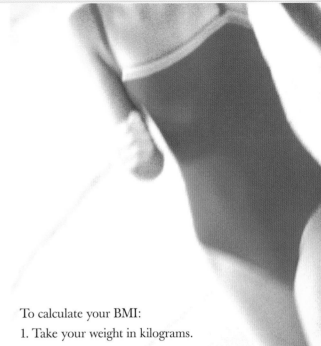

To calculate your BMI:

1. Take your weight in kilograms.

2. Divide that figure by your height in metres squared (i.e. your height in metres multiplied by itself) and you'll have your BMI.

(To work out your BMI in imperial, simply multiply your weight in pounds by 703 and then divide by your height in inches squared.)

A BMI of between 18.5 and 25 is considered healthiest. You're considered overweight if your BMI is 25 or over, and you're considered obese if it's 30 or over.

'When someone has a BMI of 25, their risk for disease goes up because their blood pressure, cholesterol, blood sugar and risk for diabetes may all go up,' Dr Foreyt says. 'We've also found that at a BMI of 30, three-quarters of all people have at least one risk factor for heart disease, such as type 2 diabetes or hypertension.'

But don't let your BMI go below 18.5 – that's too low because it's unhealthy to be that skinny.

Step 2: Measure Your Waistline

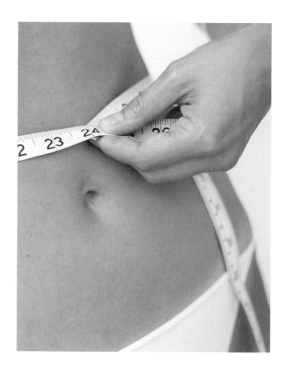

Because abdominal fat is associated with a greater health risk than fat carried in the hips, backside or thighs, your waistline is also a better gauge of your weight than kilograms or pounds. It's also a good way to double-check your weight if your BMI, measured in Step 1, isn't considered high, but it's obvious that you're heavier than you should be.

There's a right and a wrong way to measure your waist. Hold a measuring tape horizontally around the abdomen at navel level, parallel to the floor. The tape should be snug, but not pulled tight. Breathe out, and note your waist measurement.

For women, a waist circumference of 88 centimetres (35 inches) or higher is unhealthy.

WHAT WORKS FOR ME

DR MARY JANE MINKIN, clinical professor of obstetrics and gynaecology at Yale University School of Medicine, shares her secrets of weight control.

I love to eat! I've never been skinny, and I've always put on weight easily. I was the first child in my street whose mother served skimmed milk; I was drinking nearly a litre (1½ pints) of milk a day! Now I eat a sensible, low-fat diet that includes lots of fruit, vegetables and whole grains, and I still love my milk.

My fanaticism about exercise is what saves my life – and my waistline! Three or four times a week, I run 8 kilometres (5 miles) or do the equivalent on the stairclimbing or rowing machine, or I cycle for an hour. This helps me indulge my passion for food but still be able to wear a size 14.

As a child, I was never encouraged by my parents to exercise. It wasn't until I got to medical school that I adopted the exercise habit to relieve stress and get more energy.

When I gained 13 kilograms (2 stone) during my training – who had time to work out? – exercise finally helped me to lose it. Now I play basketball regularly and play football with my kids. I'd like to add weight training to my routine next.

Getting up earlier to exercise in the morning works for me. You don't have to go to a gym, either. I tell women that taking the stairs rather than the lift and walking short distances frequently during the day all adds up.

Step 3: Set a Starting Date

Once you know where you really stand, weight-wise, your next step is to set your goals and commit yourself to them. If you don't set a starting date, you could fall into the 'tomorrow syndrome'.

Make sure you're ready. Before you 'X' your calendar, make sure this is really the right time to start a weight-loss programme. You might want to wait if other responsibilities consume your life at the moment, such as a new job or a family illness.

Avoid holidays. You've probably heard that most people put on about 2 kilograms (5 pounds) from November to January. With so many Christmas dinners and parties, trying to lose weight during this time is a lofty goal. Instead, try to maintain your weight, and plan to start losing after the festive season.

Mark your calendar. Once you've established the best time to begin, make an appointment with yourself. Use the time from now until your start date to fill your kitchen with healthy foods, find a walking partner and prepare an exercise routine. 'There's a reason races have a starting point,' Dr Gullo says. The more you prepare for your goal, the better you'll perform.

Step 4: Determine Your Real Calorie Needs

Eating too much food makes you overweight, but eating too little lowers your metabolism because your body instinctively interprets a dearth of calories as a famine and shifts into low gear to conserve calories. The solution: balance what you eat with your activity. Here's a point system that makes it easy.

Consider your activity level.

- If your job or lifestyle involves a lot of sitting and you exercise rarely, give yourself 26 points.

- If you get more daily activity than light walking and you exercise aerobically for 45 to 60 minutes three times a week, give yourself 33 points.

- If you get more daily activity than light walking and you get 45 to 60 minutes of aerobic activity at least five times a week, give yourself 40 points.

Multiply your points by your goal weight in kilograms to get your daily calories. For example, if you're a 64-kilogram very active woman and you want to lose 5 kilograms, multiply 40 by 59 and get 2,360 calories.

To lose fat instead of muscle, you need to eat at least 1,200 calories a day. Problem is, the typical Western woman eats many more calories in a

WHAT TO DO IF YOU COULD CHANGE **ONLY ONE THING**

To jump-start your weight-loss programme, eat more fruit and vegetables. Besides all the nutrients that produce contains, it also plays a role in weight loss. Fruit and vegetables fill you up for a small number of calories.

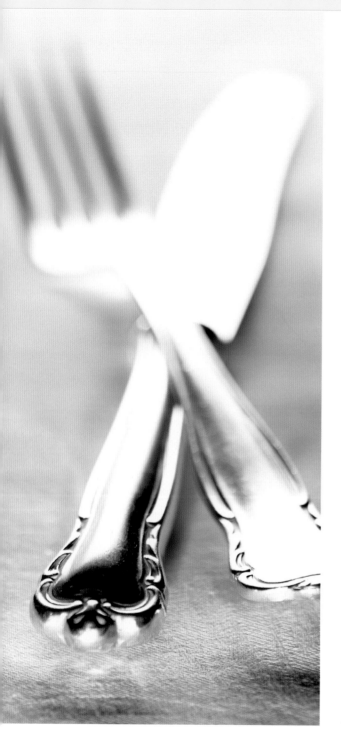

day than she needs. If you eat just 500 extra calories a day – the equivalent of a Snickers bar and a can of Coke – you'll be getting 3,500 *more* calories a week than you need. That adds up to an extra half kilo on the scales.

Step 5: Keep a Food Diary for a Week

People tend to underestimate what they eat by 20 to 50 per cent. To take stock of what you're really eating, write down your foods and portions every day for a week. Then review what you've eaten.

Your diary will help you see your eating patterns for workdays and weekends (and holidays) and pinpoint when you tend to overeat. Once you know when those periods of overeating are, you can either make sure you have a healthy snack ready or schedule an activity to keep yourself away from the fridge.

Count what you drink. A lot of people don't realize how many calories they take in from beverages. When people drank an extra 450 calories a day in one study (two gin and tonics or a cup of eggnog), they put on weight. But when they ate those extra calories in food, they ate less later in the day and lost weight. Don't sip your weight-loss goals away. Here's how to make your drinks work for you.

Drink water. There's no better thirst quencher. Water has zero calories, it fills you up and it keeps your metabolism running more efficiently.

Watch the alcohol. When you choose wine over water, you don't only get extra calories in the drink. In fact, one study found that people ate 200 more calories in food at dinner; when compared with people who drank water, those who drank alcohol ate faster, took longer to feel full and continued eating after being full.

Even if you don't drink with food, look at how alcohol can stack up the calories.

- 120 millilitres (1 small glass) of wine: 87 calories

- 120 millilitres (1 small glass) of champagne: 89 calories

- 568 millilitres (1 pint) of standard lager: 210 calories

- 568 millilitres (1 pint) of dry cider: 204 calories

- 275 millilitres (1 bottle) of Bacardi Breezer: 196 calories

Step 6: Eat More Plant Foods, Fewer Animal Foods

You don't have to count calories if you don't want to. One American study found that people who ate a variety of meals based on the dietary guidelines of the United States Department of Agriculture lost three times more weight over a year than people on a specific low-fat diet. That equates to 6 to 11 servings of grains, 2 to 4 servings of fruit, 3 to 5 servings of vegetables, 2 or 3 servings of meat, 2 or 3 servings of dairy products and a small amount of fat a day.

Eat more, weigh less. A serving of 115 grams (4 ounces) of fried chicken has 250 calories, but the same amount of lean fish, such as sole, has about 100. That's because less-energy-dense foods like sole are typically low in fat, and high in water

THREE THINGS I TELL EVERY FEMALE PATIENT

DR STEPHEN P. GULLO, president of the Institute for Health and Weight Sciences in New York, offers this advice to people he counsels about weight loss.

1 **REMEMBER THAT WEIGHT LOSS IS ABOUT LIBERATION, NOT DEPRIVATION.** It's about a change in perspective. Eat fewer calories and cut down the amount of fat you eat in the spirit of liberating yourself from the discomfort of extra weight that you've been carrying, instead of depriving yourself from certain foods.

2 **KNOW YOUR BEHAVIOUR, NOT JUST YOUR CALORIES.** If you find that you're constantly regaining weight you've lost by abusing the same types of foods, either stop buying them or find replacements for them.

3 **DON'T FORGET THAT BEING THIN IS A LIFE MANAGEMENT SKILL.** It's normal to experience setbacks and periods of feeling defeated. But in the future, when you reach 40 or 50 or 60 at a healthy weight, it won't be by accident, because ageing well is not an accident. It will be because you honed your weight management skills.

and fibre, and carry fewer calories per mouthful so they make satisfying meals.

Foods with low energy density include fruit, vegetables, stock-based soups, potatoes, fish, oatmeal, whole wheat pasta, fresh popcorn and bran cereal. Eating them instead of high-energy-density foods such as cheesecake could help you eat 20 per cent fewer calories.

So push heaps of high-energy meat to the side, and make fruit and vegetables the main attraction. Instead of a sandwich with four slices of meat, crackers and biscuits for lunch, eat just two slices of meat and add sliced tomato, cucumber and fresh spinach. Follow it with a piece of fresh fruit and a biscuit. Instead of ordering veal parmigiana at an Italian restaurant, order a large bowl of minestrone soup, a salad and half a portion of pasta with marinara sauce.

In fact, one study found that one particular food – stock-based soup – made women feel so full that they ate 100 fewer calories at a buffet than women who had had a starter of chicken rice casserole. If you follow the same logic and start eating stock-based soup before your meals, you could lose 4.5 kilograms (10 pounds) in a year.

Eating more fibre, too, could help you lose weight. Your body will quickly absorb the calories from a breakfast made of white flour and sugar, and you'll feel hungry again soon after your meal. But the calories in a bowl of bran cereal with no added sugar are absorbed slower and will keep you full longer. The same is true for fibre in other foods.

Fibre also helps move other food out of the body before the body has a chance to absorb them. For every gram of fibre you eat, you'll absorb about 4 fewer calories than if you ate simple carbohydrates.

Triple your fibre intake. Most people eat 13 grams of fibre a day. But if you eat about three times that amount – 40 grams – you could block the absorption of 160 calories a day.

Start hearty. One study found that people who had eaten high-fibre porridge for breakfast ate 30 per cent fewer calories at lunch than people who had eaten cornflakes.

Grab beans. Beans are a great way to get fat-fighting fibre, so add them to salads, soups, chilli and other dishes. Chilli has nearly 10 grams of

'Drink eight glasses of water daily. None of your body parts, from your brain to your toes, work well without adequate hydration.'

– JANE BRODY, HEALTH WRITER

fibre per serving, three-bean salad with balsamic vinegar has 12.5 grams, and red beans and brown rice has a whopping 18 grams.

Eat whole grains. Whole grains, such as brown rice, whole wheat or wholemeal bread, wholemeal flour, wholegrain and multigrain cereals, porridge oats, oat bran, whole wheat pasta and couscous, and whole wheat, wholegrain, and rye crackers not only have fibre but also have more micronutrients, such as folate, magnesium and vitamin E, than their white-flour counterparts.

Aim for nine. Fruit and vegetables are naturally high in fibre, low in fat and calories and full of healthy nutrients and antioxidant vitamins – such as A, C and E – which are important in preventing heart disease and cancer. You've probably heard advice to eat five a day, but because so many studies link diets high in fruit and vegetables with less cancer, heart disease, diabetes and osteoporosis, experts advise nine servings a day. And since they have all the components to help you lose weight, eating nine a day should be part of your weight-loss programme, too.

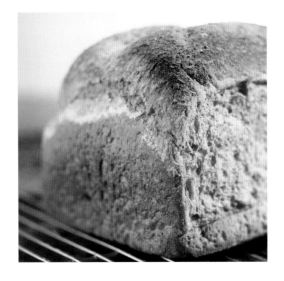

'Switch to **wholegrain** carbohydrates such as **wholemeal bread** and **brown rice**. High intakes of refined carbohydrates and sugar are the main sources of calories in the Western diet, and thus a major contribution to being overweight.'

– DR WALTER WILLETT, CHAIRMAN OF THE NUTRITION DEPARTMENT AT HARVARD SCHOOL OF PUBLIC HEALTH

Step 7: Scale Back Your Fat Intake

Fatty foods are more packed with calories than are low-fat foods. One gram of fat has 9 calories and a gram of carbohydrates has only 4 calories. So with fewer bites of a high-fat food, you'll get a lot more calories.

Fat may also affect the appetites of overweight people. In one study, overweight men who had had a high-fat meal before eating at a buffet ate 56 per cent more than lean men who had eaten the same high-fat meal. But when the overweight men had eaten a low-fat meal, they ate the same amount at the buffet as the lean men, who'd also eaten a low-fat meal. It appears that the appetite switch of overweight people is turned off slower from fat because it takes longer for their bodies to detect that fat has been ingested.

To lose weight, try to get just 25 per cent of your calories from fat. Here are some satisfying ways to do it.

Choose lean meat. Choose meat that's naturally low in fat, such as turkey breast or skinless chicken. And when you're buying any type of meat, make sure it has no more than 10 grams of fat per 90-gram (3-ounce) serving.

Look for low-fat cheese. Another great way to lower your fat consumption is to choose low-fat cheeses and yoghurt. They carry all the calcium and nutrients of the full-fat varieties.

Bake instead of fry. If you have a recipe that calls for frying – such as potato wedges for french fries – try this instead: coat the potato wedges with non-stick spray and bake in the oven at 450°F/230°C/gas 8 until they're brown and crisp.

Downsize dessert. Sweet, satisfying desserts don't have to include astronomical grams of fat. Here are some tips on making them healthier.

- Use mini chocolate chips in doughs and batters. They'll spread out more, allowing you to use fewer.

- Use only half of the baking chocolate squares your brownie recipe calls for, and replace the rest with cocoa powder, which is lower in fat.

- Use filo pastry instead of puff pastry or sweet dough – it's fat-free. Use non-stick spray, instead of butter, to moisten the sheets.

Step 8: Bone Up on Portion Size

You could count a heaped bowl of spaghetti bolognese as one portion, but your body knows how many calories you're eating. Get to know portion sizes, and you'll always have a mental picture of how much you should eat.

- 100 grams ($3\frac{1}{2}$ ounces) of raw or cooked vegetables, or about a rounded handful

- 90 grams (3 ounces) of raw or leafy vegetables, or the size of a tennis ball

- 1 medium piece of fresh fruit, also the size of a tennis ball

- 115 grams (4 ounces) cooked or tinned fruit, about a rounded handful

'Eliminate all foods containing partially **hydrogenated** oils. There's growing evidence that these **unnatural fats** are not good for us, and avoiding them and the **processed foods** that they come in would be a huge step to improving nutritional health.'

– DR ANDREW WEIL, CLINICAL PROFESSOR OF MEDICINE

- 1 slice of bread

- 40 grams (1½ ounces) of ready-to-eat cereal

- 150 grams (5½ ounces) cooked cereal, about a rounded handful

- 200 grams (7 ounces) cooked rice or pasta, about a rounded handful

- 90 grams (3 ounces) of cooked fish or meat (115 grams/4 ounces raw), the size of a deck of cards

- 90 grams (3 ounces) cooked dried beans, about a rounded handful

- 40 grams (1½ ounces) nuts, about a level handful

- 40 grams (1½ ounces) of cheese (or 60 grams/2 ounces processed); 30 grams (1 ounce) is the size of four dice

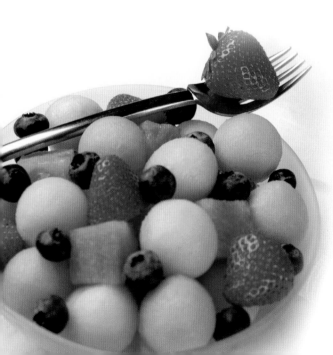

You can also follow the serving size listed on the nutrition label of your food. Or measure out your servings a few times and make a mental note of how much it covers the plate or bowl.

Step 9: Eat All Day

If you plan to skip breakfast to save on calories, your scheme will backfire. One study found that the metabolisms of people who skipped breakfast were about 5 per cent lower than those of people who ate three or more meals a day. A 5 per cent boost in metabolism could help you lose 4.5 kilograms (10 pounds) in a year.

It's also important to keep it up throughout the day. Eating more often – without increasing the amount of food you eat – will keep you full. In two studies, men who had eaten breakfast in small portions throughout the morning had a 27 per cent smaller lunch than men who had eaten breakfast as a single meal. Another good reason to avoid long stretches without food: after 4 hours, blood sugar drops, and you'll crave sweets, instead of healthier foods. Try these healthy snacks for fewer than 175 calories each.

- Half of a wholemeal bagel with jam or low-fat cream cheese

- A handful of baby carrots with a dip of 75 millilitres (2½ fluid ounces) each of salsa and low-fat sour cream

- A bowl of instant bean soup

- ½ bowl wholegrain cereal

Step 10: Sweat a Little

More than one-third of people who are overweight say they get no physical activity. But working out for 30 to 40 minutes could help you burn between 250 and 500 calories an exercise session. You could also burn as many as 50 or 100 calories more for the rest of the day after exercising.

Working out routinely can change your body's composition. Exercise helps you lose more fat, gain more muscle and regain less weight. Women who exercise also tend to follow their eating plans more closely than women who don't exercise.

And if you're one of those people with a lagging metabolism, exercise is a great way to speed it up.

Work it in. So you say you don't have time to exercise. Dr Sandra Adamson Fryhofer, a clinical associate professor of medicine, hears that all the time from her patients, but she doesn't accept the excuse. 'There's always something you can do,' she says. If you watch the morning news before work, do it while you're walking on the treadmill. 'Every little bit of exercise helps.'

If you take just 15 minutes to walk the dog in the morning, 10 minutes to walk to the shops for lunch, 5 minutes in the afternoon to stretch at your desk, 15 minutes to weed the garden when you get home from work and 15 minutes after dinner to play tag with the kids, your activity adds up to 1 hour – and 300 extra calories burned that day.

WATCH THE SWEETS, SUGAR

Eating reasonable amounts of sweets is one thing, but making sugar the main attraction of your eating plan won't help you lose weight.

Sugar may not have fat, but it certainly has a lot of calories and we're not skimping on it. On average, sugar makes up about one-third of women's diets – that's about 28 kilograms (62 pounds) a year and 151,840 calories. But it's more than extra calories that thwart weight-loss efforts: sugar also makes you hungrier. It's digested faster and its calories are stored quickly, so you'll get hungry again sooner than if you had a high-protein snack. To get down to the 7 teaspoons of sugar you should be eating a day (rather than the 19 women typically get), try to eliminate or lower your consumption of the five biggest offenders: non-diet soft drinks, baked goods, ice cream, sweetened fruit drinks and sweets. If you have the willpower to cut them out completely, you could save 78,000 calories a year – and lose more than 9 kilograms (20 pounds).

Fidget. For some people, fidgeting in their chair keeps them thin. Scientists gave 16 normal-weight people 1,000 extra calories a day for 8 weeks, but the amount of weight they put on varied between 1.5 and 7 kilograms (3 and 16 pounds). The ones who put on the least weight burned up to 692 calories a day doing everyday activities, such as walking, climbing stairs, household chores, sitting up straight, standing up straight – and fidgeting.

Can you train yourself to be a more active person naturally? 'Of course, if you make a conscious attempt' Dr Fryhofer says.

Try adding these habits to your life:

- Stand up to answer to the phone.

- Do a household chore during the adverts on television.

- Tap your feet against the floor or rotate your ankles when you're sitting.

- Dance to music as you do the dishes, iron or fold clothes.

Turn off cravings. While you work out, your body suppresses digestion and releases glucose and fatty acids into the blood for energy. You won't feel the urge to eat until you reach a state of rest and your energy fuels are back in storage. The next time you find yourself hungry out of boredom, get up and go for a walk, work in the garden or do housework. You'll curb your craving and burn some extra calories.

Turn off the TV. If you gave up one television programme a day and took a brisk walk for 30

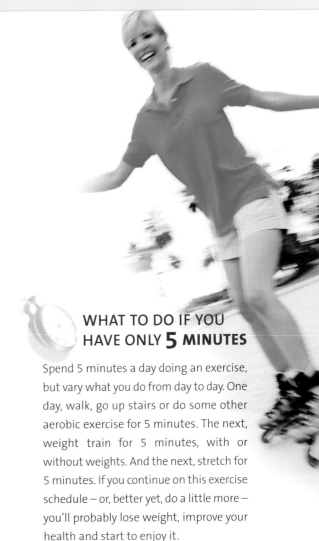

WHAT TO DO IF YOU HAVE ONLY **5 MINUTES**

Spend 5 minutes a day doing an exercise, but vary what you do from day to day. One day, walk, go up stairs or do some other aerobic exercise for 5 minutes. The next, weight train for 5 minutes, with or without weights. And the next, stretch for 5 minutes. If you continue on this exercise schedule – or, better yet, do a little more – you'll probably lose weight, improve your health and start to enjoy it.

That was the result of a study of 40 people who didn't like to exercise. They did 15 sessions a week for 10 minutes at a time at least every other day while eating a sensible diet. In 3 weeks they lost 1.4 kilograms (3 pounds), improved their strength and endurance, increased their flexibility, improved their cholesterol levels and admitted that they actually liked exercising.

minutes instead, you'd burn enough calories to lose 8 kilograms (18 pounds) in a year.

Don't stop. Once you start an exercise programme, you'll probably like it so much you won't want to stop – and that's good news when it comes to weight loss. Research shows that people who manage to maintain weight loss exercise the equivalent of walking 5 to 6.5 kilometres (3 to 4 miles) a day.

Other Helpful Strategies

If you're doing everything 'right' and still not losing weight – or losing it more slowly than suits you – these additional strategies can help you.

OUTSMART RESTAURANT FOOD

Many of us eat out regularly these days. Even when you choose the healthy options at restaurants, that's a weekly total of about 3,000 calories and 73 grams of fat.

Calories in restaurant meals stack up quickly because restaurants typically serve more than three times the amount of one serving of food.

But you don't have to become a recluse to eat healthily. You can ask for your food at restaurants to be specially cooked with no or less oil, request a menu from the restaurant in advance, or choose healthy foods at a buffet or party.

Wrap it up. According to one survey, 26 per cent of people dining out say they eat everything that's put in front of them. That's one good reason to get your waiter to wrap up half of your meal and put it in a doggy bag before it even makes it to your table.

Share with friends. Since restaurant meals are usually two or three servings anyway, ask your dinner partner if she wants to share the main course with you.

Get what you want. Don't even open your menu at a restaurant. Instead, think about what you want to eat, such as wholemeal toast and scrambled eggs, and ask the waiter for it. But don't stop there – tell the waiter you don't want sausages or bacon with it, or else he might bring it.

Think small. Try using this old standby when you are at a buffet. Take small portions of your favourite foods and refuse to go up for seconds. Then, take your time and eat it slowly so you're not left watching everyone else eat when you have finished.

***Really* party.** You don't have to stuff yourself to have fun. Instead of celebrating a birthday or holiday at a restaurant, stay at home and shift the emphasis from food to fun, with charades, board games or music and dancing.

LEARN TO TAKE YOUR TIME

Give yourself plenty of time to eat, rearranging your schedule if you have to. After looking at high-tech images of the brains of 21 adults while they ate, researchers found that their appetite switch turned off 10 minutes after they started their meal. The more time you take to eat, the fewer calories you'll inhale in the first 5 minutes of dinner, so try to spend 20 minutes at the dinner table.

Getting pleasure from your food can actually help you lose weight.

People put on weight when they're not

focusing on their food – when they're at their desks, in their car or in front of the television. But a great way to lose weight is to make a fantastic dinner and sit down and truly enjoy it. Once you get pleasure from your food this way, you probably won't need so much to feel satisfied.

CHIP AWAY AT STRESS

When you're under stress, your body releases a hormone called cortisol, which sends fat to your abdomen, where it can increase risk for heart disease. It also suppresses growth hormone and testosterone, which protect you against heart disease and gaining abdominal fat. These effects are even more dangerous after the menopause, when women's oestrogen levels drop.

You may find that you eat more when you're under stress. That's because food helps some people to relax. Stress activates your sympathetic nervous system and makes you feel on edge. Eating may activate natural painkillers in your brain, helping you to feel relaxed.

Anxiety can affect your behaviour in other ways, too. Stress from financial problems, relationship issues or just being overworked is often followed by a period of depression. And whenever you're depressed, you're probably going to eat more and be less motivated to exercise. You're also more likely to grab comfort foods, which are usually higher in fat.

A study of 1,300 people found that those who were cynical and had high levels of anxiety had the most abdominal fat. Depression also ranked high among women with the most abdominal fat.

'Watch your **portion sizes**. Most of us eat far more food than we really need, and there are many reasons to eat less, including **slowing** the **ageing** process.'

– DR KATHLEEN JOHNSON, NUTRITIONIST

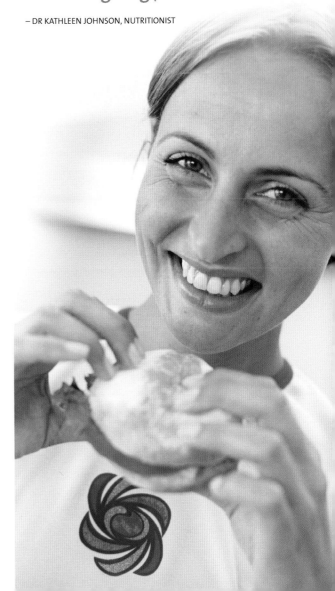

Keeping stress under control should be part of your weight-loss strategy. Here are some ideas on how to do it. (For more on stress, see chapter 6.)

Accept imperfection. The house can't be completely clean, you'll miss a deadline once in a while and your kids probably won't get straight A's. Trying not to control every aspect of life may help you lose extra flab.

Take care of you. If you make sure you are well-rested, get enough exercise and eat well, you'll feel better and hold on to positive emotions.

Turn on the radio. Listen to some soothing music, and you may ease your anxiety and even your blood pressure and heart rate under very stressful situations.

Shake, shake, shake. If you get up and dance, you'll burn calories and release endorphins in your brain, which will elevate your mood and erase stress.

Tell a joke. Humour helps ease anxiety. One study found that people who performed a stressful task after watching an episode of their favourite sitcom had lower blood pressure and heart rates than people who hadn't watched the television show.

GET SUPPORT

Pay attention to the small gains you make along the way and congratulate yourself for them. Even if you don't lose weight as fast as you wanted, remind yourself that you can bound up the stairs and not lose your breath or that you cook meals that make you feel good and keep your body healthy. Even if it's a couple of kilograms, celebrate every step you take to better health.

> '**Control** your **calorie intake**, get no more than **20 per cent** of your calories from fat, and make sure you get **five to nine** servings of fruit and vegetables daily.'
>
> – DR MOSHE SHIKE, ONCOLOGIST

Lose together. A friend may be the perfect motivator to get you out of the house for a brisk walk or to inspire you to eat low-fat meals at restaurants.

Go online. Inspiration may lie on the other side of a website link. Some research shows that weight-loss websites can help women lose weight. Check out a few chat rooms, calorie counters and exercise logs to see if this type of support is for you. Look for sites that include food diaries, personal feedback, weekly lessons and emotional support.

Swap household chores. If cleaning the kitchen puts you too close to the biscuit tin to avoid temptation, head outside and rake leaves, mow the lawn or garden. Ask your partner to do the indoor jobs.

Work together. If you want to join a support group like Weight Watchers and your partner needs a lesson on nutrition, join together and get extra support.

Hide temptation. Don't keep temptation right on the counter. If you're likely to overeat certain snacks, ask a family member to hide them on a

FORGET FAD DIETS

The best advice you'll ever get when it comes to dieting: 'Quit!'

Whether you're pigging out on pork scratchings or living on 800 calories a day, diets that don't include a variety of healthy foods or that severely restrict calories aren't good for long-term weight loss *or* your health. Some fad diets are actually more damaging to your health than obesity.

It's hard to keep up a diet low in calories, for obvious reasons: it's uncomfortable to be hungry. Think of starving as holding your breath underwater – you can do it for only so long before you gulp for air.

'Starving has nothing to do with losing weight,' says diet expert Dr Stephen P. Gullo. 'Hunger pangs are a sign that you're doing something wrong. Succeeding at weight loss doesn't mean you have to give up fine taste in food. It means you have to be a selective gourmet.'

When you lose weight from starving, your metabolism may decrease as a result. This means that even though you're eating fewer calories, you're also burning off fewer calories. It also means that instead of losing weight, you lose muscle. When you go back to eating foods higher in fat or calories, you're more likely to put on fat instead of muscle. With this new efficiency, you may put on weight more quickly, and it may take longer to lose weight in the future. Yo-yo dieting also may put your health at risk if you already have health problems. A diet of only 800 calories a day could result in lower immunity, an irregular heartbeat, irregular menstruation, a lower sex drive, lower metabolism, loss of lean body tissue, headaches, fatigue, dry skin and sleeplessness.

But even when a diet allows you to eat plenty of just a few types of food, your health will suffer. Any time you eliminate food groups, you lose out on the nutrients they provide, such as the calcium in dairy foods, fibre and vitamin E in grains, carotenoids and phytochemicals in vegetables. And some diets require you to eat foods high in saturated fat, which isn't good for your heart.

Your best bet is to stick to eating plans that include reasonable amounts of a variety of foods and don't allow you to lose more than 1 kilogram (2 pounds) a week. A satisfying meal of hearty portions of vegetables has fewer calories than some meals recommended by fad diets.

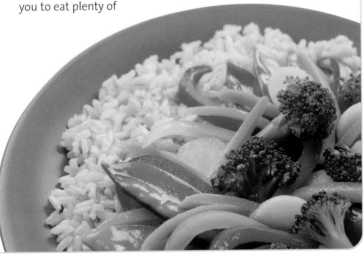

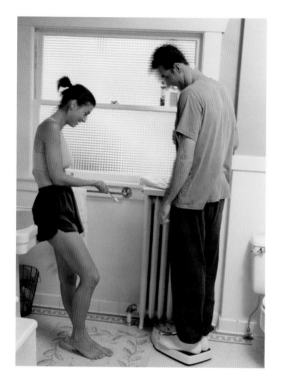

high shelf, in the back of the cupboard or some-where else you won't find them easily.

Lose a Little Weight – at First

If your BMI is 25 or higher, start out by aiming to lose between 5 and 10 per cent of your body weight. For example, if you're 162 centimetres (5 feet 4 inches) and weigh 82 kilograms (12 stone 12 pounds) your BMI is 31. To get it down to 25, you'd need to lose 35 pounds (16 kilograms/2½

stone). At first, concentrate on losing the first few pounds. Moderate weight loss will give you lower blood pressure, lower lipids, lower blood sugar and more self-esteem – and it's an easier goal than trying to lose all that weight at once.

Pace yourself. People who lose 2 kilograms (5 pounds) or more in a week lose water, not fat, so try to lose just a kilo (2 pounds) a week. Depending on how much you have to lose, it could take as long as 6 months to lose 10 per cent of your body weight in a healthy way, but that means you're more likely to maintain your new weight.

Look for other evidence. It may take a while to see results on the scales, but you'll feel your body getting stronger and healthier immediately after you start to eat well and exercise.

If you lose weight but your body mass index doesn't budge, measure your waist again. Your abdominal fat may disappear – a benefit – even if your total weight or BMI doesn't budge. It will also help keep you motivated when your weight seems to be stuck in the same 2- to 4.5-kilogram (5- to 10-pound) range despite your efforts to reduce.

Work on maintenance. Once you lose your initial goal of 10 per cent, maintaining it for 6 months will continue to improve your health and make it easier to avoid weight regain.

Do it again. If you have more to lose after your first 10 per cent, continue to set the same goals until you've reached a healthy BMI.

6

A Real-life Guide to Stress Relief

Women have more to do than ever before. At work, we skip lunch and put in overtime. At home, we're in charge of most of the housework and child care. And who takes care of parents and in-laws when they become ill? We do it all.

The result? Women are often overwhelmed and feel out of control. The unrelenting stress disrupts our peace of mind and also damages our health.

Up to 40 per cent of workers say that they experience 'a great deal' of stress on the job. And stress follows women home. Research has found that even women who are highly satisfied with their jobs have significantly elevated levels of stress hormones during and after work, due to work and home responsibilities.

Stress and the body's reaction to it can be good things. After all, you might not get up in the morning if you didn't have a job to go to. And should you ever face physical danger, your body's stress response could save your life. But when stress becomes chronic, it can damage relationships, steal restful sleep and even wear out the arteries.

It doesn't have to be this way. Stress isn't the deadline, the traffic jam or the uncooperative teenager – it's the way you react to things. That's why one woman who sees a long queue at the supermarket may feel her temper rising out of control, while another simply relaxes and browses through a magazine while she waits.

Your Body on Stress

While we tend to view stress as toxic to our minds, we generally don't consider its potentially harmful effects on the body. But the physical effects of stress are profound.

During times of stress, the nervous system triggers the release of stress hormones: adrenalin, norepinephrine and cortisol. They stimulate virtually every system in the body. For example, they cause sugars and fats to pour into the bloodstream for quick energy. Blood pressure rises, and the heart beats faster in order to boost circulation to muscles in the arms and legs. Respiration increases, which supplies the muscles with more oxygen. The blood clots more easily as a precaution against injury, and perspiration increases in order to cool the body in this energized state.

The stress response happens very quickly. It's designed to save your life in emergency situations. Once the danger is past, your body gradually returns to its normal state.

Most days, of course, stress isn't a physical threat. Stress is time pressures, traffic and the weight of responsibilities. But its effects on the body are just as profound. Stress affects immunity, which is why people who are under pressure a lot of the time tend to experience more infections, such as colds or flu. One study found that women who cared for relatives with Alzheimer's – which can be an emotionally draining full-time job – had weaker immune responses than those who weren't caregivers. Depression, which can be a major response to stress, is considered a primary risk factor for cardiovascular disease. Stress raises blood pressure, which damages the linings of blood vessels. At the same time, substances that are

WHAT TO DO IF YOU HAVE ONLY **5 MINUTES**

Find a quiet place to close your eyes. Tune out the rest of the world and rest your mind. Or go for a walk around the block if you're a physical type of person.

Even a short break from stress will help you feel better physically as well as emotionally.

released during times of stress, such as fatty acids, are trapped in the damaged areas of the blood vessels. This leads to the development of plaques, fatty deposits that can block bloodflow, increase the risk of clots and possibly lead to heart attacks.

Fat also heads to your middle during times of stress. Emotional extremes suppress the body's production of testosterone, which helps control abdominal fat. Researchers have identified dozens of physical symptoms that are associated with stress overload. They include:

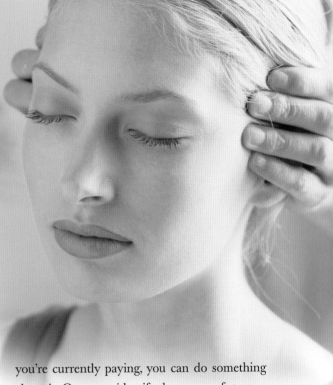

- Fatigue
- Frequent headaches or migraines
- Frequent colds or flu
- Asthma or wheezing
- Poor sleep
- Muscle tension and aches
- Nausea
- Reduced sex drive
- Hair loss
- Eating too little or too much

Apart from physical changes, constant stress also affects the emotions. You might notice frequent feelings of:

- Anxiety
- Sadness
- Frustration
- Irritability
- Anger

No matter how much stress you experience, and regardless of the physical or emotional tolls you're currently paying, you can do something about it. Once you identify the causes of stresses in your life and recognize the danger signs, you can reduce them with this six-step action plan.

Step 1: Identify Your Boiling Point

Why do some women get frazzled and irritated when they're stuck in traffic, while others stay cool even during catastrophes? Two things make the difference: the amount of control that you feel you have over your life and your basic personality.

If you're responsible for the care of your ill mother, on top of being a mum and a full-time employee, you'll understandably be stressed. A lot of things are happening in your life, and you really can't control the outcome.

RESTORING SLEEP

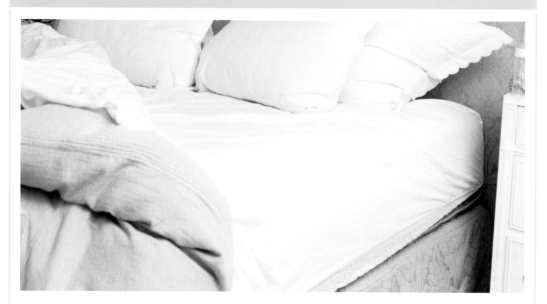

Women are feeling increasingly stressed-out – and they are losing sleep over it.

In a sleep census poll of more than 1,000 people, 62 per cent said they had a hard time sleeping, and more women than men reported symptoms of sleep deprivation. Adults as a whole lose almost 5 hours of sleep a week because of insomnia. Do that every week, and you'll lose 260 hours by the end of the year – more than a week and a half.

What's behind all this tossing and turning? Stress tops the list. When you're stressed, your muscles are tense, you have high levels of stress hormones that arouse instead of relax the body and your mind is full of troubling thoughts.

You might think you can get away with less sleep, but getting fewer than 7 or 8 hours of sleep a night affects your concentration, judgement, reaction time, memory and physical performance. Here are a few ways to ensure you get the sleep you need.

Establish relaxation rituals. Every night, take a warm bath. Or read a magazine or watch TV. Everyone should do something relaxing before going to bed. If you do this every night, your body will naturally prepare for sleep.

Avoid stimulants. The caffeine in coffee, chocolate, cola, tea, diet drugs and some pain relievers may keep you awake. If you smoke, the nicotine in cigarettes can lead to early-morning awakenings because the body is demanding the next 'hit'. Now might be a good time to give up smoking – you'll get better sleep if you do.

Stick to your workouts. People who exercise sleep better. But to avoid being too pumped up at bedtime, finish exercising 5 to 6 hours before then.

'Think of judges,' says Dr Deborah Belle, a psychologist. 'They have what seem to be extremely stressful jobs, they have a heavy workload and they make extremely important decisions.'

But they seem to live for ever. Why?

'I think it's because they have the best legal brains working for them, they can choose which cases to hear, they have the esteem and admiration of many people and they can take lavish holidays to recuperate,' Dr Belle says. 'On the other hand, their secretaries have a heavy workload without much control. They're probably under much higher levels of stress.'

Then there's personality. Women with hostile, type A personalities – they snap at waiters for making mistakes, tailgate cars on the motorway, and shout at colleagues – have a higher risk of cardiovascular disease due to stress. In a study of 276 healthy men and women, those who were less agreeable had higher blood pressures and levels of stress hormones than those who were calmer and more easygoing.

Other personality types, too, are vulnerable to health damage. In the same study, people who were introverted also tended to have high blood pressure and elevated levels of stress hormones.

Many women share a personality trait that may increase their risk for depression: rumination. Women who are introspective and passive and tend to dwell on their problems – which often makes problems seem worse than they really are – generally experience depression and unnecessary levels of stress.

All of the complexities that make people human affect the stress response.

Step 2: Recognize the Triggers

Sometimes the source of stress is obvious: driving behind a school bus or dustbin lorry that makes several stops en route is making you late for work, for example. At other times, it's not always clear if your frustration is due to your job, problems with the children, financial worries or all of the above.

You can't begin to control stress if you're not sure what's behind it. At the first sign that something's wrong, try to get to the bottom of it. One way to do that is by keeping a journal.

Sit down for a few minutes every day to write about issues that concern you. Don't waste time with the little things, like queuing at the supermarket. Try to get to the source of what's bothering you. At that point, you can start problem solving. Make a list of some of your options: getting household help, researching a new job, talking to a counsellor and so on.

Once you start identifying your stress triggers and considering solutions, you'll feel a sense of

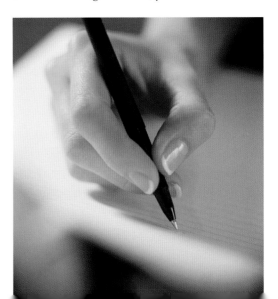

control you didn't have before, and that's one of the best ways to combat stress.

It's not uncommon for women to feel so tired and burned-out that they can't begin to muster the energy that's required for problem solving. At that point, it makes sense to see a therapist right away. You'll learn more about yourself and also discover practical ways to bring additional calm to your life.

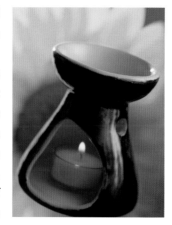

Step 3: Practise the 'Calm Response'

We've already talked about the physical changes that accompany stress. Even though these changes are a necessary part of survival, they can make life really uncomfortable a lot of the time.

Here are a few ways to control the symptoms of stress and bring additional calm into your life.

Breathe deeply. Try to make a fist while taking a deep breath. You probably can't maintain the tension for very long because breathing naturally eases tension. It's common, however, for people to breathe shallowly when they're experiencing stress – which can make the discomfort even worse. Doctors often advise women to practise breathing exercises, but simply reminding yourself to breathe deeply now and then can make a difference. It might be helpful to put little cues around the house – sticky notes on the refrigerator or in the car, for example. Every time you see one of the cues, take a moment to drop your

shoulders, breathe deeply and let go of some of the tension.

Go on holiday – in 30 seconds. Warm sand beneath your bare feet. A cool breeze against your face. The sound of a crashing ocean in your ears. Your body tenses at the perception of stress, so calm it down by thinking of something serene.

Bend with stress. When life's pressures are getting to you, put your imagination to work. Imagine that you're a strong oak tree. The trunk of the tree is your inner core, and no amount of wind will affect it. 'But your branches bend for you,' says Dr Pamela Peeke, assistant clinical professor of medicine at the University of Maryland School of Medicine. When you're faced with a traffic jam, for example, tell yourself that your core is strong and sustainable. You don't have to get upset about it.

Get some sun. Even if you don't think you have the time, get outside for a few minutes. Exposure to sunlight increases levels of serotonin, a natural hormone that reduces stress and imparts feelings of calm and well-being.

Take mini-breaks. If you let your mind rest for at least 5 minutes every hour, you'll find it easier to stay calm and focused. Close your eyes and think peaceful thoughts – or stand up and stretch. Better yet, walk briskly for a few moments: it stimulates the release of endorphins, body chemicals that neutralize stress hormones.

Distract yourself. Filling your free time with activities you love will help keep your mind off the stress of tomorrow. 'Humans are wonderful at distracting themselves,' Dr Belle says. 'And we need to feed our souls this way.'

Rewrite the script. When you find yourself believing that a bump in the road is a catastrophe, take a new perspective. Your roof sprang a leak and the car engine blew up on the same day? Instead of losing it, laugh at the irony. Turn life into a comedy instead of a drama.

Step 4: Accept What You Can't Change

Stress is never going to go away. Women have to accept that. But remember, stress isn't the issue – how you react to it is. Here are a few ways to unwind, no matter what life throws at you.

Accept the circumstances. Some types of stress, you can't solve. Breathing or taking a mental holiday might help, but nothing will take away the heartache of watching a relative become ill or the grief over the death of a parent. 'Stay in touch with the complexity of the situation, and do your best to heighten the quality of the days you have,' Dr Belle says.

Be imperfect – and calmer. When you try to achieve the unachievable – as so many women tend to do – you'll feel frustrated, anxious or depressed. So concentrate on your strengths, instead of obsessing over your flaws. The second a negative thought enters your mind, replace it with 'I'm doing the best I can' or 'I'm fine and happy and fulfilled'.

Acknowledge your mistakes and move on. Because so many people depend on them, women often feel as though they have to make the right decisions every time. It doesn't work that way, of course. Everyone makes mistakes, and the worst thing you can do is berate yourself and dwell on them.

Here's a better approach: remind yourself that within every mistake is an opportunity for growth

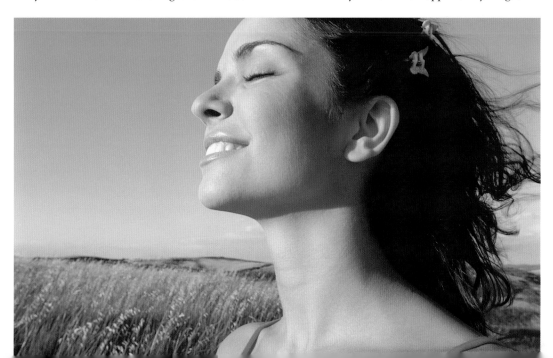

and renewal. You can't change what's already happened, but you can take the lessons you learned and apply them to the next challenge that comes along.

Step 5: Stay Socially Engaged

One thing women do well is bond with other women. Some scientists even think that women are hardwired to 'tend and befriend', to protect themselves and their children by building a social network that they can rely on for help.

'We're social creatures,' Dr Belle says. 'We're healthiest and happiest when we're part of a supportive group.'

Talking to friends about what's bothering you might help you see things in a different light. It also helps to get reassurance from friends that you're still loved and supported, despite how awful you feel.

Step 6: Practise a Lower-stress Life

If you establish certain habits every day, even when you're not under stress, you'll find that you'll naturally be a little calmer if things do go awry.

Exercise regularly. It's one of the best ways to reduce anxiety, tension, apprehension, depression and fatigue. Study after study has shown that moderate exercise reduces cortisol, the stress hormone that triggers the runaway stress response.

You don't have to be an athlete to get the benefits of exercise. Walk in the morning and again in the evening. Go the health club three or four times a week. Spend some time weeding the garden or raking leaves. Any kind of physical activity releases 'feel good' endorphins, which will help you feel calmer and more relaxed.

Have a plan B. Preparing backup plans is a great way to feel in control of life. Suppose you have to drive your daughter to football practice

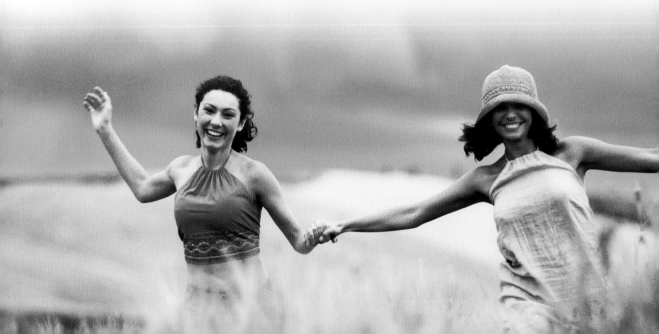

after work – but you always worry that you'll get stuck in traffic. Arrange with one of the other parents to share driving responsibilities if you get delayed. You'll worry less because you'll know that everything is covered 'just in case'.

Get a pet. Many studies have shown that having a dog, cat or other pet reduces stress. Pet owners even have lower cholesterol and blood pressure than those without pets.

Put pleasure in your diary. You can't be a great mother, wife or friend if you're burned-out and exhausted. So think about what you can do for yourself. Do you want to read the paper on Sunday mornings? Enjoy a long bath in the evenings? Put it in your diary – actually write it down. It will make you much more likely actually to keep the 'appointment'.

Keep healthy finances. Debt – credit card bills in particular – may be linked to high blood pressure, insomnia and other physical problems. When researchers surveyed more than 1,000 people, they found that those with higher credit card debts were more stressed and had the most health complaints. Get your finances in order now, and you'll enjoy better health.

Keep a low-maintenance house. Dirt won't stress you out if you can't see it. Buy rugs, sofas and chairs in earth tones, which hide stains. Choose easy-to-clean wood or linoleum floors. Put washable paint on the walls – they'll be easier to wipe down. And buy low-maintenance plants and shrubs: less work in the garden means more time for the things that are important to you.

Spend some time at the playground. If you have young children in the house, spending too

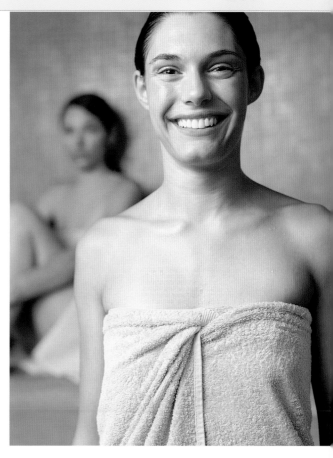

much time with them on your own is not good. Go to play groups so you have time to socialize with other mothers.

Women without children often find that it's a real kick to spend time with nieces, nephews or grandchildren. It's hard to take life too seriously when you're making up rhymes, talking in a silly voice or pushing a swing.

Cherish life. A warm breeze in the summer. The beauty of nature. The rush you feel as you ride your bike. If you believe you deserve pleasure from life, you'll be much more likely to achieve all the things that you need to be happy.

A Stop-Smoking Programme That Can't Fail

After 27 years of smoking cigarettes, Susannah Hayward crushed her last butt. Once she got over the withdrawal symptoms, she felt reborn.

'Everything smells and tastes better, my skin is pink and healthy, I can run without wheezing and I have more energy overall,' Hayward says. 'I'm also more relaxed. I don't feel agitated any more in a non-smoking environment.'

The best part for Susannah? Higher self-esteem.

'If I can give up smoking, I can do anything,' she says.

And she did. She wrote a book about giving up smoking, called *Breathe Easy*.

Many women think smoking helps them get through the day.

In reality, smoking makes you cough, lose your breath and feel *more* stressed when you can't smoke. Smoking accounts for 9 out of 10 cases of lung cancer in the UK, and women's lungs damage more easily than men's. Smoking can also cause heart disease, stroke and cancer of the larynx, mouth, bladder, cervix, pancreas and kidneys. Women risk their reproductive health as well. In fact, smoking kills 120,000 people a year in Britain, one in five of all deaths, according to Department of Health figures.

If scare tactics worked, no one would smoke. The fact is, nicotine is just as addictive as cocaine and heroin. It's never too late to give up – or to try again. Successfully stopping almost erases the damage of moderate cigarette smoking, if you quit before the age of 35 – which is when the diseases first start appearing in cigarette smokers, such as bronchitis, emphysema and periodontal disease, and circulatory disorders. Stopping may even extend your life; smokers tend to die 7 years earlier than non-smokers.

Why Smokers Smoke

Seven to 10 seconds after you inhale, nicotine releases super-normal amounts of norepinephrine and dopamine, brain chemicals that give you pleasure. You'll feel more satisfaction than you do from laughing, watching the sun set or drinking cool water on a warm day.

But after a while, your body depends on nicotine for the release of these chemicals, and it takes more nicotine to feel the same amount of pleasure. But on their way to your brain, the components of tobacco smoke *also*:

- Narrow your arteries, some of which are no bigger than a pencil lead, and allow less blood get to your heart. That constriction causes blood to move faster, which traumatizes the lining of vessels.

- Rob your heart and blood vessels of oxygen hours or days after you smoke because of the effect of carbon monoxide attaching to haemoglobin cells, which transport oxygen.

If you smoke 15 to 30 cigarettes a day, **your skin can't repair itself** from exposure to the sun's ultraviolet rays. Some doctors say **they can tell** whether or not a woman smokes **just by looking at her face.**

- Lower HDL ('good') cholesterol levels while raising LDL ('bad') cholesterol, which leads to a buildup of plaque and lipids in already damaged arteries.

- Trigger an irregular heart rhythm or heart attack if the heart becomes starved of oxygen.

- Interfere with bone rebuilding, contributing to osteoporosis.

- Damage the tiny air sacs in lungs, reducing oxygen exchange.

The effects are immediate. It's hard to breathe, let alone exercise. If you keep it up for 15 or 20 years, you'll lose 40 to 50 per cent of your lung function, called chronic obstructive pulmonary disease, and may become short of breath when having a shower or walking to your car.

Smoking a packet a day also causes 5 to 10 per cent bone loss by menopause, a significant loss considering smokers reach menopause up to 4 years earlier than women who don't smoke.

Women Take the Biggest Hit

Women who smoke (roughly one in four of us) experience more wheezing, coughing, breathlessness and asthma than men who smoke, even if they light up less often. Among men, lung cancer is decreasing; for women, this deadly disease on the rise.

Researchers don't know exactly why damage is more severe in women, but oestrogen may play a role. Researchers think oestrogen releases

PREVENT BRONCHITIS AND EMPHYSEMA

If you smoke and you've had a persistent cough for more than two years, don't dismiss it as 'smoker's cough'. A consistent cough with mucus could be chronic bronchitis.

While non-smokers can and do get bronchitis, smoking is by far the most common way to get bronchitis because smoke causes the bronchi to become inflamed and interferes with airflow. But it's also possible to get it from a bacterial or viral infection, air pollution or

industrial dusts and fumes. Bronchitis may lead to or accompany emphysema.

By all means, if you have bronchitis and you smoke, give up. Exercise may also indirectly help by strengthening the heart and body, but because exercise could make breathing even harder, consult your doctor before beginning a new exercise programme.

Like bronchitis, emphysema is accompanied by cough and shortness of breath. If the

diseases occur together, they're called chronic obstructive pulmonary disease. And as with bronchitis, smoking is the biggest cause of emphysema. Cigarette smoke damages the air sacs in the lungs so that they have trouble transferring oxygen to the blood. You'll probably notice you can't exercise as well. Even a brief walk could make you lose your breath. Stopping smoking can halt emphysema's progression in its tracks.

chemicals in the lungs that cause cells to divide. That in turn thickens the airways and stimulates cells with mutations to form tumours. Oestrogen may also help convert chemicals in cigarette smoke to carcinogens.

Smoking also affects women's reproductive health, causing:

- Lower fertility

- A doubled risk of getting cervical cancer

- Higher risk of low birth weight, sudden infant death syndrome and stillbirths among pregnant women

- Higher risk of heart disease and stroke while taking the birth control pill

If you give up smoking now, in the years to come you will erase almost all that damage. Your skin will look better and you'll breathe more easily. Your risk of cancer will go down, and after 4 years your heart attack risk will dwindle to that of someone who has never smoked.

When it comes to lung cancer, however, you'll always have higher risk than someone who has never smoked. But your risk of developing cancer will decrease every year to nearly a non-smoker's level of risk.

If you've tried to stop before and couldn't, you're not beaten yet. On average, it takes five or six tries to help stop for good. Today, smokers have more options to help stop than ever before. If one strategy didn't work for you in the past, another will. Here's a step-by-step action plan from experts who have studied smoking habits of women.

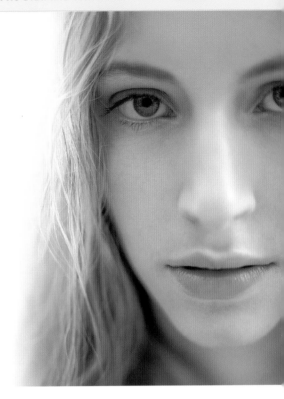

Step 1: Get Screened for Depression

Researchers estimate that one-quarter to one-third of all smokers experience anxiety or depression. They may self-medicate with cigarettes. Since women are twice as likely as men to experience depression, they're more likely to fall into this group of smokers.

'I screen all my female patients for depression and anxiety before they quit smoking, and I ask them how they are feeling after they quit so they can get treated if they have mood changes,' says Dr Hyder Ferry, an associate professor of preventive and family medicine. (For more on the symptoms of depression, see page 297.)

Step 2: Set a Stop Date

Commit to a stop date that falls some time in the next 7 to 10 days, and get rid of all your cigarettes and ashtrays by then.

'Like anything, if you don't plan exactly when you're going to do it, it doesn't get done,' says Dr Kenneth Perkins, professor of psychiatry at the University of Pittsburgh School of Medicine, who has researched smoking cessation.

The worst time to quit is during the second half of your menstrual cycle because premenstrual symptoms could make withdrawal worse. In one study, women who quit in the first 2 weeks after their period and attended group sessions experienced less severe withdrawal symptoms than women who quit smoking later in their menstrual cycle.

Step 3: Choose Your Weapon

Going 'cold turkey' is the least effective way to quit – only about 2 to 5 per cent of smokers can do so. Most others need help of some kind. If one method doesn't work, try another. Here are your options, ranked more or less from most to least effective (although this is highly individual).

Phase out cigarettes. Gradually decrease the number of cigarettes you smoke until you're down to five to 10 a day – just enough to keep from going into withdrawal. Then quit completely.

For instance, if you smoke a packet of cigarettes a day, allow yourself to smoke only half of each cigarette for a week. The next week, throw three cigarettes out before you start the pack. Continue to reduce at this pace for 4 to 6 weeks before you quit completely.

Ask your doctor about bupropion. Like nicotine, the prescription compound bupropion (Zyban) is used as an antidepressant and stabilizes the levels of norepinephrine and dopamine, two brain chemicals responsible for feelings of well-being. But while nicotine causes the chemicals to spike and then fall, bupropion releases a smaller, steady stream without causing any addiction. That means withdrawal symptoms won't bother you as much.

You can try combining bupropion with other therapies. When 4,000 people took bupropion with or without nicotine replacement therapy and had professional counselling, 40 to 60 per cent of them remained smoke-free for at least a year.

Consider nicotine replacement therapy. Although it's less effective in women than in men, nicotine replacement therapy provides enough nicotine to keep you from going into withdrawal while you break the habit of reaching for a cigarette – which takes about 5 to 10 weeks. Nicotine replacement therapy is available over the counter in the form of the patch, which could cause a mild skin rash, and gum. Prescription versions include an inhaler and nasal spray.

If you tried nicotine replacement therapy before and felt miserable, you probably didn't use a high enough dose of nicotine or you stopped using it too soon. For best results, talk to your doctor about which therapy and dose is best for you.

Look into acupuncture. Acupuncture is an ancient Chinese health practice that involves

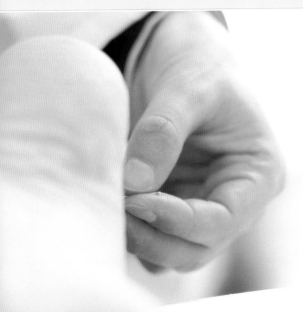

phone 01257 262124; in Australia, try the Australian Hypnotherapists' Association at www.ahahypnotherapy.org.au; in New Zealand, see the NZ Society of Clinical and Applied Hypnotherapy, www.nzhypnotherapists.co.nz.

Step 4: Start an Exercise Routine

The average smoker weighs 2.75 to 5 kilograms (6 to 11 pounds) less than a non-smoker but puts on that amount of weight after giving up. Ten to 15 per cent of women who give up put on more than 13 kilograms (2 stone). That's because nicotine curbs hunger, decreasing between-meal snacking. The elimination of nicotine reverses the weight-suppressing effect, causing women to eat more after giving up.

Research shows it's just too hard to diet *and* quit smoking, but you can exercise. Women who smoked 10 or more cigarettes a day and joined a smoking cessation programme that involved about 50 minutes of exercise three times a week put on less weight and were more likely to stay smoke-free than women who didn't exercise.

Even if you do put on weight, you'd have to put on more than 45 kilograms (7 stone) to cancel out the benefits to health of quitting.

puncturing the skin with hair-thin needles at particular locations – usually the ear for nicotine addiction.

Although there's little research that proves acupuncture works, some women who try it may experience milder withdrawal symptoms.

To find a certified acupuncturist in your area, contact the British Medical Acupuncture Society on admin@medical-acupuncture.org.uk or telephone 01925 730727, or the British Acupuncture Council on info@acupuncture.org.uk or telephone 020 8735 0400; Australian Acupuncture and Chinese Medicine Association Ltd on 1300 725 334, or aacma@acupuncture.org.au; New Zealand Register of Acupuncturists on freephone 0800 228 786, or nzra@acupuncture.org.nz.

Try hypnosis. Through hypnosis, you might increase your motivation, lower your cravings and keep from lighting up. For details of registered hypnotherapists in the UK, visit the website www.thehypnotherapyassociation.co.uk or tele-

Step 5: Quash Cravings

If you eat more to make up for not smoking, your weight will be harder to control. Here's how to deal with those cigarette cravings – during and after therapy.

Change your routine. Cues can make you want a cigarette all day long, and women may be more susceptible than men. The most common cues are the smell of cigarette smoke and drinking coffee. But there are more situations that you may not think about, such as a talking on the phone, pouring a glass of wine or unwinding after work. The solution: change your routine to miss the urge. Drink tea instead of coffee, take public transport to work if you have access and visit a non-smoking friend instead of talking on the phone. Go for a walk when you feel a craving coming on, and keep boiled sweets and lollipops handy. If possible, you might want to take a holiday from work the week you give up.

Avoid bars and alcohol. Until you've learned to cope with the craving-inducing sights and smells, and the easy availability of cigarettes, stay away from pubs, bars and alcohol. Whenever possible, stay away from people who smoke.

Breathe deeply. Take deep breaths when you get the urge to smoke. It will relax you and help you cope with cravings.

Give yourself a 2-minute massage. One study at the University of Miami found that a 2-minute hand or ear massage cut cravings, reduced anxiety and improved mood. Try these moves.

- Pinch your ear from the top down to your earlobe.

- Gently tug your earlobe.

- Use your thumb to massage the palm of your hand in a circular motion.

- Use your thumb and index finger to massage each finger from base to fingertip.

Step 6: Join a Smoking Cessation Support Group

Group sessions give you tips and support even if you're using a therapy. After reviewing several studies on smoking cessation, researchers found that people were more successful when they went to group programmes that offered behaviour techniques and mutual support than when they quit with little or no help. Maybe that's because just

---

THREE THINGS I TELL EVERY FEMALE PATIENT

1

DR LINDA HYDER FERRY, *an associate professor of preventive and family medicine, says, 'Quitting smoking is your first step to minimize ageing and slow down the skin wrinkling process.' Here are some other strategies that she emphasizes.*

- Use a mild cleanser that exfoliates your skin.

2

- Eat a diet high in natural antioxidants, which you'll get from fruit and vegetables.

3

- Wear a UVB/UVA spectrum sunscreen with an SPF of at least 15 every day.

when you think you can't go another day without a cigarette, your group knows exactly how you feel. Quality of sessions varies, so if you don't like one, try others.

Step 7: Prepare for Withdrawal

Withdrawal symptoms vary from person to person, depending on how much you smoke and your method of giving up. Knowing what to expect will help you get through it. Here's a day-to-day guide.

Days 1 and 2. Physically, you'll feel like you have a unique combination of withdrawal symptoms. You might have a headache, increased irritability or anxiety, and you'll feel uncomfortable. You might also have trouble sleeping at night and concentrating during the day.

Days 3 to 7. Your withdrawal symptoms peak on day 3 and then stabilize. Many give up at this point, but as soon as you get over this hump, you'll feel better – promise.

Days 8 to 13. Your symptoms may begin to improve.

Days 14 to 365. Physically you feel back to normal. For the first several months, you'll probably crave a cigarette occasionally, and you may have trouble sleeping. But studies show that going cigarette-free for a full year increases your chances of staying that way.

Step 8: Give Yourself a Year of Rewards

Make it easier to get to that year mark when cravings subside. Treat yourself to a new book or theatre tickets after the first day, the first week, then the first month of no smoking. Be sure to make the reward greater as time goes by.

Not only will your health improve, but your sense of taste and smell will be heightened, you won't have to clean up ash, your clothes won't smell like smoke and you'll have more time to spend on other activities or with friends and family (the average cigarette takes 5 to 7 minutes to smoke). In addition to pocketing the cash you would have spent on cigarettes, you'll probably save money on health insurance. Best of all, you won't have to rely on smoking to feel good. And remember: one slip doesn't mean you're a smoker again, so don't quit quitting.

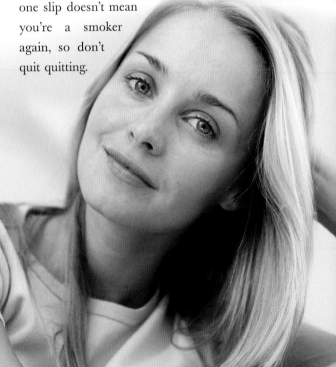

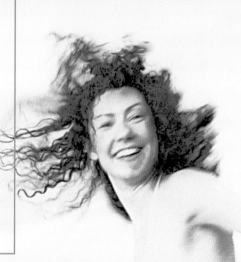

Sun-proof (and Age-proof) Your Skin

The sun can do a lot of good. It regulates sleep cycles, stimulates the body's production of vitamin D and enhances feelings of well-being. But there's also a downside: exposure to sun can lead to wrinkles, age spots and skin cancer.

In fact, sunshine is considered the single biggest cause of visible ageing. But you don't have to succumb to the damaging rays. Even if you haven't been sun smart in the past, it's never too late to start protecting your skin.

For starters, every woman should eat a diet that's rich in fruit and vegetables. They contain antioxidant compounds, which reduce the damaging effects of sunshine.

Refraining from smoking also makes a difference because cigarette smoke creates huge numbers of skin-damaging molecules.

But the most important thing you can do is shield your skin from the sun. As long as you use sunscreen, take advantage of shade and wear the right clothing, you can enjoy your favourite outdoor activities without worrying about the damaging rays.

How Sunshine Makes Skin Look Old

Every time the sun strikes your skin, the skin produces pigment that scatters and absorbs the rays. The resulting tan means your skin is defending itself from harmful radiation.

But a tan can do only so much. Over time, the ultraviolet A (UVA) and ultraviolet B (UVB) radiation in sunshine can weaken the lower layer of skin, known as the dermis, and promote wrinkles, brown spots and the development of skin cancer.

The most common (and least aggressive) form of skin cancer is basal cell carcinoma. It begins in the top layer of skin, the epidermis, and generally doesn't spread any further. While another form – squamous cell carcinoma – often remains at its original site, it is more likely to spread to other parts of the body. Both basal cell and squamous cell carcinomas can be cured if detected early. However, melanoma – a cancer that starts in the skin's pigment cells and readily spreads to other organs – can be deadly. It causes 75 per cent of all deaths from skin cancer.

How can you protect yourself from the sun's harmful rays? This three-step action plan will make all the difference.

THREE THINGS I TELL EVERY FEMALE PATIENT

DR ALAN KLING, a clinical assistant professor of dermatology, offers the following advice for maximum skin protection.

1 GET YOUR TAN IN A BOTTLE. If you don't like to have a pale complexion, try using self-tanners or bronzers. They're a lot safer than 'natural' tans. Just remember that a self-tanner does not protect you from the sun's rays, so be sure to slather on that sunscreen when you're going to be outside.

2 MAKE NO EXCEPTIONS. Skin damage can occur even on cloudy days, so apply sunscreen whenever you're going outside — even if you're planning to stay in the shade.

3 CONSIDER THE ALTITUDE. The sun's ultraviolet radiation is strongest at high altitudes. If you live at a high elevation, or if you're hiking or skiing, reapply sunscreen frequently.

Step 1: Determine Your Risk Profile

There's no way to accurately predict whose skin is most likely to show premature signs of ageing or who is more likely to develop skin cancer, says Dr Dee Anna Glaser, an associate professor of dermatology. Look out for signs of trouble, which include:

- Small pearly white bumps, or sores on the skin that bleed and don't heal.

- Red, scaly bumps that resemble a scar and have a depression in the middle.

- Dark spots that are asymmetrical, have irregular borders, have more than one colour, and are bigger than the size of a pencil rubber. These spots may be flat or elevated.

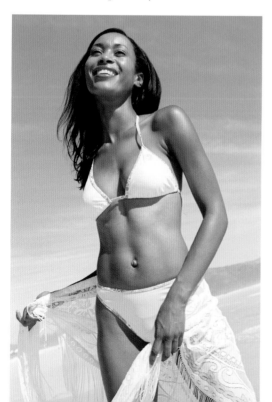

Anyone can get skin cancer, but some people have a much higher risk than others. The risk factors include:

- Fair skin. It doesn't contain as much of the natural pigment called melanin that scatters the sun's rays.

- Multiple moles or 'beauty spots'. Melanoma cells are more abundant in moles and freckles. The more beauty spots you have, the greater the risk that cancer cells will be present.

- A history of sunburns. Even if you've had only one blistering sunburn in your life, you have a higher risk for developing skin cancer.

Step 2: Choose (and Use) the Right Protection

Wearing sunscreen is essential. You should use it every day, especially when you're spending time outdoors. To get the most benefits from sunscreen, here's what Dr Glaser advises.

Choose products with a high SPF. It stands for 'sun protection factor', and it's a measure of how well sunscreen protects your skin.

SPF refers to the length of time that sunscreen protects the skin. Suppose your skin naturally starts to burn in 20 minutes. If you use sunscreen with an SPF of 15, you won't begin to burn for 5 hours – 15 times longer. Always use a sunscreen with an SPF of 15 or higher.

Apply it often. In real life, sunscreens aren't always as effective as the SPF would indicate. If you're swimming, sweating a lot or rubbing your skin with a towel, the sunscreen is going to dissipate.

Reapply it every 2 hours – more often if you're swimming or perspiring a lot.

Buy a broad-spectrum sunscreen. These sunscreens will help block UVB and UVA rays. UVB light is the primary cause of sunburns, and protecting skin against UVA light plays an important role in preventing wrinkling and signs of ageing. Choose a product that contains zinc oxide, titanium dioxide or avobenzone, also known as Parsol 1789.

Apply it with your makeup. If you use moisturizers or other skin products in the morning, it's fine to apply sunscreen at the same time.

First, apply topical medications if you use them. Let them dry, then apply alpha hydroxy acid or other anti-ageing creams if you use them.

WHAT TO DO IF YOU HAVE ONLY **5 MINUTES**

Use a moisturizer that provides UVA and UVB protection. It may not block radiation as completely as normal sunscreen, but it provides good protection, and it's fast and convenient to apply. Most cosmetics companies make facial moisturizers with UVA and UVB protection – check the label to make sure.

Make sure you follow with a moisturizer, especially if you're using alpha hydroxy acids, which may have a drying effect on the skin. Then apply the sunscreen, followed by any makeup you're going to wear.

Give it time to work. In general, sunscreen is most effective when it's absorbed into the

TREAT PSORIASIS WITH SUN – SAFELY

Most people are advised to avoid the sun, but doctors have found that sunshine is among the best treatments for psoriasis, a skin condition that results in itchy red patches or silvery scales on the face, elbows, knees and other parts of the body.

The sun's ultraviolet rays kill T cells, which are a type of white blood cells that trigger the unattractive flare-ups.

To get the benefits of ultraviolet light while minimizing the risks, here's what doctors advise.

Cover unaffected areas. Apply sunscreen to areas that aren't affected by psoriasis. Since your face and hands get an abundance of sunshine naturally, wear gloves and put a towel over your face during 'light therapy' sessions, suggests Dr Gerald Kruger, a

dermatologist. Light therapy sessions are prescribed by a dermatologist and involve using a tanning bed or a home ultraviolet light system to treat psoriasis.

Stick to the schedule. Some ultraviolet light is helpful, but excessive amounts can harm the skin. Your dermatologist will prescribe how much light you should be getting.

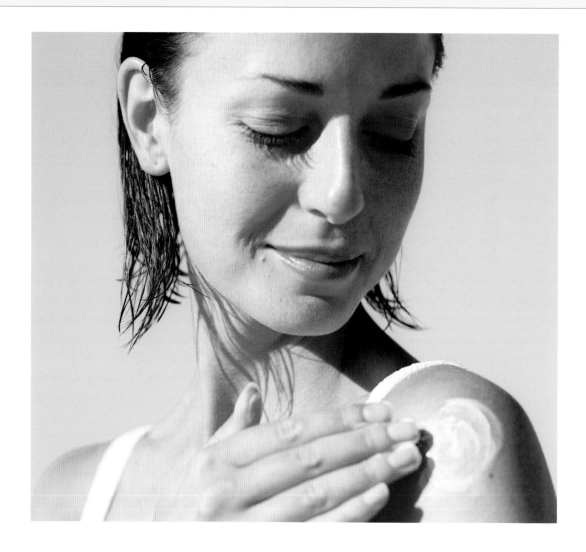

WHAT WORKS FOR ME

DR T. SHAWE, a dermatologist, knows all too well what happens with excessive sun exposure – which is why she's careful to protect her own skin.

I always use the best sunscreens I can find. I look for sunscreens that contain transparent zinc oxide, like SkinCeuticals Ultimate UV Defense SPF 30, which contains 7 per cent transparent zinc oxide.

When I know I'll be spending some time outside, I wear a sunscreen with an SPF of 30. But when I'm going to be inside most of the day, I use a sunscreen with an SPF of 15.

skin. Rub it on at least 30 minutes before you go outside.

Use the right amount. It takes about 30 grams (1 ounce) of sunscreen to cover the average person's body. That's about the amount that would fill a shot glass. You should be fully covered in cream before venturing out into the sun.

Step 3: Add Extra Protection

Wearing sunscreen helps to decrease the incidence of wrinkles and prevent the development of skin cancer. But sunscreen isn't enough by itself. Here are some additional ways to protect the skin.

Always wear shades. Sunglasses protect the delicate skin around the eyes from wrinkles. They also help prevent cataracts and macular degeneration, the leading causes of vision loss in the elderly. Wear shades whenever you go outside, even on hazy days.

The best sunglasses block 99 to 100 per cent of UVA and UVB rays – look for ones that have labels claiming 100 per cent or even total UV protection. Wraparound sunglasses and styles that fit close to the eye are especially good because they prevent the sun's rays from coming in through the sides.

Wear a hat. A tightly woven hat made of canvas, with a 10-centimetre (4-inch) brim all the way around, helps shade your face, ears and the back of your neck.

Wear long-sleeve shirts. And wear long trousers. They offer the best protection from the sun's burning rays.

Forget about tanning salons. For some people, the UVA rays in tanning salons can produce a tan faster than the sun can. That's because the rays are intense – and damaging.

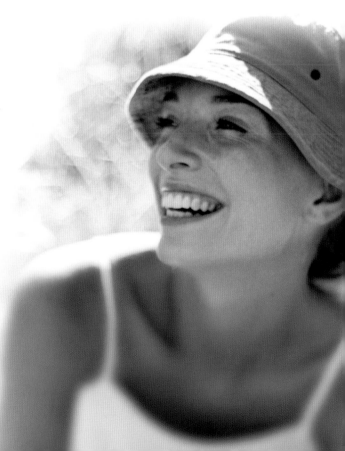

WHAT TO DO IF YOU COULD CHANGE **ONLY ONE THING**

Women should stop associating a tan with beauty and health, says Dr Dee Anna Glaser, associate professor of dermatology at a leading medical school. It may take time to become accustomed to a paler complexion – but *not* having a tan means that you're healthier.

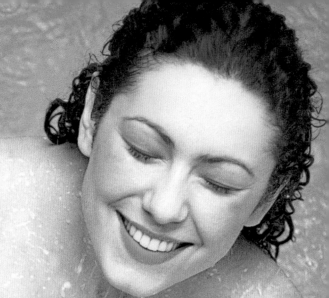

Beauty Products That Rejuvenate

The next time you browse around the cosmetics counter at the pharmacy or department store, take a moment to check out some of the 'anti-ageing' lotions and potions. You'll be amazed at how many there are. Cosmetics companies have developed hundreds of products for protecting and preserving the skin. A few may even reverse some of the visible signs of ageing, such as wrinkles and age spots.

Before reaching for specific skin-care products, you should keep in mind that your skin reflects your life.

If you smoke, sunbathe for a tan, eat junk food, put on too much weight or experience a lot of stress, your skin will pay for it. If, on the other hand, you relax often, eat healthy meals and generally maintain positive lifestyle habits – as outlined in chapters throughout this section – you'll be rewarded with skin that's smooth and firm, even in your later years.

Drinking a lot of water – at least eight large glasses daily – is especially important because it helps plump the cells of the skin, making them look smoother and younger, says Dr Kathy A. Fields, clinical instructor of dermatology at the University of California. Equally important to making the skin look plump, she adds, is good humidity in the air around you.

Sunscreen, of course, is essential. It's the only way to prevent future damage because it blocks the sun's ultraviolet radiation. This is important because sun exposure accounts for about 90 per cent of all skin cancers. Doctors advise applying sunscreen lavishly after your moisturizer but at least 30 minutes prior to sun exposure and reapply every 2 hours. Choose products that block both UVA and UVB rays and that have a sun protection factor (SPF) of at least 15. (For more information about sunscreens, see chapter 8.)

Wearing sunscreen and generally taking care of your health are just the beginning for healthy-looking skin. The skin naturally breaks down over time, especially after menopause, when declines in oestrogen cause the skin to lose elasticity.

Genetic factors also play a role: if other family members have a lot of wrinkles, you have a higher chance of developing them, too.

This doesn't mean that you're at the mercy of time, however. In the past few years, cosmetics companies have created hundreds of rejuvenating products that really can protect the skin, reverse wrinkles and generally make you look younger.

Some products have been exhaustively tested and proven to work. Others look good in the bottle and the labels make them *sound* effective, but there's little evidence that they make a difference. The only way to know which products to take seriously is to understand a little bit of the science behind them. To make things easy, we've created an easy-to-follow six-step plan.

You'll learn which products to look for, and how to use them to get the best results.

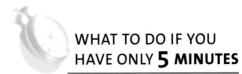

WHAT TO DO IF YOU HAVE ONLY **5 MINUTES**

Rather than experiment with dozens of anti-wrinkle products, go straight to Retinova, which has been proven to work.

Available only on prescription, Retinova is used for severe acne scarring and discolouration and excess pigmentation due to sun exposure. It may be available from a private dermatologist. It is a better moisturizer than Retin-A (also only available on prescription) because it is in an emollient base, and it works just as well at removing fine wrinkles.

Step 1: Start with a Cleanser

The skin needs to be clean to be healthy, so it's important to use cleansers to gently wash away dust, makeup and surface oils.

Use soap-free cleansers. They're much less drying than normal soaps. Try Neutrogena Deep-clean Cleansing Lotion or Johnson's pH 5.5 Facial Wash.

Exfoliate after the age of 40. The skin naturally sheds its top layer, uncovering the fresh, youthful-looking layer underneath. In women under 40, this shedding occurs every 30 days. After about 40, it slows to every 60 days, which makes the skin dry, the pores clogged and enlarged, and the skin dull and sallow. You can, however, speed up the process by using a scrub.

Scrub soaps contain tiny polyethylene beads, which gently remove dead cells and moisturize the skin. Don't bother with scrub soaps that contain pits from almonds or walnuts, though. They can actually damage the skin.

If you're aged 40 or older, you can use gentle scrub soaps every day. If you're under 40, use them only once a week or as needed.

Step 2: Use a Moisturizer

Before using any anti-ageing skin product, it's worth giving moisturizers a try. They add moisture and plumpness to cells on the surface, which makes the skin softer.

Use oil-free products. They contain an ingredient called dimethicone. It's a type of silicone

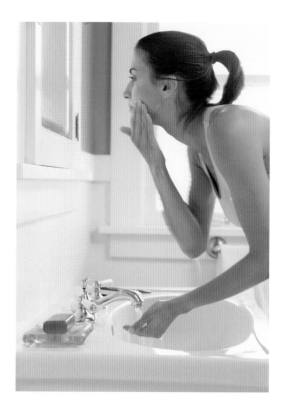

that gives moisturizers a light feel. A good example would be Oil of Olay.

Keep your moisturizers simple. If you have sensitive skin, avoid moisturizers loaded with fragrances and extracts. Check the label: it should list fewer than 10 ingredients. Eucerin and Almay products are a good choice as moisturizers for sensitive skin.

If you still want the luxurious feel of moisturizers made with green tea or other extracts, but you aren't sure how your skin will react, test them on a small area of skin on your neck near the ear. Apply the moisturizer a few nights in a row. If you don't have any irritation, redness or itching, it will be fine to use on your whole face.

Moisturize after showers or baths. The moisturizer will form a barrier over the moisture that's already on your skin, which gives it time to be absorbed by the cells.

Step 3: Fight Wrinkles Naturally

Many anti-ageing products claim to 'erase' wrinkles and make the skin look years younger. Some of this is marketing hype, but there's good evidence that products that contain natural acids (alpha or beta hydroxy acids) really can erase fine lines or brown spots, at least temporarily. They work by exfoliating the superficial layers of skin and can actually stimulate collagen production, which plumps up the skin and makes it look softer and fresher, says Dr Lisa Kates, a leading dermatologist.

Alpha hydroxy acids come in moisturizers, eye creams and many other products. Terms to look for on labels include glycolic acid (derived from sugar-cane), lactic acid (from milk), tartaric acid (from grapes), citric acid (from citrus fruits), malic acid (from apples) and mandelic acid (from walnuts). You may want to look for products that contain salicylic acid, which is a beta hydroxy acid. In women with sensitive skin, some of these products can be irritating.

Use a mild product first. Over-the-counter (OTC) products can have acid concentrations up to 10 per cent, while stronger versions, usually available by prescription only, have concentrations up to 30 per cent, says Dr Ira Davis, assistant professor of dermatology at a leading medical college. The acids can be irritating, so it's a good idea to start with a low-concentration product, then move up to something stronger if you need to. Be patient. It may take 6 to 8 weeks to see a difference.

THREE THINGS I TELL EVERY FEMALE PATIENT

Dr KATHY A. FIELDS, is a clinical instructor of dermatology. She offers women the following advice for achieving fresher and younger-looking skin.

1 **ALWAYS USE SUNSCREEN.** Choose a product that blocks both UVA and UVB light. Don't be afraid to use too much. Apply a thick, even layer 30 minutes before you go outside, and reapply every 2 hours if you are in the sun all day.

2 **USE AN EXFOLIANT SCRUB.** It's fine to use normal soap on your hands, but for your face, use a gentle scrub. Use it once a week or as needed if you are under 40 and every day if you are over 40. It really makes your skin glow.

3 **USE A MOISTURIZER DAILY.** It's among the best ways to keep the skin looking healthy. You may want to buy a moisturizer that contains either alpha hydroxy acids, retinol or kinetin, which will remove old skin cells and brown spots and hydrate the skin.

Products with alpha or beta hydroxy acids make the skin more sensitive to sunshine because the top layer of skin is thinned, which allows more ultraviolet radiation to penetrate. Although other factors, such as the amount of melanin, also affect the skin's tendency to reflect or absorb harmful rays, it's essential to use a sunscreen and avoid excessive sun exposure when using these products. Chemical-free sunscreens, such as those containing titanium dioxide or zinc oxide, may be the best choice since other sunscreen ingredients may irritate the skin.

Use furfuryladenine. It's a plant compound that moisturizes the skin, and research suggests it can help improve fine lines or even out skin tone.

Look for products that contain N6-furfuryladenine or kinetin (its chemical name). Almay Kinetin is one brand you may find at your local chemist.

Try something stronger. Over-the-counter ageing products usually have such low concentrations of active ingredients that the benefits may be minimal. To change the structure of the skin, you may want to try prescription products that contain tretinoin, such as Retinova or Retin-A. These medicines have been studied for more than a decade, and excellent clinical studies have shown that they enhance the structure and function of the skin. They increase collagen production, lighten brown spots, slough off dead skin cells, decrease fine lines and improve overall

THE NEW WRINKLE FIGHTER

Reducing fine lines and regaining a smoother, younger complexion: those are the promises of alpha hydroxy acids (AHAs), one of the main ingredients in most age-erasing cosmetics. The downside: these ingredients tend to be harsh on skin.

But you won't find this side effect in products containing the next generation of wrinkle fighters. Researchers say amphoteric hydroxy complexes (AHCs) will give you all the benefits of AHAs, with virtually none of the common side effects, such as stinging, irritation and redness.

'The stinging associated with AHAs is thought to be caused by the rapid absorption of the acid into the skin,' says Dr Barbara Green, who worked on the clinical studies with NeoStrata and Cognis, the companies that first developed AHCs. These new complexes are AHAs combined with an amino acid that slows the release of the active ingredients into the skin, making them less likely to irritate, explains Green.

'I'm finding that AHCs are great for people with sensitive skin who have had problems using AHAs in the past,' says dermatologist Dr Linda K. Franks. They can also be great for use on particularly delicate skin, such as the eye area, she says.

This combination of AHAs with amino acids is currently available in Exuviance skin products, available over the internet.

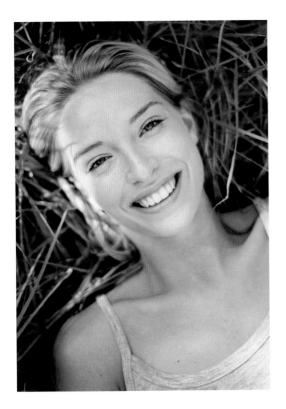

Step 4: Bleaches for Skin Spots

After decades of sun exposure, nearly everyone will develop pigment-related problems, such as age spots or freckles. It isn't always possible to eliminate them completely, but they can almost always be faded to the point of invisibility with bleaching creams.

These products contain active ingredients such as hydroquinone or kojic acid, which interfere with pigment formation. Kojic acid is found in Natural Skin Lightening System and other products. For the most part, kojic acid doesn't work as well as hydroquinone. Prescription-strength hydroquinone (over 2 per cent) tends to give better results than over-the-counter products (up to 2 per cent).

To get the best results, use prescription hydroquinone in combination with products containing kojic acid. Use daily or twice per day as tolerated and avoid the sun, or the brown spots and age spots will return within hours. People with black skin should not use lightening creams because of the danger of a dramatic change of skin colour where they are applied. The cream leaves unsightly patches that are hard to disguise. There is no safe way to lighten dark skin.

texture and tone. Products with tretinoin can dry or irritate the skin, so start slowly, using it just 2 or 3 nights a week, and increase usage to nightly as tolerated.

Pharmacies carry OTC products with retinol, which is lower in strength than tretinoin and generally well-tolerated. Retinol is converted to active retinoids in the skin and is an excellent start for improvement in texture, tone and pore size. One of the myths regarding retinol and tretinoin is that they cannot be used if you are trying to tan. Research shows that they are helpful in preventing collagen damage while you're in the sun and therefore can be used daily with good sun protection.

Step 5: Freshen Up with Masks or Peels

Over the centuries, women have used an incredible number of natural products to make masks – skin-coating slurries – that remove oils from the

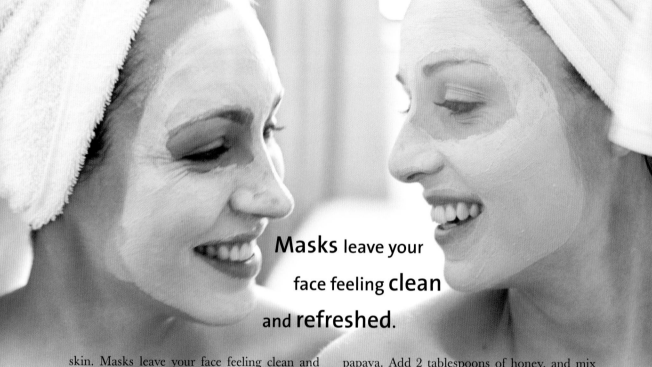

Masks leave your

face feeling clean

and refreshed.

skin. Masks leave your face feeling clean and refreshed. Peels are somewhat different. They remove the top layer of skin, as well as lighten some brown spots.

Choose the right mask. When you're shopping for mask products at the cosmetics counter, it's important to find one that matches your skin type. If you have dry skin, buy a hydrating mask. For oily skin, use clay masks or 'deep cleansers'. For acne, use a sulphur or 'purifying' mask.

Make your own. If you enjoy the feel of fresh ingredients on your skin, it's easy to make your own masks. One you may want to try is this Tropical Fruit Masque. It includes pineapple and papaya, natural sources of alpha hydroxy acids.

To make the mask, use a blender or food processor to purée a quarter of a fresh, medium pineapple and half a medium, slightly green fresh papaya. Add 2 tablespoons of honey, and mix thoroughly.

Test a small amount on your inner arm to be sure you aren't sensitive. Leave it on for 20 minutes. If your skin doesn't get red or itchy, go ahead and apply. Wash your face thoroughly, spread the mixture evenly over your face, avoiding the eye area and leave it on for 5 minutes. Then rinse with cool water. You can repeat the treatment once a week.

Get a glycolic acid peel. Performed by qualified beauticians or, less commonly, by dermatologists, this is sometimes called the 'lunchtime peel' because it works so quickly. The beautician will apply glycolic acid to your face, which removes dead cells and quickly uncovers the younger, smoother skin underneath. The peel tingles, but it isn't uncomfortable. Peels cost from

£75. For qualified practitioners, contact the British Association of Dermatologists (020 7383 0266). Or, in Australia, contact the Australian College of Dermatologists (02 9879 6177).

Try a chemical-free peel (micro dermabrasion). A qualified beautician will use a very fine brush to exfoliate the top layer of skin. It's very relaxing, takes 10 to 15 minutes, and your skin will look (and feel) younger almost instantly. A series of five treatments is recommended.

Get longer-lasting results. Many women want to have fresher, younger-looking skin, but they don't want to spend a lot of time on home or professional treatments. One option is to have a peel called the trichloracetic peel. It's performed at a specialist clinic or hospital by a dermatologist, and it will improve the appearance of the skin for as long as a year, says Dr James W. Goodnight, director of the Facial Plastics Center in New Jersey. The procedure takes under an hour.

This is one procedure that you won't want to have done during your lunch break. The skin will burn during the procedure, and it will peel off in large pieces in the days to come. Women who have this treatment usually plan to stay close to home for about a week, until the peeling process is complete.

Step 6: Say Goodbye to Puffy Eyes

Few things can make you look more tired (or older) than puffy eyes. They're usually caused by such things as fatigue, water retention, allergies, or even a reaction to eye makeup. To quickly tighten the skin and help your eyes look younger, here's what doctors advise.

Try grape seed extract. It's found in Caudalie's products and the Lancome Vinéfit range. Some people report good results from their personal experience, and preliminary studies suggest that applying grape seed extract to the skin can reduce eye puffiness caused by water retention or poor circulation. As a bonus, it helps smooth the complexion and may protect against the sun's harmful rays. It can be used nightly.

Reduce puffiness with tea bags. Brew a cup of tea using two tea bags. Set the bags aside until they're cool, then place them on the puffy areas of your eyes for a few minutes. The cool moisture can reduce swelling for up to 24 hours. In addition, tea contains tannins, compounds that reduce eye inflammation.

You can get similar effects by placing cool cucumber slices or even cooled spoons on the puffy areas.

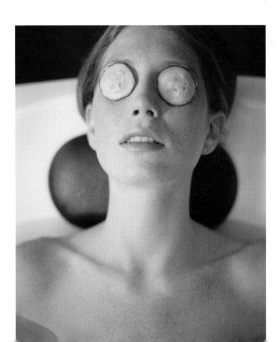

Balancing Your Emotions

Imagine a time when you felt at peace. Relaxed. Content. Free of worry. Now imagine that you could feel that way every day.

Sounds impossible? It's not. You can balance your emotions.

Although psychologists have different views of what constitutes emotional balance, they agree that it involves spending more time at peace than blowing up in anger, writhing with jealousy or being dragged down by sadness.

Internally, we all have a central home base. It's a state of normal calm and contentment.

No one spends all their time in that peaceful zone, of course. Life is full of conflicts. But a reasonable goal – one that any woman can achieve – is to return to that soothing home base after a setback, such as a clash with a colleague or a disagreement with your husband.

You'll feel better immediately, but that's not the only benefit. You'll also enjoy better health. Negative emotions such as anger and anxiety can weaken the immune system and leave you vulnerable to illness. Stress and tension also increase the risk of high blood pressure, heart disease and dozens of other serious conditions.

Experts don't suggest that women should never get mad, jealous or sad. What you can do is minimize the amount of time that you spend experiencing these or other negative emotions. In just six steps, you can strengthen your ability to handle any situation with calm and confidence.

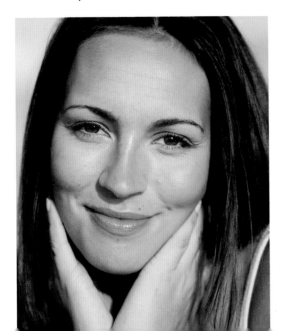

Step 1: Take an Emotional Inventory

Before you start working on your emotional skills, it's helpful to know just how balanced you already are. Start with a quiz.

1. How often do you feel physically healthy, energetic and well rested?

    A. Almost every day

    B. About 50 per cent of the time

    C. Rarely

2. How often do you experience the gamut of emotions: sadness, guilt, fear, joy, love and excitement?

    A. Every week

    B. Every month

    C. I can't remember the last time I felt some of those emotions

3. How often do you express your emotions to other people?

    A. Only when I think it's appropriate

    B. Only when the emotions are strong

    C. All the time

4. How often do you feel physically or emotionally numb after an activity, such as watching television, exercising, working, browsing the Internet or reading a book?

    A. Hardly ever

    B. Once in a while

    C. Every day

5. When you're sad, what are you most likely to do?

    A. I look for people to be with

    B. I spend time with others, if it is convenient

    C. I'd rather stay at home when I'm sad

6. How often do you find yourself struggling to do things that were easy in the past, such as home accounts or completing projects on time?

    A. Only when stress is very high

    B. Once in a while, but not regularly

    C. Regularly

7. Do your spouse, family, children and close friends support you?

    A. Every day

    B. Only when I really need them

    C. Not enough

8. How often do you ask friends and family for help?

    A. Daily or weekly

    B. Monthly

    C. Only when I'm desperate

9. Do you have hobbies?

    A. Yes, and I do them regularly

    B. One or two, which I tend to neglect

    C. There's no time for hobbies

Step 2: Identify Your Emotional Strengths and Weaknesses

If you answered all of the quiz questions honestly, you'll have a pretty good sense of how good a job you're doing staying balanced. If most of your answers were A, congratulations: you're on the right track. If most of the answers were B, you need to do a little work – and this chapter will help. If most of your answers were C, you're going to have to try harder to find your emotional centre.

Let's take a moment to look at each of the quiz questions to see how they measure emotional health and wellness.

Question 1. Negative emotions frequently result in physical symptoms. It's normal, for example, for people to feel tired or lethargic before they actually feel the underlying emotions, such as anger or rage. When you're feeling physically 'off' and there's no good reason for it, it's likely that your emotions are out of balance.

Question 2. Many people don't feel comfortable with certain emotions, such as anger or jealousy. These feelings still have to come out, however.

What people often do is transfer their energy to another emotion, such as guilt, says Dr Vivien D. Wolsk, a clinical psychologist. Soon guilt will overwhelm you because it's the only emotion you allow yourself to feel.

Question 3. Expressing emotions to others is important. This doesn't mean blowing your top at the slightest provocation, of course. Nor does it mean you should always say exactly what's on your mind.

In healthy human relations, emotions have to be expressed appropriately. Suppose, for example, that your husband says something that annoys you. If it's a minor issue, the healthy thing would be to respond to it as if it *is* a minor issue. If you overreact and go into a rage, your emotional balance is a little off, and your relationships are going to suffer.

Question 4. Most people have ways of coping with emotional troughs. A common strategy is to numb negative emotions, such as guilt or anger, by engaging in routine activities – watching television, working extra-long hours or even exercising long past the point at which you'd normally give up, says Dr Lisa Firestone, a clinical psychologist. When you're in this defensive state, you push away the people who can help you through rough times.

Question 5. Negative thoughts become more powerful when you're alone. And the more powerful the thoughts become, the less likely you are to seek out human contact. That's why therapists advise people who are feeling blue to spend time with others. Even if you decide not to talk about

A QUICK COURSE IN ANGER MANAGEMENT

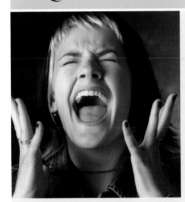

In the traditional view, women aren't supposed to get angry. It's not seen as a very 'feminine' way to behave. Maybe that's why women often cry instead of confronting the person who is bugging them. Why they're nice to people who have insulted them. Or, in some cases, why they blow their tops at the slightest provocation – because the pent-up anger just has to come out.

Whether you express your anger or suppress it, there are a number of ways to understand it and keep it at healthy levels.

Use anger as a signal. Rather than push anger away, work out what it's telling you. Say to yourself, 'I'm angry because something's wrong.' It will help you work out what needs fixing.

Think before you act. Feeling the emotion isn't the same as acting on it. When you're boiling with rage, ask yourself if this is the time and place to express it. You may want to go to a private place to vent it. Or take a long walk to think things over.

Confront the source. There's nothing wrong with confronting people who have made you angry.

Wait until you cool off. Then explain how their words or actions made you feel.

As long as you approach people calmly and with a genuine desire to work things out, they'll usually work with you to find a solution.

your problems, the simple human contact will boost your mind and even relieve mild depression.

Question 6. When you're emotionally out of balance, concentration and focus diminish. Tasks that should be easy become increasingly difficult and fatiguing.

Question 7. Women are responsible for a lot these days. They keep the house clean. Take care of children. Do the shopping. And all this is often on top of working outside the home. If you aren't getting a lot of support in your life, your emotions – and your health – are going to suffer.

Question 8. Women expect themselves to be able to handle everything. They haven't given themselves permission to ask for help.

Feeling uncomfortable with or overwhelmed by your workload is a red flag. Not only does it mean that your physical and emotional resilience is needlessly being sapped, but it also means that you're not taking responsibility for getting the help you need.

Question 9. Hobbies – such as collecting antiques, bird-watching or writing short stories – are a great way to incorporate downtime into your life. If you don't have a few hobbies that you enjoy, there's a good chance that you're spending too much time working, caring for others or generally assuming the burdens of the world.

Step 3: Keep a Journal

If you completed the quiz above, you have a pretty good sense of your emotional strengths and weaknesses. But that's just the beginning. Inside everyone are vast, subterranean networks of emotions. These emotions guide everything you do – and everything you think and feel. To find and maintain your emotional balance, it's essential to understand what's happening deep inside – and keeping a journal is a great place to start.

Studies have shown, for example, that people who write in journals, especially about the traumas in their lives, report feeling better about themselves. An increasing number of psychologists and psychiatrists have begun incorporating journal writing into their practices as a treatment for depression and anxiety disorders.

There are no formal rules for keeping a journal. In fact, the opposite is true – your personality and desire for creativity should be your guides. To get started:

Please your personality. Your journal can be leather-bound or made of recycled paper. It might have leopard-print designs or flower petals on the pages. It can be as simple as a spiral notebook. Everyone has different tastes – and this is your chance to indulge them.

Write as much or as little as you like. You don't have to write in a journal every day to achieve emotional balance. There isn't a prescribed number of words you should write. Keeping a journal is simply a tool, and it's up to you to decide how it works best for you.

On one day, for example, you might sit down to write – and realize that you don't have a lot to say, maybe only a sentence or two. That's fine. On another day, especially one with a lot of emotional challenges, you might find yourself writing page after page as you think about what

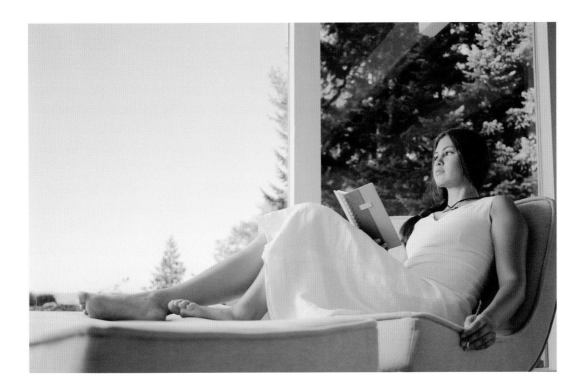

THREE THINGS I TELL EVERY FEMALE PATIENT

DR LISA FIRESTONE, a clinical psychologist, offers this advice for achieving emotional balance.

1 **ACCEPT ALL YOUR EMOTIONS, THE GOOD AND THE BAD.** Nobody chooses to feel a certain way, she says. Allow yourself to experience all of your feelings – including emotions typically labelled as negative, such as hostility and anger. Accept all your emotions, but understand that you choose your behaviour in response to them.

2 **MOVE BEYOND NEGATIVE THOUGHTS.** Everyone is self-critical at times. Pay attention to how you criticize yourself, and expose these thoughts to a more rational evaluation. Write them down or tell them to a friend. It is important to act in your own self-interest, not on negative self-critical thoughts.

3 **MAKE A LIST OF THE ACTIVITIES AND PEOPLE THAT BRING YOU JOY.** Then make a list of those that bring negative emotions. Look at the lists daily – and do everything you can to embrace the 'good' and avoid the 'bad'.

happened, what people said and how you reacted to everything.

Put it on your schedule. While it's best to avoid feeling obliged to write in a journal, it's often helpful to set aside certain times when you're going to write – first thing in the morning, for example, or right after dinner. If you miss an 'appointment', fine – but setting a schedule will make it easier to keep at it.

Date the pages. Some journals have the dates already on the pages. If yours doesn't, jot down the dates, including the year, you're writing. When you review your journal entries months or even years later, the dates will provide fascinating insights into what you were thinking or feeling at different stages of your life.

Write anything. Nearly everyone experiences writer's block when they first start keeping a journal. This might be the time to remind yourself that you're not trying to create literature but only trying to explore and understand your innermost feelings.

Still blocked? Close your eyes for a moment and imagine a stressful situation in your life. That's your topic: describe the situation in as few or as many words as you wish. Once you start, you'll probably find that the words will flow faster than you can write them down.

GETTING A GRIP ON GUILT

Guilt is what you feel when you've done something wrong or when you are toying with the idea of doing something wrong. It's what you feel when you call in sick at work to go shopping with a friend or fantasize about having an affair with an attractive man.

Women suffer from guilt to a disproportionate degree. It tends to come from feeling as though they can never do enough.

Women are brought up to be caretakers. As a result,

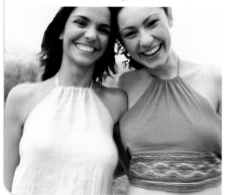

women focus on the needs of others. And when the other person isn't happy, for whatever reason, women can feel responsible, thinking either that they caused the unhappiness or that they must fix it or solve it – or both.

As with many emotions, guilt can easily take on a life of its own, especially if you don't talk about it.

One of the best ways to come to terms with guilt and to shrink it to a manageable size is to discuss your feelings with others, be it a friend, family member or therapist. The guilt that looms so large in your own mind will probably appear pretty small to others. Plus, your friends can share their own guilty secrets – which will put your own in perspective.

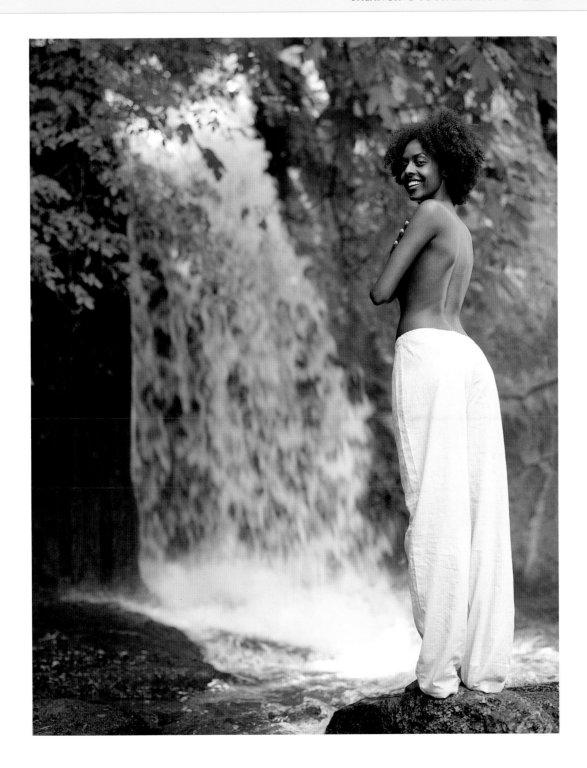

NEW HELP FOR BIPOLAR DISORDER

We all experience emotional ups and down – feelings of elation followed by troughs of sadness. For most of us, these emotional swings are triggered by real-life events: getting a pay rise at work or a compliment from a supervisor might be followed by finding out a roof needs repair. We deal with the emotions, then get on with our lives.

For people with bipolar disorder, however, the emotional swings come out of the blue – and the emotions may be so extreme that it's almost impossible for people to function normally without medical help, says Dr Francis Mark Mondimore, an assistant professor of psychiatry and behavioural science.

People with bipolar disorder – an estimated 1 per cent of the population have this condition – may go from being profoundly depressed to being wildly elated or manic. During the depressive stage, they may lose their appetite and have little interest in their normal activities. When they're manic, they almost seethe with energy. They can't keep up with their own thoughts, they have little need for sleep and they may have hallucinations.

A generation ago, there weren't a lot of treatments for bipolar disorder. Today, with a combination of medications and lifestyle changes – such as avoiding alcohol, getting enough sleep and exercising regularly – many people with this condition are able to keep it under control.

Step 4: Create Pockets of Tranquillity throughout the Day

In today's busy world, it's easy to get so caught up in responsibilities that you never set aside quiet times for yourself. Women who don't take time to recharge their physical and emotional batteries will experience ever-escalating amounts of stress and tension.

It may feel like an indulgence to give yourself some daily quiet time, but it's not: it's as important for good health as eating nutritious foods or getting a good night's sleep. Here are some places to start.

Take the time to breathe deeply. According to a proverb, 'He who half breathes, half lives'. It's extremely common for women to briefly hold their breath when they're under stress – or to breathe shallowly throughout the day. Apart from the fact that shallow breathing doesn't supply the body and brain with the necessary oxygen, doing so also makes it more difficult to experience emotions fully.

Aim to set aside a few minutes each day to do nothing but breathe deeply. Breathe in through your nose, and keep taking in air until your abdomen swells. Hold the breath for just a moment, then slowly exhale through your mouth. This technique, called diaphragmatic breathing, floods the tissues with oxygen and makes it possible to get in touch with your emotional life.

Find a safe place. When you're overwhelmed

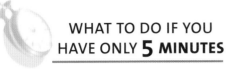

WHAT TO DO IF YOU HAVE ONLY **5 MINUTES**

Set aside at least 5 minutes every day to meditate and get away from the distractions of the world.

Find a quiet place. Close your eyes, or maybe look at the flame of a candle. Allow your thoughts to float through your mind, but don't dwell on them. If you practise this regularly, you'll find that you'll be able to disregard self-critical thoughts and self-destructive emotions, no matter where they come from or when they arrive.

with a negative emotion, it helps to have a private room or place to let the emotion out. When you're feeling sad or depressed at home, for example, you might want to retreat to the bathroom and have a long, hot shower. At work, people often retreat for a few moments to an empty office or even to their car. Giving yourself the time to escape makes it possible to release negative emotions as they accumulate, rather than allowing them to build throughout the day.

Move your body. Any kind of exercise – walking up and down stairs, raking a few leaves, jogging on the spot – increases your breathing rate and triggers the release of endorphins, chemicals in the brain that help regulate mood.

Don't wait until you're stressed to start moving. Women who do some aerobic exercise four or more times a week will feel physically and emotionally stronger.

Give yourself positive messages. Everyone deals with a lot of negativity throughout the day, and it's normal to feel overwhelmed and frustrated. Over time, however, these negative feelings can begin to take over – which is why it's so important to remind yourself of how strong and special you really are. It could end up being a self-fulfilling prophecy. When you're having a tough time, say to yourself, 'This is hard, but I have the strength to get through it.'

Step 5: Plan and Conquer

Emotional stress and negative emotions come in infinite forms, and they're often unpredictable. But that doesn't mean you can't anticipate them – and plan ahead to deal with them.

Imagine, for example, that you're knocked off course at work – by a difficult colleague or an unexpected problem with a supervisor. On top of the challenge of working things out, you'll also have to deal with the rush of adrenaline and other stress hormones that are released when the unexpected hits. Multiply this by a few dozen times a day, and it's easy to see why so many women feel embattled and exhausted.

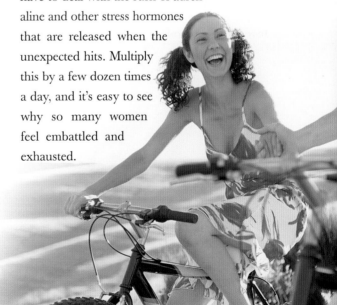

You can't anticipate all the specific problems you're likely to face every day, but you probably have a few emotional hot buttons in your life – things that consistently sap your strength and batter your emotions. If you take a few minutes to plan your coping strategies in advance, you'll be less likely to be taken by surprise – and you may be able to circumvent the problems alto-gether. Whatever the issue is, plan ahead for it by identifying at least three alternative ways to approach it.

When you plan your options, you'll be much more likely to achieve your goals – and you'll also feel stronger and more confident.

Plan your words. Confrontation is a fact of life. Hardly a day goes by when you don't have to

PUT THE BRAKES ON ANXIETY

Anxiety is a normal reaction to threatening situations. For some women, however, the emotion is so intense that they find it difficult to go about their lives. Doctors estimate that one in four people, a majority of them women, suffer from anxiety disorders at some time in their lives. These can result in panic attacks, a racing heart, nausea, chest pain, dizziness and other symptoms. The attacks can be so severe that people rush to casualty departments because they think they're having a heart attack. A fully-fledged anxiety disorder is a serious problem that requires medical attention. In most cases, however, women can control mild-to-moderate anxiety with a few simple steps.

Prepare yourself. Some things in life, like job interviews or talking to groups of people, are especially likely to provoke anticipation anxiety. One of the best ways to control it is to be as prepared as possible – by rehearsing a presentation in advance, for example, or by learning more about the company you're applying to.

Take some deep breaths. It's one of the best ways to reduce shortness of breath, a speeding heart or other anxiety symptoms.

Stop irrational thoughts. People often feel anxious because of what experts call 'catastrophic thinking' – the belief that the worst is about to happen.

When this is happening to you, imagine a red flashing light – and mentally shout 'Stop!' At the same time, distract yourself – by counting backwards from 100, for example. Your mind will find it difficult to return to the same troublesome thoughts.

deal with uncomfortable situations: a mail-order parcel that didn't arrive when it was supposed to; a friend who always says something inappropriate; a neighbour who plays loud music late at night. Just thinking about it gets you upset – and the tension keeps building.

Plan in advance what you'll say. You'll be less likely to respond in the heat of the moment (which can make a bad situation worse), and you'll also feel more confident about your ability to handle it.

You can't eliminate confrontation, but as long as you plan for it and give yourself choices, you'll always feel you are in charge – and that's an essential part of keeping your emotions in a healthy balance.

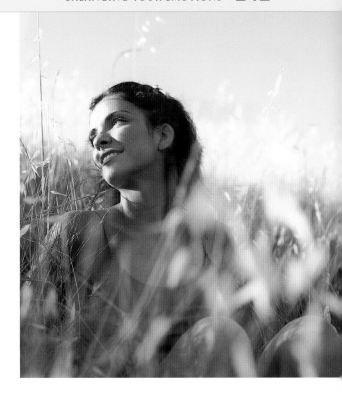

Step 6: Practise the Art of Acceptance

Women who achieve a sense of control in their lives are often amazed by how much stronger and confident they feel. Unfortunately, there are thousands of things we all wish we could control – everything from our dress size to the behaviour of teenagers – but can't. Sometimes you just have to accept that some things are out of your hands.

Allow yourself to feel your emotions. Emotions are going to come and go whether you want them to or not. Instead of pushing uncomfortable emotions away, be honest and allow yourself to feel them. Cry when you're sad. Don't automatically say 'fine' when someone asks how you're doing. Admit it when you're depressed or anxious.

People believe that if they feel an emotion, it will take over. But being aroused emotionally can last only so long. The sooner you allow yourself to feel an emotion, the sooner it will go on its way.

Be good to yourself. And say it with words. Every morning, look in the mirror and say something positive: 'I appreciate you' or 'I love you'. Saying things out loud helps them become real.

Remember the anchors in your life. When things feel like they're spinning out of control, take an inventory of all the things that you know are solid and reliable: your child is safe on the bus; your car will get you to work on time; your computer will turn on and work. When you realize how much in your life is dependable, you'll have more trust in your ability to work through life's problems.

Healthy Sex at Any Age

Sex therapists say that most women – whether they're young or old, single or married – have one thing in common: they want to be more in touch with their sexuality.

Sex helps women feel intimacy. Intimacy creates passion, and passion is sexually satisfying.

Sex also helps women feel more feminine, more attractive and closer to their partners.

For many women, living without an intimate sexual relationship is like living without chocolate or their favourite meal.

Low energy, stress, menopausal discomfort and side effects from medications are just a few of the factors that may get in the way of good sex – but they don't have to. Here's a three-step plan that will help keep your passion at healthy and satisfying levels.

Step 1: Accept Your Sexuality

Some women were brought up to think of sex as something 'forbidden' or improper. Some feel that it's inappropriate for a woman to express her full range of sexual desires – or even to admit them to herself. These and other emotional barriers may prevent women from fully exploring – and enjoying – their sexuality.

Open your mind to possibilities. Sexuality is a natural part of who you are. You may choose how much or how little sex you have, but the feelings will always be there. Many people aren't entirely comfortable with their sexuality. One solution is to browse your favourite bookshop or online catalogue. There are literally hundreds (if

DRUG 'COCKTAILS' ARE THE CLOSEST THING TO A CURE

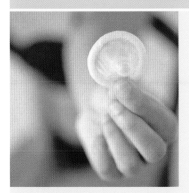

It's hard to imagine that until about 20 years ago, no one had ever heard of AIDS. Although scientists first identified the human immunodeficiency virus (HIV, the virus that causes AIDS) in 1959, it wasn't until the late 1970s that it made its appearance. Today an estimated 42 million people worldwide have HIV/AIDS.

People continue to think of AIDS as a 'male' disease, but the rate of infection in women has increased steadily.

Most women get the virus from having sex with men who are infected or from injecting drugs with a contaminated syringe. Women who have other sexually transmitted diseases have a higher risk of being infected with the AIDS virus.

HIV can survive in the body for years without causing symptoms. In the early stages, the only way for a woman to know she's been exposed to the virus is to have a blood test.

Scientists have made tremendous progress in understanding the AIDS virus, but there still isn't a cure. However, it's often possible to dramatically reduce levels of the virus in the body by giving people a combination of antiviral drugs. There are many medications to choose from, so when one combination doesn't work, another probably will.

Until doctors find a way to beat the virus, the best strategy by far is prevention. For women who aren't in long-term, committed relationships, this means always using a condom during sex. Sex with a condom isn't as spontaneous as some women would like, but it's among the best ways to stay healthy and infection-free.

DEALING WITH HERPES

When a woman is first diagnosed with herpes, she'll probably assume two things: that she'll suffer from frequent outbreaks and that her current partner hasn't been faithful.

Neither is necessarily true. Although there isn't a cure for herpes, many women can live most of their lives free of outbreaks.

And it's not uncommon for men and women to unknowingly harbour the virus for years or even decades without having symptoms.

The herpes virus often lives silently in the mouth or genitals. When an outbreak starts, a woman may experience itching or burning, pain in the legs or buttocks, or a feeling of pressure in the abdomen. After a few days, she may develop small, painful sores.

The first outbreak usually lasts for 2 to 3 weeks, but future episodes tend to be less severe. However, the virus is highly contagious during the active phase.

Here are a few ways to ease the discomfort.

- **The prescription drug acyclovir (Zovirax)** can reduce the discomfort of outbreaks and shorten their duration. A prescription drug called famciclovir (Famvir) also treats herpes outbreaks, and may help prevent future attacks.
- **Try aspirin**. Taking 125 milligrams of aspirin at the first sign of cold sores (caused by the herpes virus) may speed their healing time.
- **Take soothing baths.** Or gently dab the sores with a warm, moist towel. Applying moist heat is one of the best ways to reduce irritation.

not thousands) of informative books that explore all aspects of female sexuality. You'll discover many emotional and physical possibilities that you may want to explore for yourself.

Love your body. Research has shown that body perceptions, positive as well as negative, strongly affect sexual satisfaction.

Few women are completely satisfied with their bodies – but don't let this hold you back. When you're with your partner, focus on the parts of your body that you feel good about. It might be your soft skin or delicate hands, or the gentle curve of your neck. When you think about the things that please you most, you'll feel more attractive, and feeling attractive will make you more confident and assured.

Conquer old memories. Negative feelings about sex are often caused by early experiences. For some women, it was sexual abuse; for others it was the outcome of having sex before they were fully ready. As a result, they see sex more as a service than as a means to self-fulfillment.

One way to overcome these feelings is to let your partner know that you want more control in the bedroom. This might mean that you'll be the one to initiate sex, and you'll also take charge of setting the pace. Limit touch to only what is comfortable for you. As you gain a greater sense of control, your enjoyment will also increase.

Step 2: Keep Your Body Healthy

It's hardly a coincidence that the line 'Not tonight, I have a headache' has become a catch-all cliché for avoiding sex. If you don't feel good physically, you aren't going to want to have sex – and you probably won't enjoy it very much when you do.

How do you maintain or improve your 'sexual fitness'? By doing the things that promote your health overall.

Eat a healthy diet. Apart from preventing illnesses and improving energy, a diet that's high in essential nutrients and low in fat will make you feel better – and maybe sexier – overall.

Stay physically active. Regular exercise will relieve stress, improve your mood and help you feel great about your body. When researchers looked at women aged 50 years and older, they found that those with the highest levels of physical fitness were also the ones who enjoyed intimacy more often.

Protect yourself. Nothing dampens ardour faster than the thought of sexually transmitted diseases. Your best move: always use a latex condom, whether or not you use other forms of birth control.

If you're in a long-term, committed relationship, of course, condoms probably aren't necessary unless you're using them for birth control or if one of you already has a chronic condition, such as herpes, that is transmitted through sexual contact.

Step 3: Give Nature a Helping Hand

Lack of desire is the most common sexual problem for women. This may be caused by relationship issues, but it can also result from physical changes or underlying health problems.

THREE THINGS I TELL EVERY FEMALE PATIENT

DR MICHAEL PLAUT, is an associate professor of psychiatry. Here's what he advises women who want to explore and renew their sexuality.

1

ALLOW INTIMACY TO HAPPEN. It's easy to get so caught up in life's responsibilities – overdue bills, looming deadlines, problems with the children – that you never really let yourself go. During intimate moments, try to focus entirely on the moment at hand. Deal with the responsibilities later.

2

COMMUNICATE WITH YOUR PARTNER. Men aren't mind readers. The only way your mate will know what pleases you – and what you don't like – is if you're honest and forthright about your preferences.

3

BE OPEN TO NEW THINGS. The sex that you enjoyed when you were 20 may not be what you enjoy today. Men and women are constantly changing, and there's no reason for sex and intimacy to stay the same.

When women approach menopause, the body's levels of oestrogen begin to decline. This can result in vaginal dryness and more irritation. It can also result in hot flushes, insomnia or other physical factors that can lower libido.

Start with lubrication. The vagina naturally produces less lubrication as menopause approaches; women who take low-dose birth control pills also may be too dry for comfort. Don't let this slow you down. Pharmacies stock a variety of water-based lubricants, which are safe and comfortable to use.

Look into side effects. A number of medications – including some antidepressants, birth control pills and drugs for controlling blood pressure – may inhibit sex drive in some women. If you've noticed a dip in your libido, ask your doctor if switching to a different prescription would be helpful.

Ask about hormone tests. If your thyroid gland is underactive, you may have decreased levels of androgens, hormones that fuel the sex drive. Conversely, high levels of prolactin, a female hormone, also can cause libido to diminish. Your doctor can check hormone levels with a simple blood test – and if they're lower (or higher) than they should be, you may need medication to restore the proper balance.

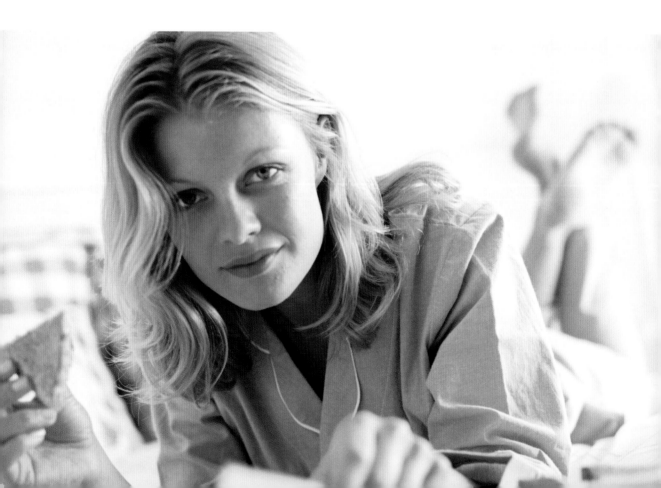

THE PILL VERSUS LIBIDO

When researchers from the Kinsey Institute for Research in Sex, Gender and Reproduction followed 79 women who took birth control pills for a year, they found a life-altering side effect that women and their doctors usually don't mention:

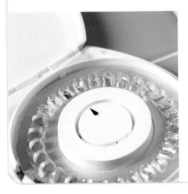

lowered libido and less sex. 'There's currently no way to predict which women will experience adverse sexual or emotional side effects or which pills are more likely to cause them,' says Dr Stephanie Sanders, associate director of the institute. 'The important message is this: if you like the convenience and reliability of oral contraceptives, you can usually work with your doctor to find a pill that's right for you.'

Here's how to preserve your sex life without discontinuing the Pill.

Discuss your symptoms with your doctor. Research shows that health professionals rarely discuss the emotional and sexual side effects of the Pill with their patients. Speak up.

Don't skip a dose. In addition to the obvious – an unplanned pregnancy – missed doses or irregular timing may cause hormonal fluctuations that could dampen your mood and sex drive.

Consider a change. There are many varieties of birth control pills. If one pill causes side effects, try another with a different type or amount of progestin.

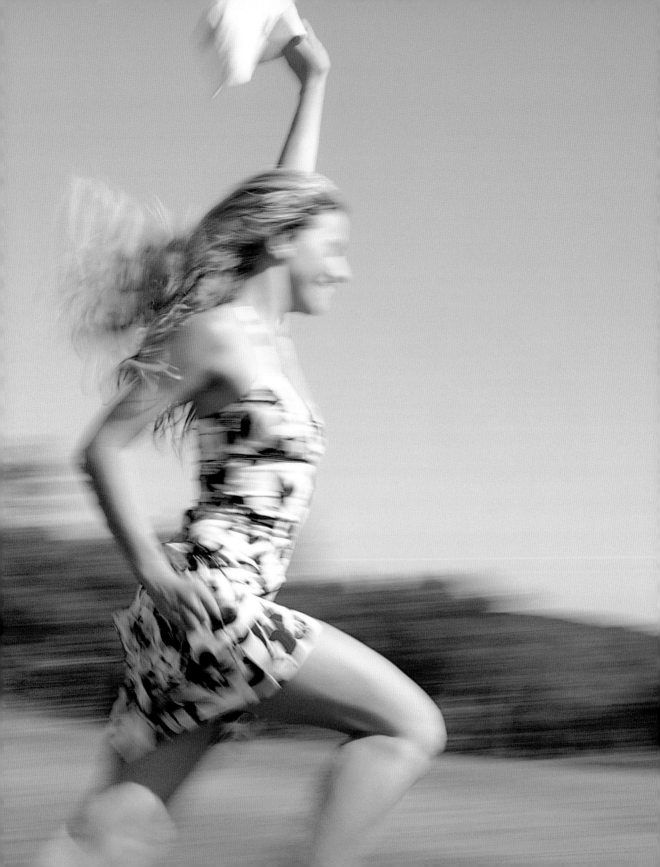

PART 3

Hormonal wellness: the best-ever life-stage strategies

CHAPTER

12

PMS and Menstrual Discomforts

Each month during your reproductive years, a flurry of activity takes place within and around your reproductive organs. A single egg passes from an ovary to a fallopian tube, where it lies in wait for sperm.

While the egg waits, the ovary releases oestrogen and, a bit later, progesterone, in order to create a nourishing and protective nest in the lining of the uterus.

Some say a woman peaks at this premenstrual time of the month – that is, she is not only physically 'ripe' but also emotionally and intellectually at her best.

Should the egg remain unfertilized, the uterine lining begins its monthly regenerative ritual by trickling out blood vessel–constricting substances called prostaglandins. The chemicals stimulate contractions that release the uterine lining – and trigger cramps that may start as early as a week before the period begins and continue until menstruation is done.

Because prostaglandins have inflammatory and pain-causing effects, many women also experience a range of unpleasant symptoms, such as a touch of nausea, bloating, headaches, diarrhoea or breast tenderness.

What's Normal and What's Not

The cramps, fluid retention and occasional moodiness that many women experience before and during their periods are nothing more than signs that their reproductive systems are following their normal, healthy patterns, says gynaecologist Dr Ronald Young.

But there may be other changes that aren't so healthy. Severe menstrual pain, called dysmenorrhoea, for example, warrants a checkup with your doctor because it could be a sign of endometriosis, uterine fibroids or pelvic inflammatory disease.

Emotional changes can be just as telling. A little moodiness is one thing, but the onset of menstruation shouldn't leave you feeling morose or out of control. Severe emotional swings are often signs of physical problems, including diabetes and thyroid disorders.

More than 150 physical and emotional changes have been linked to the menstrual cycle. When women are otherwise healthy, menstrual-related changes in their physical or emotional health are often caused by lifestyle factors, such as stress, nutritional deficiencies or a lack of sleep, says Dr George J. Kallins, a gynaecologist.

Because the menstrual cycle can trigger such a wide range of signs and symptoms, there is no cure-all. However, doctors have identified more than 300 treatment options for menstrual or pre-menstrual discomfort. It's worth being optimistic because you're sure to find some simple remedies that will work for you.

Home Remedies

 Sometimes even small changes can have profound effects on the way you feel. Women have always treated **PMS** and menstrual discomfort with home remedies – simple, time-tested strategies that can make a difference. Here are some things you may want to try.

Take ibuprofen straight away. Ibuprofen blocks the body's production of pain-causing prostaglandins – and it's much less likely than other painkillers to cause side effects.

If you start taking ibuprofen at the first sign of symptoms, you'll have protective levels of the medication in the bloodstream, which will prevent the discomfort from getting worse later on, says gynaecologist Dr Melvin V. Gerbie.

He advises taking 400 milligrams of ibuprofen three times daily. Start taking it 2 days before your period, and keep taking it until the time in your cycle when the cramps usually stop – usually about the second day after menstruation begins.

Water down bloating. Fluid retention caused by high hormone levels can cause uncomfortable swelling in the abdomen, breasts and ankles. It sounds paradoxical to drink a lot of water when you feel like a sponge, but water acts as a diuretic and removes excess fluid from the body. The advice is to drink at least eight large glasses of water daily before and during your period.

Avoid cigarette smoke. Research has shown that even second-hand smoke can make premenstrual discomfort worse. In one study, Chinese researchers looked at 165 female non-smokers, all newlyweds. None of the women had a history of menstrual discomfort. In the months after marriage (and their exposure to second-hand smoke by household members), there was a significant

when to see a doctor

If you're experiencing so much discomfort before or during your period that you can't function normally: make an appointment to see your doctor. Mild menstrual discomfort may be normal, but if it's interfering with your life, there's probably an underlying problem that needs to be addressed.

If you've been having depression, anxiety or irritability for more than 3 months, or if the feelings aren't limited to the 7 to 10 days before your period: you could be confusing clinical depression with PMS. Make an appointment to see a psychologist or psychiatrist, or discuss it with your doctor.

If you're having cramps as well as irregular or heavy bleeding, or if the blood is coming out in clots: you could have physical problems that need looking into.

increase in premenstrual lower-back pain and abdominal discomfort.

Nutritional Treatments

Oestrogen regulates the body's metabolism of a variety of nutrients, and it also affects the body's ability to absorb them. New evidence suggests that levels of calcium, vitamin D, iron and other key nutrients may rise and fall in synchrony with oestrogen fluctuations. Some researchers believe that short-term nutritional deficiencies are responsible for some of the premenstrual symptoms that have perplexed doctors for decades.

More than 10 major studies, for example, have shown that supplementing the diet with calcium or vitamin B_6 can relieve menstrual or premenstrual symptoms in women who usually don't get adequate amounts of these nutrients.

Supplements can only do so much, of course. Every woman should eat a healthy diet and maintain adequate levels of vitamins and minerals throughout the month, not just before and during the menstrual period.

'Don't think about getting enough fresh fruit and vegetables – and avoiding processed foods – only when your symptoms hit,' says Dr James G. Penland, a research psychologist and PMS researcher. As extra insurance against PMS discomfort, however, it's fine to use supplements containing no more than the daily recommended intakes.

Get enough magnesium and vitamin B_6. 'One of the reasons that these two nutrients are so highly recommended for PMS is that they help assure a healthy supply of the mood-regulating brain chemicals serotonin and dopamine,' says Dr Kallins. Research suggests that these chemicals, called neurotransmitters, also play a role in easing or preventing physical symptoms, including bloating, headaches, acne and cramps.

You can get a lot of magnesium and vitamin B_6 from figs, raisins, sweetcorn and bananas.

The B vitamins work together, which means that supplemental B_6 won't be helpful unless you also have adequate amounts of the other B vitamins. So it's a good idea to take a multivitamin or a B-complex supplement, he says.

Ease breast pain with a nutritional combination. If your breasts get tender as your period approaches, you might want to try a remedy suggested by Dr Mary Jane Minkin, clinical professor of obstetrics and gynaecology at Yale University School of Medicine.

Take 1,000 milligrams of evening primrose oil, 400 to 800 IU of vitamin E and no more than 10 milligrams of vitamin B_6 daily. This supplement combination reduces the pain and inflammation that are triggered by surges in prostaglandins during the menstrual cycle.

Focus on the 'top four' proteins. Many of the foods that Westerners depend on for protein – mainly meat and dairy foods – are also high in fat, which has been linked to menstrual cramps. Better sources of protein include fish, soya foods, egg whites and pulses.

These foods provide more than just protein. Soya foods and pulses are rich in phyto-oestrogens, plant-based chemicals similar to the

WHEN BAD THINGS HAPPEN TO HEALTHY WOMEN

Her Monthly Discomfort Led to a New Life

When Charis Lindrooth was a schoolteacher, she found that any stress and disappointments that she felt during the month would climax in the days before her menstrual period.

'I'd feel fine the rest of the month, and then, a few days before my period, I'd habitually dwell on everything so much that I'd make myself physically sick,' says Charis. 'When depression set in really hard, it sent me off on a crazy sugar binge.'

She finally found the discipline to stop eating sweets – and it made a remarkable difference in how she felt.

She also consulted a herbalist, who gave her black cohosh and black haw for her moodiness, and ginger and cardamom for her digestive problems.

'I also started on chamomile and lemon balm tea, which really helped resolve my anxiety,' she says. 'After taking these herbs for a month, it felt like suddenly something was really healed inside me.'

Charis was so inspired by the changes that she decided to study nutrition and body work. Eventually she left her job as a teacher and went on to become a chiropractor – and she's getting ready to complete a degree in herbal medicine.

'I sometimes tell people that the call to my vocation came through my uterus,' she laughs.

---

oestrogen that women produce naturally. Fish is rich in omega-3 fatty acids, which help regulate mood, and egg whites provide an abundance of protein with virtually no fat.

Don't give in to cravings for sugary food. Many women crave chocolate, cakes and other sweet foods before and during their periods. Indulging in these foods causes a rapid rise in blood sugar, which in turn can cause your energy and mood to crash. Highly processed carbohydrates, such as crisps and fizzy drinks, aren't much better because they supply a lot of calories and not a lot in the way of important nutrients. If you fill up on 'empty' calories, you may find that you're not getting enough important nutrients to prevent menstrual discomfort.

It's fine to give in to cravings on occasion, but only if your diet consists mainly of fresh fruit and vegetables, whole grains and other nutritious foods. The fibre in a plant-based diet is especially helpful because it helps remove excess oestrogen from the body, which will go a long way towards reducing menstrual and premenstrual discomfort.

Take advantage of healing oils. We mentioned earlier that chemicals called prostaglandins are responsible for some of the pain and discomfort that occur before and during your period. But there are actually several types of prostaglandins, including some that inhibit pain and inflammation. Flaxseed (linseed), hemp and borage oils, available in health food stores, stimulate the body's production of 'good' prostaglandins.

Adding these oils to your diet may inhibit cramps, bloating and breast tenderness. These oils aren't used for cooking, but you can add them to salads or other foods. Try to get a total of 3 teaspoons of one or more of these oils daily all month.

Alternative Therapies

Most women experience some degree of premenstrual stress. As it turns out, stress is not only a symptom of PMS but also a cause of it.

When we experience stress, the adrenal glands take progesterone and make cortisol, a stress hormone, out of it. This results in low levels of progesterone – and low progesterone is thought to be a primary cause of menstrual cramps and PMS symptoms.

To reduce your risk of suffering from stress-related PMS, try to develop and practise stress reduction strategies every day.

Each woman has a different approach to reducing stress. Some of the most helpful are meditation, taking hot lavender-scented baths and getting at least 8 hours of sleep every night. Other helpful strategies include the following:

Press away symptoms. For centuries, Asian healers have practised reflexology, a technique in which one 'adjusts' the body's internal organs by pressing certain points on the feet, hands and ears. In one study, women with PMS underwent foot, hand and ear reflexology sessions in which

THREE THINGS I TELL EVERY FEMALE PATIENT

DR GEORGE J. KALLINS, a gynaecologist, offers the following tips for controlling PMS and menstrual discomfort.

1

EXERCISE OFTEN. 'I see in my patients that those who exercise regularly experience fewer menstrual symptoms than those who don't,' says Dr Kallins. Natural chemicals called endorphins are released during exercise. Known as 'feel good' chemicals, endorphins can help ease cramps, breast tenderness and other types of menstrual discomfort.

For the best endorphin 'rush', Dr Kallins advises women to focus on aerobic exercises, such as fast walking, bicycling or swimming. Try to exercise for 20 to 30 minutes at least four times a week.

2

DON'T TAKE ANTIDEPRESSANTS UNLESS YOU'VE TRIED CALCIUM FIRST. Scientific studies have shown that calcium supplements – about 1,200 milligrams daily – can reverse menstrual-related mood swings, depression and anger. The mineral also reduces the discomfort of cramps and headaches.

3

LIMIT INDULGENCES. Women who eat a lot of sweets or fast food, or who consume caffeine or alcohol regularly, tend to have more menstrual and premenstrual discomfort than those who eat a healthier diet. 'Don't think of it as depriving yourself,' Dr Kallins advises. 'Think of it as a gift you're giving yourself to feel more balanced on every level.'

practitioners manipulated the trigger points that correspond to the uterus and ovaries; other women in the study were given 'sham' treatments at inappropriate trigger points. The women who received the real treatment had a significant reduction in symptoms, says Dr Terry Oleson, expert in behavioural medicine.

To find a professional reflexologist in your area, go to the Association of Reflexologists' website at www.aor.org.uk, Reflexology Association of Australia at www.reflexology.org.au, or Reflexology New Zealand at www.reflexology.org.nz.

Practise progressive relaxation. An easy way to relax and let go of tension is to tense and then relax each muscle in your body. The technique, known as progressive relaxation, is simple. While you're lying down, contract the muscles in your feet. Hold the tension for a moment, then relax. Then move up to the calves . . . the knees . . . the thighs . . . and onwards up to your head. It takes about 15 to 20 minutes to work through the whole body.

At the end of each session, you'll find that your levels of physical and emotional tension will be substantially reduced.

Imagine a beautiful light. Another way to practise progressive relaxation is to lie down and visualize a golden-white light running down like a waterfall, says Dr Oleson. Imagine that the light is pouring through your head, then through your face, the back of your head and your neck. Gradually let it pass down through each region of the body until finally it runs out from your feet.

'Give yourself a good 15 minutes to settle your

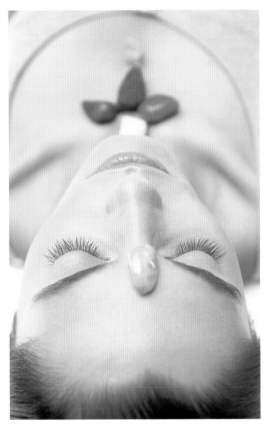

body down,' says Dr Oleson. 'Remind yourself that you deserve this gentle self-care every day.'

Combine exercise with meditation. Women who exercise tend to have less PMS or menstrual discomfort than those who are sedentary. To get even more benefits from exercise, Dr Kallins recommends making it 'mindful'. In other words, focus all your thoughts on your body – the stretching of your muscles, the slap of your feet on the mat or pavement, the breath going in and out of your lungs – and not on the things that are troubling you.

The idea, he explains, is to use your movements to put yourself into a kind of mild trance.

WHEN BAD THINGS HAPPEN TO HEALTHY WOMEN

A Meat-free Diet Banished Menstrual Pain

Barbara Swanson is an energetic and healthy woman, but for a long time she had such unbearable menstrual cramps that she routinely missed 2 days of work a month.

'When my period hit, I couldn't do anything but lie uncomfortably on the sofa in front of the television,' says Barbara. 'I had to take a lot of over-the-counter painkillers, which only seemed to make me sleepy.'

In 1997, Barbara was asked to participate in a university study that was looking at the link between vegan (meat- and dairy-free) diets and pain-free periods. She volunteered – and several cooking classes, a restocked pantry and two menstrual cycles later, her cramps were markedly reduced, she could function at work, and she was up off the sofa and jogging.

Barbara has stuck with the vegan diet ever since. 'I have some great cookbooks that I use for making simple dinners,' she says. For desserts, she enjoys soya ice cream and soya yoghurt, and she has even found vegan versions of fast foods, like burgers and hot dogs.

She was also pleased to get an additional bonus from the vegan diet: soon after giving up meat and dairy, she lost 2 kilograms (5 pounds) – and the weight never came back.

When your mind is relaxed, you'll be more in touch with your body and feelings – and that's the first step to managing them more effectively.

Prevent cramps with dang gui. A herb traditionally used by Asian healers, dang gui (or dong quai) appears to improve circulation, which helps remove pain-causing chemicals from the body. It also boosts levels of magnesium, iron and B vitamins. This herb, also known as Chinese angelica, works slowly and can be used safely long term. Use it for a month before judging its effects. Take three doses a day, with meals, in any of these forms: dried root, 1 gram boiled in water; tincture 1:5, 1 teaspoon; tincture 1:1, 20 drops; tableted root, one 500-milligram tablet. You can find angelica tincture and tablets at most health food shops. Avoid products made from the leaves or seeds – buy only products made from the root. And don't buy a product containing other herbs.

Use Agnus castus supplements. The fruit of the chaste tree, Agnus castus (vitex) is a popular folk remedy for PMS – and one study suggests that it may work. In a German study, women suffering from PMS were given 20 milligrams of dried Agnus castus extract daily. After taking the supplements for three menstrual cycles, more than half of the women reported a dramatic reduction in headaches, irritability and other symptoms of PMS.

Agnus castus is available in health food shops and some pharmacies. Try taking two 500-milligram tablets twice daily for a few months to see if it helps. (The seeds – also called the berries – are the most effective part.) If it does, you'll have to keep taking it: in the study, women who took Agnus castus and then gave it up had a return of symptoms within 3 months.

Try black cohosh. If you're approaching the menopause and your menstrual and premenstrual symptoms are getting worse, black cohosh, a herb, may help. It helps modulate the effects of a woman's hormones and may prevent the extreme 'swings' that cause discomfort. It seems to be especially helpful for women who are approaching the menopause, says Dr Kallins. If you're postmenopausal, check with your doctor before taking this herb, as it may cause bleeding. And don't use black cohosh if you're taking oestrogen in any form.

Take two 500-milligram dried root tablets three times a day. And don't take this herb if you're already on hormone replacement therapy.

Medical Options

Most women can control menstrual or premenstrual discomfort with changes in lifestyle or diet – but some can't. Since there are other causes of severe pain, consultation with a knowledgeable doctor is imperative before you start taking medication for pain. If your symptoms aren't getting better, here are some medical options that might make the difference.

Take high-dose ibuprofen. Available by prescription, ibuprofen tablets that contain 800 milligrams appear to be more effective than taking four over-the-counter pills containing 200 milligrams each.'It's a mystery why, but it seems to make a difference,' says Dr Gerbie.

Try contraceptive pills for 6 to 12 months. 'For some women, the Pill ends all the discomfort because it stops the hormone fluctuations that occur with ovulation – and it stops the lining of the uterus from building up so much,' says Dr Gerbie.

In many cases, taking the Pill for 6 months to a year will balance the hormones and relieve symptoms for good. Let your doctor know if you're using the Pill only for menstrual or premenstrual discomfort, and not for birth control, because you'll need a different dosage.

Consider antidepressants. Some women have a severe form of PMS known as premenstrual dysphoric disorder, which has the same force as major depression. A number of prescription antidepressants have been shown to reduce symptoms of this serious condition by more than 50 per cent.

A medication that seems to be especially helpful is fluoxetine (like Prozac). You'll probably be advised to take it during the time between ovulation and the onset of your period, or you will take it for the entire month.

CHAPTER

13

Contraception

Contraceptives are incredibly effective. When used correctly and consistently, all of the leading contraceptives have been shown to prevent pregnancy more than 99 per cent of the time.

So why is it that 50 per cent of unwanted pregnancies occur in those who use contraceptives?

In most cases, it's because people are using products that really aren't right for them, says Dr Mitchell Creinin, an associate professor of obstetrics, gynaecology and reproductive sciences. When contraception seems inconvenient, for example, or when it causes worrying side effects, people simply won't use it.

There are many different types of contraception. By knowing what's out there and choosing products or practices that suit your personality and lifestyle, you'll be able to get maximal protection without sacrificing comfort.

Every woman knows what's best for her, so don't let doctors or other health care advisors limit your options in advance, says Dr Creinin. 'Your doctor doesn't pay your bills, take care of your kids, deal with your in-laws, or have a relationship with your husband or partner,' he adds.

Don't put too much weight on hearsay, either. Just because your sister or mother or most of the women in your book group prefer a certain method does not mean that it's the right one for you. With so many options to choose from, don't accept anything less.

The Right Match for Every Woman

Start by asking yourself if you need protection from just unwanted pregnancy or if you also need protection from sexually transmitted infections (STIs). Some STIs cause infertility, some increase the risk of uterine cancer and still others can threaten your life. You have to recognize that they're out there, and if you have any doubt in your mind that your partner has undisclosed relationships, your safest bet is clearly the male or female condom.

If condoms aren't for you, other 'barrier' methods of birth control, such as a diaphragm combined with spermicide, work much better than nothing. On the other hand, contraceptive pills or other methods of hormonal contraception, along with intra-uterine contraceptives, may increase your risk for STIs because they alter the cervical mucus.

If you are in a mutually monogamous relationship and can use hormonal methods of birth control, you'll have to educate yourself about the pros and cons of using these products. We'll discuss this more below.

Another concern to keep in mind is whether you're planning to get pregnant in the future – and how soon you'll want it to happen. Fertility will usually return immediately upon stopping use of the Pill or a barrier method; even an intrauterine contraceptive or implant can be removed and assure a relatively quick return of fertility. However, the injection method of contraception known as Depo-Provera, which is given every 3 months, may delay pregnancy for 10 months after it's discontinued.

Your Guide to Contraceptive Options

As you review your options, here are some other questions to ask yourself.

- Do I have the discipline and personality for this method?

- Does this method take away from or add to the pleasure of sex?

- What are the short-term and long-term costs?

BARRIER METHODS

Barrier methods are among the oldest and safest form of birth control. A barrier contraceptive's mission is to prevent a sperm from ever meeting up with an egg. Barrier forms of contraception include the diaphragm, cervical cap, sponge and condom. The chemicals in spermicidal foams, jellies and films also act as barriers.

Perhaps the most exciting evolution in barrier contraception was the female condom (femidom), which has been available since 1992.

Many women like the female condom because it makes them feel in control. You place the closed end – an inner ring – up in the vagina as far as it will go, then guide your partner's penis into the outer ring. When used correctly, it can prevent pregnancy as effectively as the male condom, and it may be even more effective in preventing disease since it covers more of the female genitalia.

Another promising development is an improved version of the cervical cap, a thimble-shaped cone that is placed in the vagina and held in place with suction against the cervix. Softer and smoother silicone caps are replacing the original rubber ones, and you will also soon see caps with a one-way valve that lets out a woman's natural secretions but doesn't allow other secretions to get in. Older caps can be worn for 2 days, but the newer models can stay in place for 5 to 7 days. The increase in convenience makes them a very attractive option.

Barrier contraceptives haven't proved in studies to be quite as effective as the Pill or other hormonal methods, but as long as they're used in combination with spermicides or other barrier chemicals, they're nearly as good.

Here's some expert advice on using barrier contraception.

Get the proper fit. Diaphragms and caps come in different sizes. If yours feels uncomfortable or loose, ask your doctor for a refit. Always assume you will need a different size after childbirth, abortion, or putting on or losing 4.5 kilograms (10 pounds) or more, which changes the size of your cervix.

Select safe lubricants. Many barrier methods are designed to be used with spermicides or lubricants. Lubricants can increase pleasure. They also provide additional protection against pregnancy and may decrease the odds that a condom will break. Be sure to use commercial lubricants, such as K-Y Jelly and Astroglide. Don't use household products, such as Vaseline, cooking oil or whipped cream. They can cause condoms to break down, and they provide no spermicidal effects.

Get ready in advance. If you find that fussing with a contraceptive disrupts the moment, remember that a diaphragm can be inserted 6 hours in advance. The female condom can be inserted up to 8 hours in advance, and the cervical cap can be inserted 2 to 3 days before a romantic encounter.

Remember to remove them. More than a few women have left diaphragms or caps in place long past their allotted time, which can result in bladder or even blood infections. It may be worth writing a note to yourself and putting it on the bathroom mirror or somewhere else where you'll see it.

ORAL CONTRACEPTIVES

The Pill has been in use for more than 40 years, and it's getting safer all the time. That's because the dose of hormones in the Pill has been falling as practitioners have become wiser about deciding who can and cannot use it. In fact, doctors have found that contraceptive pills can even offer some health benefits that are unrelated to contraception.

There are two basic forms of oral contraceptives: the combination pill and the mini-pill (progestogen-only pill or POP). Combination pills contain synthetic oestrogen and progestogen, which are hormones similar to those already produced in a woman's ovaries. These pills prevent ovulation from taking place. Combination pills are available as monophasic pills, which provide oestrogen and progestogen at the same doses throughout the pill pack, and as biphasic and triphasic pills, which vary the amount of hormones over the course of the month.

Mini-pills contain progestogen only. They do not consistently stop ovulation. They do, however, thicken the mucus over the cervix to prevent sperm from entering the uterus. They also stop the uterine lining from growing, which makes it more difficult for the egg to get implanted. These pills are usually used by women who are concerned about the possible health risks – such as heart disease, stroke or breast cancer – of oestrogen-based pills.

It's important for women to weigh some of the risks of using contraceptive pills with some actual health benefits. For example, women who use contraceptive pills may have a reduced risk of colon, endometrial and uterine cancers. The oestrogen in the Pill also protects against the bone-thinning disease called osteoporosis, says Dr Joseph Goldzieher, a professor of obstetrics and gynaecology.

Because combination pills prevent ovulation, they can relieve or prevent menstrual pain, ovarian cysts or fibroids. They can also prevent the hot flushes, headaches, irregular bleeding, vaginal dryness and other symptoms that may occur in the years preceding menopause.

Contraceptive pills are very effective – but only if you remember to use them. Here are few ways to keep with the programme.

Pack your pills. Carry extras in a pill pack just in case you forget your morning dose. You can keep the pills in your purse, wallet or backpack, where you'll always have easy access to them.

Take them on a strict schedule. Progestogen-only pills prevent pregnancy by thickening the cervical mucus. This effect lasts only for 24 hours, so it's important to take the pills at the same time every day. If you doubt your ability to stick to a regular schedule, you may want to choose another type of contraceptive.

LONG-ACTING HORMONAL METHODS

For many women, the nicest thing about long-acting hormonal methods of birth control is privacy. Nobody will find your pills, your partner won't feel an IUD string or the rim of a diaphragm and there's no messy spermicide, says Dr Robert Hatcher, a professor of gynaecology and obstetrics.

Depo-Provera has been available since 1992. The amount of hormones is higher than in other hormonal contraceptives, and it contains only progestogen, rather than a combination of oestrogen and progestogen. It may cause unpredictable menstrual spotting, and it's also been linked to weight gain and bone loss in some women.

However, if you're one of the women who can use Depo-Provera without side effects, consider yourself lucky: it's the most fuss-free contraceptive available, offering 3 months of protection with one injection.

Ask about needle-free options. Long-acting hormonal contraceptives are available in patch or implant forms (such as Norplant), but they are not popular. If you want the protection of

when to see a doctor

If you're taking the Pill or other hormone-based contraceptives and you experience chest pain, blurred vision or leg pain: call your doctor immediately. The symptoms could be caused by inflammation, a blood clot or even a stroke. Women who take the Pill have a slightly increased risk of developing these conditions, compared with women who don't use hormonal contraception, although the actual risk is still very small.

If you're developing acne or have unpredictable bleeding: these are common side effects of contraceptive hormones, and changing the dosage (or the medication) will probably resolve the problem.

If an intra-uterine device becomes visible: the device has fallen out of position, and you'll want to get it repositioned immediately to prevent damage to the uterus or intestine. Avoid sexual intercourse or use an alternative method (such as condoms) until you can talk to your doctor about other contraceptive options.

hormonal contraceptives but could do without the injections, ask your doctor if one of these products would be right for you.

INTRA-UTERINE DEVICES

There's a good reason why many women appreciate an intra-uterine contraceptive. Once it's inserted, it can be left alone for 5 years or more. It virtually stops monthly bleeding and cramps, and it's more effective than getting your tubes tied – and it's totally reversible. A recently approved product called Mirena contains a slow-release hormone called levonorgestrel, which mimics the effects of progesterone. This intra-uterine contraceptive is more than 99 per cent effective.

'The hormone is released locally in the uterus,' says Dr Creinin. 'The amount of hormone that gets into the rest of your body is only about 10 per cent of the amount that comes from taking birth control pills. This means that there's less potential for side effects.'

You can also use an intra-uterine contraceptive that contains no hormones. Instead, it contains a lot of copper, which sterilizes any sperm it encounters. In fact, it has the unique ability to prevent pregnancy even if it's inserted 5 to 7 days after unprotected sex. If you're in a fix, ask your doctor to insert one immediately. If you like it, you can leave it in for 5 to 8 years. The copper intra-uterine contraceptive is more than 99 per cent effective. The one drawback is that it may increase menstrual bleeding or cramping.

OTHER CONTRACEPTION OPTIONS

Tubal sterilization, a permanent procedure, is reserved only for those women who know that they don't want to have any (or any more) children. A small incision is made in the abdomen. The surgeon then seals the fallopian tubes, thereby creating a permanent roadblock on the egg–uterus highway.

Women who are most likely to regret getting their 'tubes tied' are those under the age of 25, those who have divorced and then remarried, and those who rushed into the procedure after pregnancy or an abortion.

Even if you already have children, don't discount the possibility that you may want to have more later on, especially if you happen to divorce and then remarry. Long-term, reversible methods, such as an intra-uterine contraceptive, or a vasectomy for the spouse of a woman in a mutually monogamous relationship, might be better for you.

Some women depend on the 'withdrawal method' for birth control, which can be a very

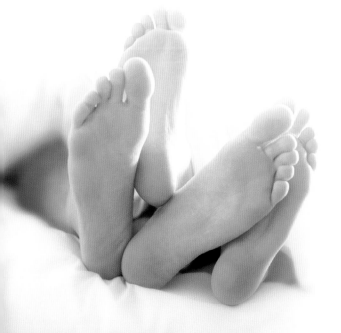

unreliable method. However, some women learn to practise the symptothermal method. It's a system of observing menstrual cycle patterns and abstaining from sex before and during ovulation. The more data you take using this method (such as body temperature, the appearance of vaginal mucus, self-cervical examinations and urine tests), the more effective it becomes.

It's a valuable educational tool for every woman to learn. It can also be quite moving to be so aware of your body's changes throughout the month.

EMERGENCY CONTRACEPTION

Emergency contraception is based on the reality that a woman, no matter how careful she tries to be, might find herself getting pregnant against her will. She might be forced to have sex; condoms can break; and a diaphragm can slip. And sometimes passion dissolves a firm 'no' into 'oh, yes'.

The first thing to know about emergency contraception pills (ECPs) or 'morning-after' pills is what they are not. They are not meant to be a regular contraceptive method. Nor are they used to terminate pregnancies. As with some other contraceptives, ECPs either prevent ovulation or alter the uterine lining to prevent the implantation of an egg. You can think of them as very strong, fast-acting birth control pills.

To be effective, the pills have to be taken according to strict guidelines. You might be told to take the first dose within 72 hours (the sooner the better) after unprotected sex, followed by another dose 12 hours later. However, for maximum effectiveness you may well be told to take both tablets together. The pills are unlikely to cause serious side effects, but some women may experience nausea, vomiting, abdominal cramps, headache, breast tenderness or dizziness.

You can get emergency contraception from your doctor or family planning clinic, or direct from the chemist or pharmacist.

Here are some additional emergency strategies to keep in mind.

Get checked for infection. If you had unplanned sex outside of a mutually monogamous relationship, you might be at risk for an STI. The symptoms don't always show up right away (or at all). The only way you'll know you're infected is to ask your doctor to give you an examination.

Go to the source. If you want information about emergency contraception, ring the Family Planning Association (now fpa) helpline on 0845 310 1334 (9 a.m.–7 p.m. Monday to Friday) or visit www.fpa.org.uk. Or, in Australia, call FPA Health on 1 300 658 886 or visit their website at www.fpahealth.org.au.

Get emergency pills in advance. 'The effectiveness of ECPs drops off every minute after unprotected sex, and then drops off very rapidly after 72 hours,' says Dr Goldzieher. Since your doctor may not be able to see you immediately or the pharmacy may be closed, you may want to get the pills in advance and keep them in a safe place.

14

Pregnancy

Every single day of your whole pregnancy, you are contributing to your child's well-being. You do so by what you eat, how you stay fit and relaxed, and how you practise prenatal care.

You're doing more than supporting a developing baby over 9 or 10 months. You're also growing as a woman and a mother-to-be, says Dr Deborah Issokson, a psychologist specializing in reproductive mental health.

'The most important advice I can give is not to rush through 40 weeks trying to get everything ready for the baby,' she says. 'Focus instead on your personal development. Pregnancy is an incredibly reflective time when your sense of being a woman, a wife or partner, and even an employee is evolving to a new level. Make the time and space for that natural shift, and you'll feel emotionally your best before, during and after pregnancy. Emotional well-being can also translate into physical well-being.'

Get the Best Support

Whether you are having your first child or your fourth, getting good prenatal education is one of the smartest parenting decisions you'll make.

Birth preparation (or antenatal) classes allow you to gain vital new information. Plus, you'll have the chance to talk about the experience with other pregnant women. The more you learn about the physical and emotional changes that other women undergo during pregnancy, the better prepared you'll be to cope with your own.

Government-funded classes are free, run by a health professional and usually held in hospitals or health centres. Groups can be quite big. Private classes are usually held in someone's home or at a community setting, and will be run by a teacher trained by the organization running the classes. There is normally a charge, which may be waived in certain cases. The biggest network of private antenatal classes in the UK is operated by the National Childbirth Trust (see their website at www.nctpregnancyandbabycare.com). In Australia, contact the Maternity Coalition and ask about their Choices for Childbirth programme (www.maternitycoalistion.org.au). Classes should prepare you, physically and emotionally, for anything that might come up. The class should offer instruction on a variety of relaxation and breathing techniques, as well as discussions and role playing for you and your partner.

Concerns for Older Mums and Higher-risk Pregnancies

Many women today are getting pregnant when they're in their thirties and forties, and for the most part the pregnancies are uneventful. 'Even women in their early fifties today are expected to have routine and normal pregnancies,' says Dr Ronald J. Wapner, a high-risk obstetrician and medical geneticist.

However, women who are over 35 do have a slightly increased risk for foetal chromosome abnormalities. There's also a higher risk if they've had children with a birth defect or a chromosome abnormality such as Down's syndrome, says Dr Wapner.

If you fit this profile, see a specialist in genetics to assess specific risks before you conceive. You'll also want to consider additional screenings once you get pregnant, such as the chorionic villus sampling (CVS) test at or after 10 weeks, or an amniocentesis procedure in your fourth month.

Here are some additional issues older women may face.

- **Diabetes.** The body produces anti-insulin hormones during pregnancy, which can result in a temporary condition called gestational diabetes. It can also aggravate pre-existing diabetes.

  Women who are 40 years or older have a 7 per cent chance of developing gestational diabetes, compared with 1.7 per cent for a woman in her twenties. To avoid the complications that can be caused by uncontrolled blood sugar – such as an over-sized baby – be sure to get dietary advice from a nutritionist or a perinatal specialist.

- **High blood pressure.** If you have hypertension, it's important to get it under control before you conceive, says Dr Wapner. Since your heart will be pumping more blood when you're pregnant, you may develop high blood pressure for the first time. You'll need extra rest to avoid a serious complication called pre-eclampsia, which can rob a foetus of blood-flow.

- **Premature or low-birth-weight babies.** Both are common among older mums because they're more likely to be carrying twins or triplets. There are also pre-term births because of maternal illness, such as high blood pressure. Uncontrolled blood

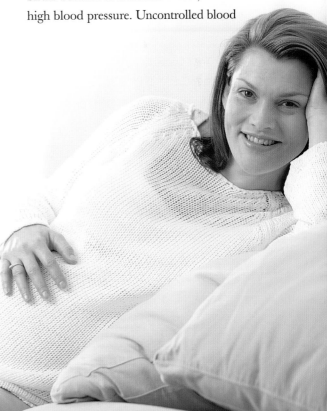

pressure or unhealthy lifestyle factors can also increase the risk of premature or low-birth-weight babies.

- **Repeated miscarriage.** Losing a baby may be your body's way of coping with genetic abnormalities. As a woman gets older, miscarriages occur more frequently because there are more genetic abnormalities of pregnancy. It may also be a sign of irregularly shaped reproductive organs, a hormone imbalance or an immune system disorder.

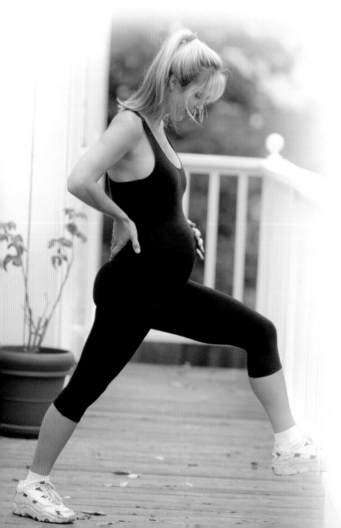

A Healthy Pregnancy

Regardless of your age when you conceive, the following advice will help ensure a safe and healthy pregnancy.

Take folic acid supplements. All women who are thinking about getting pregnant should take a minimum of 400 micrograms of folic acid daily. Folic acid helps prevent spinal cord defects.

Stay fit before and during pregnancy. Regular exercise can keep blood sugar under control, and women who are fit generally have lower blood pressure. In addition, getting in shape will improve your stamina to push out a baby. Check with your doctor first, but if you aren't currently exercising, you might want to start by walking. Start at an easy pace – so you don't break into a sweat – for 10 to 15 minutes at a time the first week. Add a few minutes each week as you feel comfortable, gradually working up to an hour most days, if possible. Stop walking and contact your doctor immediately if you become short of breath or have uterine cramping. And be sure to drink plenty of water before, during and after exercise to prevent dehydration and overheating.

Put on a healthy amount of weight. You should aim to put on 2.5 to 3.5 kilograms (5 to 7 pounds) in the first 13 weeks of pregnancy; 4.5 to 6.5 kilograms (10 to 14 pounds) in the second 13 weeks; and 4.5 to 6.5 kilograms (10 to 14 pounds) in the last trimester. Being too thin or overweight can complicate pregnancy, especially if you have gestational diabetes or high blood pressure.

Don't smoke, and avoid alcohol. Smoking and drinking can raise the risk of miscarriage, birth defects and low-birth-weight babies. Ideally, women should avoid alcohol and tobacco even before they conceive.

Eat nutritious foods. Every pregnant woman needs to do her best to get a nutritious diet. It should include lots of fruit and vegetables, whole grains and other healthy foods. You'll certainly want to avoid excessive amounts of sweets or highly refined (and nutritionally 'empty') foods.

Get enough rest. Women who are at risk for pre-eclampsia or other health problems will usually be advised by their doctors to curtail their working hours. But regardless of risks, listen to your body – and be prepared to slow down when you're feeling fatigued.

Feeling Well on Every Level

Between the time your future child is conceived and the time you deliver, your uterus will expand to 1,000 times its prepregnancy size. Your body will be producing 25 per cent more progesterone and 100 per cent more oestrogen. These tremendous physical changes can result in nausea, backache, headaches, digestive difficulties and fatigue – not to mention potentially overwhelming emotional ups and downs.

Women who mentally prepare themselves for motherhood generally feel better physically as well as emotionally.

'Women need to stay connected with their bodies and natural rhythms, with their partners, and with other women who want to talk about the birth and mothering experience,' says Dr Issokson. 'Things like journal writing, yoga, swimming, gardening, good self-care, connecting with other women and talking about what they envision for themselves as mothers are all activities that reflect where women are spiritually and physically when they are pregnant. If they ignore the reflective and spiritual aspects of pregnancy, then women often end up feeling disconnected from themselves – and they feel disconnected from their bodies as birth approaches.'

To get in harmony with your mind and body during this important time, here are a few worthwhile strategies.

Allow yourself to feel ambivalence. 'I don't think there's any way to go through a life-altering event such as childbearing without some internal conflict, even in the most planned and wanted pregnancy,' Dr Issokson says. It's normal and healthy for women to acknowledge their anticipated losses – like how much they're going to miss sleeping late on Sundays, or giving up a degree of sexual intimacy or the loss of freedom and spontaneity that comes with a child-free life. Admitting and coming to terms with these and other losses and changes will help a woman accept the entire experience of having a baby – the difficulties along with the joy.

Give yourself time to bond. When you're pregnant, set aside time to bond – not only with your spouse but also with your baby-to-be. Try a 'story time and music box' ritual every night. Here's how it works.

You and your husband take turns reading. It can be anything from children's books to football scores, as long as you are addressing your future child. Afterwards, play a music box on your stomach. As the foetus matures, it will respond with a flurry of activity when it recognizes these sounds. Later, as soon as your baby emerges from the womb, playing the music box will orient and comfort your newborn child.

Reduce nausea naturally. One study found that 90 per cent of pregnant women had less nausea when they took ginger. Fresh ginger tastes great when it's added to stir-fries, soups and spicy biscuits, and it's entirely safe during pregnancy.

Because nausea usually increases when the stomach is empty, it's important for women to eat frequent, small meals during pregnancy, says Dr Mary Lake Polan, professor and chairperson of the department of gynaecology and obstetrics at Stanford University.

Don't lose sleep because of back pain. 'During pregnancy, the tissues that support the spine and pelvis naturally get soft in order to allow the pelvis to open for delivery. This, along with the extra strain from her changing centre of gravity, strains a pregnant woman's back,' says Dr James Cable, a back injury specialist.

He advises pregnant women to sleep on their side with the knees slightly bent. Put one pillow between your legs and another beneath your abdomen for extra support.

Know when to consider therapy. 'Mental health services should be a routine part of everyone's prenatal care,' says Dr Issokson. 'Pregnancy and birth trigger a lot of issues for women. Some issues are old ones that have never been resolved or that have crept back up, and some issues are new. While not everyone needs therapy, a few sessions with a counsellor or therapist can create a wonderful opportunity for women to sort through these issues. For a woman who has a history of depression or anxiety, trauma, violence or eating disorders, a prenatal session with a therapist can help her evaluate her risk factors for postnatal difficulties, like postnatal depression,' she says.

Therapists can help with many different issues: the previous loss of a child, anxiety about birth or the sense of vulnerability that so many women experience. If you suffer depression after giving birth (postnatal depression), working with a therapist is among the wisest things you can do.

Increase communication with your partner. 'Discuss what you both think parenthood will ultimately be like, and what your fantasies are. Along with these ideal expectations, understand what you both perceive as your roles and responsibilities,' suggests Dr Issokson.

You might, for example, discuss who will be responsible for getting up in the middle of the night when the child cries. Or you might discuss the types of discipline you believe in or who will take days off from work when it's time to visit the doctor. If your relationship has problems, this is the time to seek couples counselling and commit to getting your relationship as a couple in good working order, adds Dr Issokson. 'Don't fall for any fantasies that a baby will make your marriage better. Babies add stress to every relationship. The stronger, healthier and more communicative a relationship is, the better it is able to handle the stress of new parenthood.'

15

Childbirth

No two births are exactly alike. Every woman creates in her mind the ideal situation and circumstances for giving birth. Things can always change, of course, sometimes at the last minute. Planning for childbirth is important, but so is maintaining a spirit of flexibility.

Conceiving a Birth Plan

Women use words like 'peaceful', 'powerful' or 'beautiful' to describe their birthing experiences, but there are also practical considerations: the kinds of support you get, which procedures you do or don't want, and the type of setting that you feel comfortable in.

Creating a birth plan will help you think through the decisions that will one day come together to create the optimal scenario. It's a way of clarifying your expectations and ensuring that everyone is working together to fulfil your needs.

To create a birth plan that will help make your childbirth dreams come true, here are some points to keep in mind.

Get information from a variety of sources. Read about the kinds of births that are offered in hospitals, at birthing centres or at home. Learn about the pros and cons of different medical interventions, from 'natural' vaginal births to Caesarean sections. Ask the mothers in your life to tell you their birth stories. Always discuss your birth plan with your midwife or doctor during your pregnancy, and be realistic about their response. If either is reluctant to accommodate your plan, you need to find out why and either revise the plan or look for a person who is comfortable with your wishes.

Look into Caesarian section rates. There are many situations when surgical delivery, known as Caesarean section, is essential. But if a hospital or clinic has a Caesarian section rate that approaches one in four births, it may be a sign of overuse of medical interventions, says Dr Mindy Smith, a professor in family practice.

Understand the pros and cons of medication. Epidural anaesthesia is highly effective at relieving discomfort in your pelvic area, but it reduces the amount of control a woman has during delivery – and it increases the odds that you'll need a Caesarian or a forceps delivery. Drugs that induce labour can decrease the anxiety of waiting, but may increase your need for pain relief, which carries some risk to the unborn child.

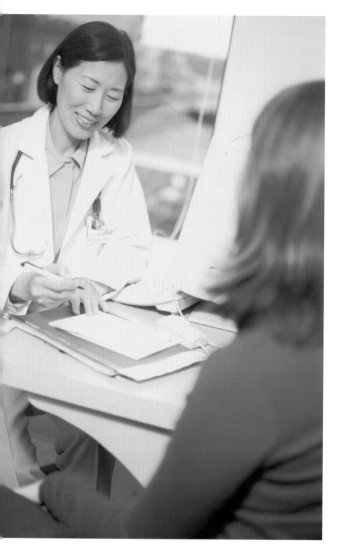

Many women want to avoid the use of drugs during childbirth, and that's fine. Just be sure to plan ahead. If you want to utilize acupressure to manage pain, or nipple stimulation to increase uterine contractions, consider making it part of your birth plan.

Decide about episiotomy. A surgical incision made in the area between the vagina and anus, episiotomy can be performed to make more room for the baby to pass. Some doctors feel that even though episiotomies may take several months to heal, it's a safer option than risking tissue tears, which sometimes occur during childbirth.

Other doctors, however, maintain that natural tears heal as easily as surgical incisions and are less likely to extend into the rectum. They also cite statistics that indicate that about 20 per cent of first-time mums can make it through childbirth without tearing. This soars to 80 per cent for subsequent births.

If you're adamant about not having an episiotomy, there are a number of non-surgical options, such as using a warm compress to soften the tissue prior to delivery or having a daily perineal (the area between the vagina and the anus) massage during the last 6 weeks of pregnancy. Perineal massage works best for first-time mothers, who are more likely to tear.

Women sometimes indicate in their birth plans that they want to try non-surgical measures first – but they'll opt for the incision if there's too much distress to them or their babies.

Discuss the birth plan with your doctor or midwife. Plan on doing this around the sixth or seventh month of pregnancy.

Create an easy-to-read outline. It's not uncommon for women to create birth plans that fill an entire journal. But when it's time for the birth, the doctor or midwife isn't going to have time to read all of your thoughts. To make things easy, condense the birth plan into a one- or two-page outline that can be read at a glance. Make duplicates so that everyone who will be present will have a copy.

Help During Labour

The early part of your labour typically lasts between 6 and 18 hours. You might experience painful, irregular contractions or regular, non-painful ones. The early phase doesn't result in cervical dilation, but it can hurt, keep you awake and seemingly go on for ever. At this time, you want your birth partner to be nearby, and you may feel better if you stay busy around the house, says Dr Mary Lake Polan, professor and chairperson of the department of gynaecology and obstetrics at Stanford University.

Following the early stage, you'll have approximately 4 to 8 hours of active labour. That's when the contractions increase in intensity and the baby makes its way down into the birth canal. Once you are fully dilated, expect to deliver in less than 6 hours – or in as little as 30 minutes.

Labour needs a lot of support, both physically and emotionally. Here's what the experts advise.

Fill your mind with positive images. Try to clear your mind of worry and all the clutter that you normally carry around. Try to visualize the baby coming through – and imagine how healthy the baby is.

Find out about birth balls. These air-filled physiotherapy balls are often used to help women feel more comfortable and to gain control, throughout their labour. Getting on your hands and knees and leaning over the ball helps reduce back pressure, while sitting on the ball opens the

when to see a doctor

When contractions settle into some sort of a pattern, it's time to ring the hospital, doctor or your midwife. Labour is about to begin.

When contractions noticeably increase in strength and occur about every 4 to 5 minutes for 60 seconds at time, and this pattern has continued for 30 to 60 minutes: you may be entering the final phase of labour, and you'll need professional assistance.

When your waters break: it's time to get to the hospital or birthing centre – or, if you're giving birth at home, to get the assistance of your midwife.

pelvis for babies who are having a more difficult time getting through.

Water down discomfort. Labouring in a pool of water can significantly reduce your pain. Immersion supports the mother's weight, reduces the opposition to gravity and reduces pressure on the abdomen. It also relaxes the pelvic floor muscles. In addition, labouring in water can increase the rate of dilation. If a birthing pool isn't available, you can use the shower while sitting on a birth ball.

Create a soothing environment. Take full advantage of relaxation aids, such as aromatherapy mists in a scent you find relaxing, your favourite music, soothing 'hot pads' made from rice-filled socks gently warmed in a microwave or simply your comfiest nightdress.

CHAPTER

16

Infertility

Women naturally have a drop in fertility starting around the age of 30, when there's a reduction in the quantity and quality of eggs. Research has shown that one out of seven women between 30 and 34 will have trouble conceiving. Between 35 and 39, the odds change to one in five, and by the time a woman reaches 40 to 45, they're one in four.

While 'infertile' has come to mean a delay or difficulty getting pregnant, it rarely means a woman is unable to conceive, says Dr Ken Gelman, a reproductive endocrinologist.

Lifestyle factors play a surprisingly large role in a woman's ability to conceive. Losing or putting on weight, giving up smoking or giving up alcohol, for example, can increase the chances of conception. When self-care isn't enough, medication or surgery can often make the difference.

For more difficult cases, assisted reproduction wonders such as in vitro fertilization and artificial insemination can make parents out of people who at one time would have been considered sterile.

How aggressively a woman chooses to treat infertility depends largely on how much cost – in terms of time, money, risk and emotion – she is willing to invest.

Regardless of the medical options, every woman who is trying to get pregnant needs to maintain a diet and lifestyle that will push the odds in her favour.

Lifestyle Strategies

Hit a hormone-safe weight. Fat cells in the body stimulate an over-abundance of oestrogen, which inhibits ovulation. Not enough fat, on the other hand, also inhibits oestrogen. 'Fertility is not supported by extremes at either end of the weight spectrum,' says Dr Gelman. 'A body mass index (BMI) between 20 and 27 seems to be the best range to foster fertility.' To calculate your BMI – and to take steps to achieve the appropriate weight – see chapter 5.

Exercise moderately. Women who exercise especially vigorously – by running marathons, for example – may experience delays or disruptions in ovulation. 'Limit yourself to 45 minutes of daily workouts, such as strength training, walking, cycling or aerobics,' says Dr Gelman.

Keep your environment pure. Limit your exposure as much as possible to photography chemicals, pesticides, solvents, dust from treated wood or heavy metals, such as mercury or lead. Environmental toxins have been linked to infertility in women and sperm abnormalities in men. If you or your spouse has to work with these or other toxins, wear a respirator or breathing mask, and protective gloves and clothing, and always ensure that there's adequate ventilation.

Don't smoke – and avoid second-hand smoke. It reduces the production of eggs as well as sperm.

Drink lightly. One study has shown that among women who consumed alcohol while trying to conceive, the probability of conception dropped more than 50 per cent when compared with women who abstained from alcohol.

Giving up alcohol is a good way to promote fertility. If you continue to drink, limit yourself to three drinks a week. On specific days when you're trying to conceive, avoid alcohol altogether.

Switch to decaffeinated coffee or tea. Studies have shown that beverages with caffeine can cause delays in conceiving, and they may increase the risk of early miscarriage.

Nutritional Treatments

Take prenatal supplements. They contain a number of conception-supporting nutrients, including magnesium, B vitamins, and vitamins C and E. In fact, the chemical name for vitamin E, tocopherol, means 'to bring forth offspring'. Supplement manufacturers don't make specific prenatal formulations for men, but there are a few key nutrients that can help boost a

---

THREE THINGS I TELL EVERY FEMALE PATIENT

DR ALICE DOMAR, director of the Mind/Body Medical Institute for Women's Health, gives this special advice to women who are trying to get pregnant.

1 **RALLY SUPPORT.** Infertile couples often feel isolated and alone. Ask your doctor to recommend a local support group. Or visit www.repromed.co.uk/infertility (the website of the Centre for Reproductive Medicine) for details of organizations supporting infertility patients throughout the UK. Australian Infertility Support Group (AISG) is a support group for people in Australia and New Zealand, who are dealing with infertility: www.nor.com.au/community/aisg.

2 **SET PARAMETERS BEFORE YOU START TREATMENT.** Infertility treatments are expensive and time-consuming, and sometimes risky to the health of the woman and the baby. Couples should set specific time (and cost) limits based on how far they want to go to achieve pregnancy. Knowing these limits in advance will help reduce long-term stress.

3 **TRY TO RELAX DEEPLY FOR AT LEAST 20 MINUTES A DAY.** Some of the most restorative techniques are prayer, guided-meditation tapes and deep abdominal breathing.

man's fertility. They include zinc (25 milligrams daily), copper (3 milligrams daily), L-carnitine (0.5–2 grams daily) and vitamin C (1,000 milligrams daily but don't continue this dose for more than a few weeks at a time, and diminish the level gradually to avoid rebound scurvy).

Men who want to be parents shouldn't take more than the recommended daily amount of vitamin E, Dr Gelman adds. It may lower sperm counts when it's combined with vitamin C. It's always best to check with your doctor before taking any new supplements.

Eat natural foods. To support overall health and fertility, not only do you need the full spectrum of required daily nutrients, but you also need good digestion to absorb them.

Experts advise women who are trying to conceive to eat three to six daily servings of digestion-friendly whole grains, such as brown rice, oats and barley, and nine daily servings of fresh fruit and vegetables. Make sure that you get 70 grams of protein daily. The protein can come from beans, nuts, eggs, lean meats or cheese. Buy organic foods whenever possible; it will reduce your exposure to hormone-disrupting chemicals that may be used by non-organic farms.

Mind-body Techniques

Women who are facing infertility often feel anxious, depressed and discouraged. Apart from disrupting their peace of mind, these and other negative emotions can also disrupt the way the body functions.

'Emotional distress can impair ovulation or cause the fallopian tubes and uterus to contract to the point where an egg is prevented from implanting,' says Dr Alice Domar, assistant professor of medicine at Harvard Medical School.

Studies have shown that women with a history of depression run nearly twice the risk of having trouble conceiving. As a result, Dr Domar and her colleagues at Harvard Medical School have developed a behaviour-oriented fertility treatment programme. On average, about 44 per cent of the women in the programme get pregnant – a success rate that's comparable to women who are in their reproductive prime.

The programme stresses stress management, esteem issues and positive thinking. Some of the most important things women can do include:

Try visualization. A woman might be angry because she had a miscarriage. She might resent her husband for failing to understand her despair,

when to see a doctor

Young couples who have not achieved pregnancy within a year should see their doctor: there's a good chance that either you or your partner has a physical problem that's going to make getting pregnant a challenge, says Dr Ken Gelman, a reproductive endocrinologist.

If your periods are painful or irregular, or if the bleeding is unusually light or heavy: these are common symptoms of endometriosis, uterine fibroids, pelvic inflammatory disease or polycystic ovary syndrome, all of which can lead to infertility.

and she'll probably be angry with the doctors who can't 'fix' the problem. The more frustration she feels, the more likely she is to have trouble conceiving.

Women need to release their negative emotions – not by venting, which can make them feel worse, but by filling their minds with positive thoughts and images.

Here's an example of how it works. Take a few minutes every day to imagine that a magic carpet has arrived to take you away from your troubles. As you sail through the clouds above mountaintops, mentally place the day's disappointments inside a stone – then gleefully hurl the stone away from you.

This type of imaginative thinking, called visualization, is an excellent way to cope with anger and anxiety and to replace the emotions with feelings of strength and power.

Permit yourself to lie low. Women who are infertile often say that they find it difficult to be around children – or around people who are always asking whether they're making 'progress'. You can't isolate yourself for ever, but you shouldn't feel obliged to maintain a busy social life at times when you'd rather be alone.

Confront destructive ideas. Women who are trying without success to get pregnant often link their self-worth to their ability to have children – and they may blame themselves for having 'waited so long' to start a family.

Try to put these feelings behind you as much as you can. They distort reality and needlessly cause frustration or fear. Try writing down your thoughts in a diary or talking to a supportive friend or family member. If these techniques don't help, you should consider talking to your doctor about counselling.

MULTIPLE BIRTHS EQUAL MULTIPLE NAPPIES!

Women who undergo assistive reproduction procedures, such as in vitro fertilization and gamete intrafallopian transfer – which involves the injection of one or more eggs mixed with sperm directly into the fallopian tubes – will have multiple births about 38 per cent of the time. Among those who use ovulation-inducing drugs, 20 per cent of the children are twins or triplets or other 'multiples'.

Fertility specialists advise women that multiple births have higher risks of birth defects or delivery complications, especially in older mums.

Then there's the sheer workload. Women who are considering fertility treatments should ask themselves if they have the energy and tolerance that's required, say, for the more than 1,000 monthly nappy changes required by a set of triplet newborns. That comes to three new nappies (one for each of three little bottoms) every 2 hours for a whole month.

Medical Options

✚ When you're having trouble getting pregnant, the first order of business is for your partner to see a urologist or fertility specialist, who will probably perform a semen analysis to rule out a low sperm count or sperm abnormalities. You should visit your doctor or a fertility specialist, who will ask about your menstrual history and perform a complete physical examination.

Both of you may need further evaluation of your reproductive organs to check for problems such as blocked tubes or scar tissue in the woman.

Infertility often occurs when a woman is ovulating irregularly or not at all. These cases are often easy to correct because for more than half of couples, the use of drugs leads to pregnancy after 6 months if there are no other problems requiring treatment.

Assisted reproduction technologies, such as in vitro fertilization (IVF), manipulate eggs and sperm outside the womb to improve the chances of pregnancy. According to the Human Fertilization and Embryology Authority (HFEA), about 25 per cent of women aged under 38 achieved a birth per treatment cycle with IVF, while the success (live birth) rate for women under 38 treated with donor insemination was about 11 per cent.

Women are usually advised to progress from the easiest treatment options to the most aggressive, giving each treatment at least three menstrual cycles to take effect; after six menstrual cycles, it's probably time to move on to another approach.

'It may be important to move more quickly through your options if you feel that your proverbial reproductive clock is ticking,' says Dr Gelman. 'Some couples in their forties want to bypass medications and elaborate testing and go straight to in vitro fertilization. It's always an individual choice.'

For more information about infertility, visit the websites of the HFEA at www.hfea.gov.uk or the National Fertility Association at www.issue.co.uk. Australia's National Infertility Network www.access.org.au. Fertility NZ is New Zealand's national network www.nz.infertility.org.nz.

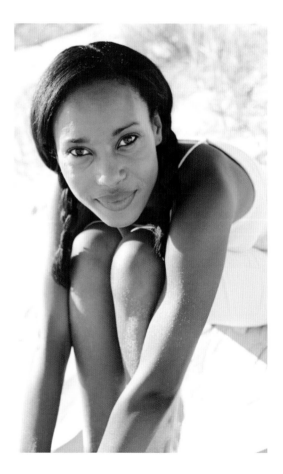

CHAPTER
17

Polycystic Ovary Syndrome

When ovaries are stimulated by high levels of hormones, they sometimes develop blisterlike growths, called cysts. The cysts themselves are unlikely to cause problems, but the hormones that trigger their growth may cause problems elsewhere in the body.

Some women suffer with lots of tiny ovarian cysts as a result of a condition called polycystic ovary syndrome (PCOS). Women with PCOS may develop unwanted hair growth on the face, torso, chest and/or buttocks – and thinning of the hair on the head. They may put on weight or develop acne as adults. PCOS can interfere with menstrual cycles and fertility as well.

All women produce a small amount of testosterone, the 'male' hormone, but women with PCOS produce relatively high amounts. The extra testosterone disrupts levels of other hormones in the body. It may cause irregular menstrual cycles and stop ovulation. Because of this, the body continues producing oestrogen but stops producing progesterone.

Many women with PCOS don't know they have it. All they know is that they're unhappy with the appearance of their bodies – and they often don't suspect that there's an underlying physical reason, says Dr Walter Futterweit, an endocrinologist and an advisory board member of the US Polycystic Ovarian Syndrome Association.

In young women, PCOS is the leading cause of infertility. It may not be discovered until a woman tries to conceive but cannot.

Luckily, most women with PCOS can control the symptoms with a combination of medication and home care.

Lifestyle Strategies

Exercise regularly and keep an eye on your weight. In women who are overweight, testosterone is converted in the fat tissue to female hormones. An effective way to restore hormones to their proper levels is to maintain a healthy weight. Talk to your doctor about appropriate exercise and diet plans. As you lose fat tissue, your oestrogen levels will naturally decline.

Nutritional Treatments

Control insulin levels. The majority of women with PCOS develop a condition called insulin resistance. Insulin is the hormone that carries glucose (blood sugar) into cells where it's needed. If the cells become resistant to insulin, the body produces more of it – and this in turn stimulates the production of more testosterone by the ovaries.

There are a number of ways to overcome insulin resistance. In addition to helping to control weight, exercising regularly – it can be walking, bicycling, hiking or even gardening for 20 to 30 minutes most days of the week – will help the body's insulin become more efficient. You also may be told to follow a low-glycaemic (low-carbohydrate) diet. (For more information on low-glycaemic eating, see chapter 25.)

Curb your sugar cravings. Sugar increases your insulin levels, which causes weight gain and aggravates hormone imbalances, says Dr Lila Amdurska Wallis, a clinical professor of medicine. Replace sugary treats with foods like grains, fresh fruit and vegetables. Without those sweets taunting your hormone levels, you'll feel healthier and more energetic.

Eat small amounts at a time. 'If you are in the habit of eating two or three heavy meals a day, switch to five to six light meals,' Dr Futterweit advises. Each meal should contain between 250 and 300 calories. That's about all that insulin-resistant cells can handle at one time.

Enjoy protein or low-carbohydrate snacks. Women are usually advised to enjoy rolls, bread or other high-carbohydrate foods. For women with PCOS, however, foods that are high in carbohydrates may cause surges in insulin. Better snack choices include protein (such as plain yoghurt, cheese or nuts and seeds), or low-starch vegetables, such as cucumber or broccoli.

Drink water – but avoid fruit squashes. Squashes are generally too sweet for women with

THREE THINGS I TELL EVERY FEMALE PATIENT

DR WALTER FUTTERWEIT, an endocrinologist, advises women with polycystic ovary syndrome to follow these recommendations.

1

GET SERIOUS ABOUT LOSING WEIGHT. Many women with PCOS are obese. The good news is that losing as little as 7 to 8 per cent of the weight is often enough to lower excess hormone levels.

2

SEE AN EXPERT. PCOS can be complicated to control. Your family doctor can help, but women with PCOS really need to be under the care of an endocrinologist, an expert on the body's hormones.

REARRANGE THE FOOD GUIDE PYRAMID. The standard for healthy eating, the food guide pyramid, recommends getting the bulk of calories from complex carbohydrates, such as whole grains. Women with PCOS, however, should get about 40 per cent of calories from lean protein, such as lamb, fish or legumes. About 30 per cent of calories should come from vegetables and only about 30 per cent should come from complex carbohydrates. Some women have even more success when only about 10 to 20 per cent of calories come from carbohydrates.

3

when to see a doctor

If you have a history of skipped menstrual periods that are followed by serious acne outbreaks: make an appointment to see an endocrinologist. This is a classic symptom of polycystic ovary syndrome (PCOS).

If you have hair growth on the face or body and thinning hair on the head: in women this usually means that the balance of hormones has been disrupted, and you could have PCOS.

PCOS. The ideal beverage is water. It's also fine to drink unsweetened almond milk or skimmed or semi-skimmed milk.

Medical Options

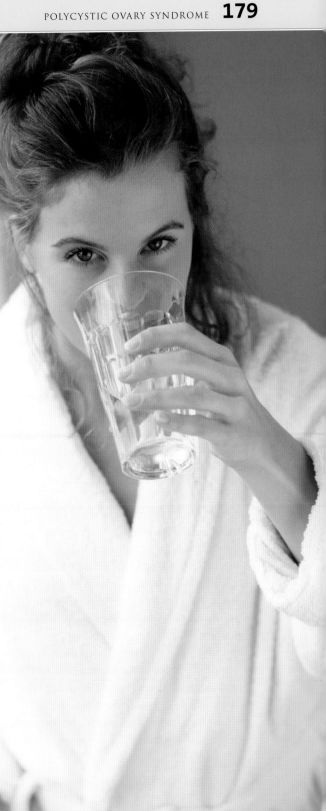

Lower insulin with medication. Doctors often advise women with PCOS to take metformin (Glucophage), an insulin-regulating drug that's commonly used to treat diabetes. Women who take it can often normalize their menstrual cycles. They also may see a reversal in weight gain or unwanted hair growth.

Consider the Pill. Oral contraceptives may be used to restore a normal menstrual cycle and help reduce hair growth and acne. Anti-androgen (male hormones) pills such as spironolactone (Aldactone), which block the effects of testosterone, can also be helpful in conjunction with the Pill.

Shut down the source. When the symptoms of PCOS can't be controlled with other medication, your doctor may recommend that you take drugs called GnRH agonists (such as Synarel), which 'turn off' the ovaries.

Once the ovaries stop functioning, the troublesome hormones will gradually return to more normal levels. This is not used often in view of the loss-of-bone effect, which may occur after 6 months of use.

For more information on polycystic ovary syndrome, see the website of the Polycystic Ovarian Syndrome Association at www.pcosupport.org.

WHEN BAD THINGS HAPPEN TO HEALTHY WOMEN

She Was Eating All the Wrong Foods

Christine Gray DeZarn had kept her weight at 64 kilograms (10 stone) throughout her adult life – so she was understandably alarmed when it suddenly jumped to 90 kilograms (14 stone 4 pounds) when she was 27. She responded the way a lot of women do: by going on an ultra low calorie diet. But even when she was eating a meagre 800 calories daily, she continued to put on weight.

'The doctor I was seeing was convinced I was cheating on my diet, but I was practically starving,' she remembers.

At about the same time, she began getting acne along her jaw. She also discovered hair growing on her face and stomach, and when she and her husband tried to have their first child, they had no success after 6 years and 11 trials of assisted reproduction treatments.

Christine first heard about polycystic ovary syndrome (PCOS) on an online infertility support group. 'I read everything I could get my hands on about metabolism, and how blood sugar and hormones are affected by the different foods you eat. I found out what a mistake I had made by following a low-fat, high-carbohydrate diet. It doesn't work for people with insulin resistance. I was actually triggering my condition by eating a lot of processed grains and cutting back on protein.'

As soon as Christine eliminated sugar, pasta, rice and other high-carbohydrate foods from her diet, the weight started to naturally drop off. She lost 13 kilograms (2 stone) in 3 months, and 22 kilograms (3½ stone) within the first year. 'Within 2 years, I was down to 61 kilograms (9 stone 6 pounds), which is better than where I started,' she adds.

As a busy travel industry trainer, Christine had to maintain her eating plan while staying in hotels and eating on aeroplanes and in restaurants. She always eats the same breakfast: scrambled eggs and fresh fruit. Most restaurants serve chicken Caesar salad, and it's also easy to find her favourite snack – celery with blue cheese dressing.

Today, a decade after she was diagnosed, Christine, 38, continues to follow a strict diet because it controls her weight and other symptoms of PCOS. 'I will eat this way for the rest of my life because it works,' she says.

CHAPTER

18

Fibroids

The thought of uterine fibroids – benign growths of the uterine muscle called leiomyomas – is enough to rush many women into action. As a rule, however, if fibroids aren't causing symptoms, they may not need treatment at all.

Around 20 per cent of women of reproductive age have fibroids; African-Caribbean women are at least twice as likely to have fibroids as other women. You can have one fibroid or a whole cluster. Most fibroids are between the size of a pea and a tennis ball, although they can potentially grow much larger.

It's not uncommon for women with fibroids to be unaware of them. They're often discovered during routine examinations, when a doctor feels them while pressing on the abdomen.

Most women with fibroids will experience a dull ache in the abdomen, pelvis or back. Fibroids may also cause abnormal menstrual bleeding.

In many cases, however, they cause no symptoms at all – and doctors advise women to simply get used to the idea that there are harmless guests inside the pelvis.

If you are having symptoms, your doctor may simply advise you to wait: fibroid growth is stimulated by the female hormone oestrogen. Once a woman approaches menopause, and oestrogen levels decline, the symptoms will usually disappear, says Dr Sam Jacobs, a reproductive endocrinologist and associate professor of obstetrics and gynaecology.

In the mean time, you may want to take a few steps to manage fibroids naturally.

Home Remedies

Manage your weight. Excess body fat leads to excess oestrogen, which can increase the size of fibroids. The best way to maintain a healthy weight is to take regular exercise. A combination of weight training and aerobic activities – such as running, cycling or fast walking – decreases fat tissue and adds muscle, which can help lower excess levels of oestrogen in the body. (For a complete guide to maintaining a healthy weight, see chapter 5.)

Ease the ache. Applying heat to the abdomen will often relieve discomfort, especially when you're having your period. Some doctors advise using a castor oil pack.

Pour 120 millilitres (4 fluid ounces) of castor oil on a thick piece of cotton cloth. Fold the cloth in half and put it on your abdomen. Cover it with plastic wrap and a thin towel, then put a heating pad or hot-water bottle on top.

You should leave the pack on your tummy for up to an hour a day, and repeat the treatment daily.

Nutritional Treatments

Eat less meat. 'The oestrogenic additives used in the beef industry can disrupt your hormone levels enough to signal fibroids to grow,' says Dr Jacobs.

In one study, Italian researchers compared the diets of 2,400 women. They found that women with fibroids ate more beef, ham and other red meats than those without fibroids. A plant-based diet is beneficial because fruit and vegetables contain natural plant compounds called isoflavones, which help prevent oestrogen from fuelling fibroid growth.

Alternative Therapies

Try an Eastern remedy. Asian practitioners of traditional Chinese medicine (TCM) have many approaches for treating fibroids, including herbal and dietary treatments that are designed to remove excess oestrogen in the body. Seaweed has been shown to be very effective in treating fibroids. Eating liver or taking liver organ supplements has been shown to be most effective in removing excess oestrogen, reducing fibroids and regulating the menstrual cycle. In addition, an Asian doctor may advise women with fibroids to perform healing movements, such as t'ai chi or qigong, which are said to restore healthy circulation to the pelvic area.

For registered practitioners of Chinese herbal medicine, visit the Register of Chinese Herbal Medicine (RCHM) at www.ichm.co.uk. The Australian Acupuncture and Chinese Medicine Association Ltd is at www.acupuncture.org.au.

THREE THINGS I TELL EVERY FEMALE PATIENT

DR LYNN BORGATTA, an associate professor of obstetrics and gynaecology, offers this advice to women with fibroids.

1

DON'T BE FRIGHTENED. Fibroids are tumours, but they're benign and won't increase your risk of cancer. They're almost always harmless, and the symptoms (if there are any) will probably be easy to manage, possibly with medication that shrinks fibroids, among other options.

2

BE CONSERVATIVE. If you need relief from fibroid symptoms and you're planning to have children, talk to your doctor about medication before considering surgical procedures.

TALK TO YOUR DOCTOR ABOUT HYSTERECTOMY OPTIONS. If you need a hysterectomy, let your doctor know that you don't want the ovaries and cervix removed along with the uterus unless it's absolutely necessary. A supracervical hysterectomy is less traumatic and healthier in the long run.

3

Acupuncture Saved Her from a Hysterectomy

After an casualty visit for abdominal pain, Sharon Saunders, a cookery writer, discovered that she had a fibroid the size of a 16-week pregnancy. The fibroid had grown so fast and was causing so much discomfort that her doctor recommended a hysterectomy.

Sharon wasn't convinced that surgery was her best option, especially because she knew that fibroids often shrink with the onset of menopause. At 48, she was hoping to find a treatment that would tide her over for a few years. After reading an article about the use of acupuncture for treating fibroids, she decided to give it a try. She made an appointment with a practitioner of traditional Chinese medicine, who recommended weekly acupuncture treatments, along with medicinal herbs.

After 4 months, she checked back with her doctor, who reported that the fibroid had shrunk by a third.

'I got to keep my uterus, and the pain went away entirely,' says Sharon, who continues to have regular acupuncture treatments. 'I go back once a month for what I call wellness maintenance,' she says. 'It has really helped my allergies, too.'

Medical Options

Fibroids need to be treated when they're causing heavy or abnormal menstrual bleeding, chronic pain, bowel or urinary obstructions or other symptoms, says Dr Lynn Borgatt. You'll also need treatment if you're trying to conceive and the fibroids are interfering with pregnancy.

The treatment options include:

- **Gonadotropin-releasing hormone (GnRH) agonists (Lupron/Lupron Depot).** These are treatments that shrink fibroids temporarily. Their main use is to shrink fibroids prior to surgery. The drawback to these treatments is that they may cause menopause-like symptoms, such as hot flushes and vaginal dryness. Over time, they can also raise cholesterol levels and increase the risk of osteoporosis, so they are usually not used for longer than 6 months.

- **Myomectomy.** This means removing fibroids surgically. Small fibroids can be cauterized with a laser or electrical needle; larger fibroids are cut away from the uterine wall. Depending on the location of the fibroids, surgery may be done through the abdomen or through the vagina. The surgery is usually successful, although there's a small chance that a hysterectomy will be needed to finish the surgery. Also, there's a 30 per cent chance that the fibroids will return. Fertility is usually preserved, but pregnancy can sometimes be complicated.

■ **Hysterectomy.** This means removing the uterus. Once the uterus is removed, the fibroids are also gone and won't come back. The problem with hysterectomy is that it's major surgery – there may be a long recovery time. Also, women who have this procedure won't be able to have children afterwards. A supracervical hysterectomy is limited to removal of the uterus only, leaving the ovaries and cervix intact.

■ **Uterine artery embolization.** This is a surgical procedure in which the blood vessels that supply the fibroids are destroyed with a bombardment of plastic particles. The advantage of this procedure is that it's less stressful than other forms of surgery, and it's unlikely to interfere with a woman's ability to conceive. It's a relatively new procedure, however, and experts aren't sure how effective it will prove to be over time.

when to see a doctor

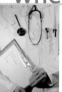

If your periods are heavier than usual, or you're having irregular bleeding: see your doctor. This is often the first symptom of fibroids.

If you're having trouble urinating or moving your bowels: it can mean that fibroids are getting large enough to exert pressure on the bladder or intestine.

If you've been diagnosed with fibroids, whether or not they're causing symptoms: you'll need to have them monitored regularly: 3 months after the diagnosis, and every 6 months thereafter.

When medical intervention is necessary, ask your doctor about all your options. There are many considerations, including the severity of symptoms, whether you'll want to get pregnant in the future, and how close you are to the menopause. The size of the fibroids and where they're growing can also affect your treatment options as well as your risks.

CHAPTER

19

Endometriosis

The uterus is lined with a spongy tissue called the endometrium, which provides a soft nest for fertilized eggs. Normally, an egg is released each month, and if it isn't fertilized, the endometrium swells, breaks down and sloughs off, exiting the body as menstrual fluid.

Sometimes, however, the cells that make up the endometrium grow outside the uterus on nearby organs, such as the fallopian tubes or ovaries. The cells also sometimes implant themselves on the outside of the uterus. They can even spread to the lungs, digestive tract or other parts of the body. This disease is called endometriosis, and it can result in painful, and potentially serious, symptoms.

Because endometrial cells are sensitive to the hormonal changes of the menstrual cycle, the symptoms often flare up during the menstrual period. Women may experience severe, even incapacitating pain, fatigue and many other unpleasant symptoms. Endometriosis also can result in gastrointestinal symptoms, painful sex or, during periods, painful urination. More than 30 per cent of women with endometriosis also face infertility.

Endometriosis sometimes can be controlled with the use of birth control pills or other hormone-altering medication. Surgery to remove the tissue is another treatment that can help. But for about one in three women, the renegade tissue will eventually come back, says Dr Carolyn R. Kaplan, an assistant clinical professor of obstetrics and gynaecology.

Doctors aren't sure what causes endometriosis. Evidence suggests that the cells get 'scattered' around the pelvis when menstrual blood doesn't effectively make its way out of the body. The immune system should recognize and destroy these errant cells, but for some reason it doesn't.

There are a number of treatment options for endometriosis. A good starting place is for women to strengthen their immune systems and do everything possible to keep their hormones in the proper balance, says Dr Deborah A. Metzger, associate clinical professor of reproductive endocrinology and obstetrics and gynaecology at Stanford University.

Some women with endometriosis will require medical treatment, either to remove the tissue or to manage the monthly flare-ups. In many cases, however, women can control the discomfort with home care.

Home Remedies

🏠 **Treat yourself to heat.** Applying warmth to the lower abdomen is a very effective way to soothe the uterus, says Dr Toni Bark, an expert in integrative medicine. Taking warm baths or applying a hot-water bottle or a heating pad is the easiest approach. For longer-lasting heat, your doctor may advise you to use a patch that releases heat for long periods of time, such as Robinson FemEase therapeutic heat wraps, available direct by mail order in the UK, telephone 01909 735009.

Exercise when able. Walking, swimming and other forms of exercise increase circulation, which helps the body remove excess oestrogen from the blood. Exercise also stimulates endorphins, natural chemicals that help reduce pain.

Avoid pollutants. The hormones in a woman's body are exquisitely balanced, but

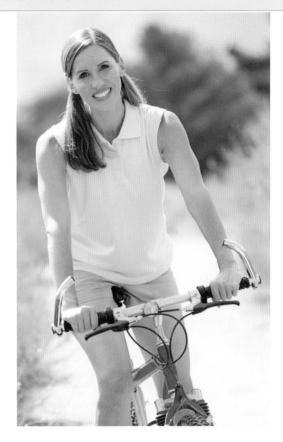

THREE THINGS I TELL EVERY FEMALE PATIENT

DR TONI BARK, an expert in integrative medicine, has seen great success when women with endometriosis do the following things:

1

TAKE 1 TABLESPOON OF GROUND FLAXSEED (LINSEED) DAILY. Linseed contains an oil that reduces painful inflammation. It's also high in fibre, which can help remove excess oestrogen. 'I recommend having it for breakfast every morning,' says Dr Bark. 'You can mix it with sunflower seeds, fruit and almond milk.'

2

USE EVENING PRIMROSE OIL. Available as a supplement, evening primrose oil reduces inflammation and often relieves pain within a month, says Dr Bark. The recommended dose is 500 milligrams twice daily.

3

TAKE A MULTI SUPPLEMENT THAT CONTAINS B VITAMINS AND VITAMIN E. Vitamin E carries oxygen to tissues and helps reduce scar formation in women with endometriosis. The B vitamins are particularly important because they help balance the body's hormones, says Dr Bark.

modern society has thrown a spanner into the works. Humans have introduced more than 70,000 industrial chemicals into the environment, and some of them suppress immunity and disrupt the natural balance of hormones.

Dioxin, for example, a waste chemical that's widespread in the environment, might have profound effects on a woman's hormones. In one 13-year study, female rhesus monkeys were exposed to dioxin, and 79 per cent developed endometriosis. These studies were in monkeys, not humans, but something similar may occur in humans. We don't know for sure without more studies.

An important place to start is to avoid food that may have high amounts of dioxin in it, but more about that later. Products that have been bleached with chlorine may contain dioxin and other chemical contaminants. Although a survey did not show a connection between tampon use and endometriosis incidence, some women like to use non-chlorine-bleached tampons and sanitary towels.

Some people may find it's also helpful to use dioxin-free toilet paper, cosmetics and other products whenever possible. Opt for cloth towels and cloth serviettes instead of paper.

Nutritional Treatments

Eat organically. Commercial livestock typically is injected with growth hormones and antibiotics – and women who eat meat may suffer the effects. 'In my opinion, an immediate way to protect your hormone balance and immune system is to make sure that you don't eat meat and dairy products that aren't certified as organic,' says Dr Bark.

Filter your drinking water. Use water purifiers that filter out lead, mercury, chlorine and other hormone-disrupting contaminants. Look at the labels for the specific substances that each type of filter will remove.

Alternative Therapies

Relax as much as you can. Stress management helps to improve immune function and may also decrease pain. Every woman has her own ways of coping with stress, including meditation, yoga and relaxation exercises. Or try more creative approaches: take an art class; do voluntary work; get more engaged with your hobbies. Women who nurture their creative sides will naturally experience less stress.

when to see a doctor

If you have abdominal pain that increases with your period, around ovulation or with intercourse: there's a good chance that you have endometriosis, and it may get worse without prompt treatment.

If you're having trouble getting pregnant: endometriosis is a common cause of infertility. Endometriosis may cause scarring around the tubes and ovaries that could lead to infertility. If other women in your family have had endometriosis, you have a higher risk of getting it as well.

WHEN BAD THINGS HAPPEN TO HEALTHY WOMEN

Natural Treatments Gave Her Control

Menstrual periods are rarely as regular as the textbooks would have you believe, but for Karen Susag, they were unusually erratic from the beginning.

'My periods varied greatly. Sometimes I would only have a period every 6 months, and when I did, I'd be immobilized with pain. There also were times that I would end up in casualty,' says Karen.

At one point, the pain was so severe and frequent that she missed a whole term of college. That's when a doctor finally recognized that her symptoms were caused by endometriosis.

In the next 10 years, she had surgery six times for endometriosis and to remove scar tissue. She also tried a variety of hormone treatments, which invariably brought on headaches, nausea and fatigue.

On the advice of a practitioner specializing in immunotherapy, Karen eliminated dairy products, sugar, yeast, alcohol and caffeine from her diet. In addition to immunotherapy, she underwent acupuncture and took Chinese herbs under supervision of a traditional Chinese medicine practitioner. And she did everything possible to reduce the stress in her life.

'I have a completely different way of approaching things,' she says. 'I listen to my body, and know when I'm pushing myself too hard. If I work late, then I take the morning off.'

The treatments have worked, Karen says. Her pain level is right down, and she generally has a lot more energy. 'The hardest thing about having endometriosis is knowing that it's a chronic problem. But I've discovered that if you keep your life in better balance, you can keep it in check.'

Medical Options

Consider drug therapy. 'Gonadotropin-releasing hormone (GnRH) agonists and antagonists, such as leuprolide (Lupron) and nafarelin (Synarel), turn off the signal to ovulate, leading to a reversible "medical menopause",' Dr Kaplan says. This causes oestrogen levels to drop. Menstrual periods stop, and over time the errant endometrial cells will shrink.

Look into IUDs. Intra-uterine devices (IUDs) were once discouraged for women with endometriosis or other pelvic problems, but a new type of IUD, called Mirena, releases a synthetic hormone called levonorgestrel into the uterus. It appears to suppress endometrial growth.

A Finnish study looked at 56 women who were considering hysterectomies to relieve excessive uterine bleeding. Half of them were asked to use the Mirena IUD to see if it helped. Two-thirds of the women experienced so much relief that they decided to cancel the surgery. Although this was only one small study of women who were considering hysterectomies for 'excessive uterine bleeding', not endometriosis, the Mirena might be considered an option for endometriosis.

CHAPTER
20

Pelvic Inflammatory Disease

If you suspect that you may have contracted a sexually transmitted infection (STI) – symptoms include a foul-smelling discharge, painful urination and a dull ache in the lower abdomen; pelvic pain; or fever and chills – don't wait to see if it will go away. Contact your doctor straight away.

You have to act quickly if there's even a hint that you have an STI. That's because untreated STIs can lead to pelvic inflammatory disease (PID), a broad term that refers to infections of the upper genital tract, usually involving the fallopian tubes and sometimes the ovaries and even the lining of the uterus. As with many infections, intensive treatment with antibiotics is necessary to destroy the bacteria that are making you ill. Delays in treatment, on the other hand, can allow the harmful organisms to rage out of control, potentially damaging your reproductive organs beyond repair.

Unfortunately, women don't always see a doctor at the first sign of symptoms. A quarter of PID cases require hospitalization and the use of intravenous antibiotics; in rare cases emergency surgery is needed, to drain infectious fluid from the abdomen or repair organ damage. Because the infection can scar and block the fallopian tubes, PID may result in infertility. Blocked tubes can also put a woman at higher risk for ectopic pregnancy, a dangerous condition in which a fertilized egg grows in the fallopian tube instead of in the uterus. About 1.7 per cent of women have PID and this is a conservative estimate. It's a common result from STIs. It doesn't have to be, though; the vast majority of cases can be prevented by taking precautions against sexually transmitted infections by using condoms.

Unwelcome Infections

The organism that results in PID is usually chlamydia or, less commonly, gonorrhoea (or both). These STIs are especially prevalent among sexually active women with multiple partners. If you've had unprotected sex and suspect that you may have been exposed to an STI, get tested right away. One reason that STIs are so dangerous is that one in five people infected with chlamydia or gonorrhoea doesn't have symptoms. Women can carry the disease for weeks, months or even years before the infection spreads or results in full-blown PID. PID isn't always caused by sexually transmitted infections. Some women may develop infections after childbirth, abortions or other types of pelvic surgeries. These types of infections are rare, however. In most cases – 99.9 per cent – STIs are to blame.

Home Remedies

Allow yourself some downtime. Your body has taken a beating, and you need time to recover. Drink a lot of fluid, eat lightly and get some rest.

Avoid sex until the antibiotic treatment is complete. Otherwise, you could pass the infection to your partner. When you do resume sexual activity, be certain that your partner has been tested and treated for STIs. You don't want to be exposed to the same harmful organisms that made you ill in the first place.

Steam away infection. Sitting in a hot environment – a steamy shower, for example, or a deep bath – increases body temperature, which boosts the activity of the immune system and creates an unfavourable environment for harmful germs. The moist heat will also reduce discomfort in the abdomen and back.

Don't be hard on yourself. Because of the link between PID and sexually transmitted infections, women often feel guilty, embarrassed or ashamed. Put the feelings behind you. It's fine to acknowledge that you may have made some mistakes, but it's more important to look forward to the future.

Alternative Therapies

Use live-culture supplements. Antibiotics kill beneficial bacteria in the body along with the bad. To replenish 'good' bacteria, take probiotic supplements, which contain live cultures of *acidophilus* and *bifidus*. Probiotics can improve digestion, assist the immune system and help prevent yeast infections in women who are taking antibiotics.

THREE THINGS I TELL EVERY FEMALE PATIENT

DR SAM JACOBS, a reproductive endocrinologist, gives the following advice for preventing pelvic inflammatory disease (PID).

1

USE PROTECTION. If you and your sexual partner aren't mutually monogamous, or if you haven't both been tested for sexually transmitted diseases, use condoms, even if you're on another form of birth control, says Dr Jacobs.

2

INTRA-UTERINE CONTRACEPTIVES AREN'T FOR EVERYONE. 'Although intra-uterine contraceptives are an excellent form of birth control, they're not appropriate for women with a history of multiple partners, STIs or pelvic inflammatory disease,' says Dr Jacobs.

3

DON'T DOUCHE. It pushes bacteria up into the reproductive tract, which can increase the risk for PID, says Dr Jacobs.

Take 1 teaspoon of probiotic powder three times daily for as long as you're taking antibiotics. Continue taking the probiotic for an additional 3 weeks. Look for probiotics that are kept in the refrigerated section of health food shops. They contain the highest concentration of beneficial bacteria.

Savour spicy stir-fries. The spices ginger, turmeric and cayenne contain chemical compounds that reduce inflammation, pain and congestion in the abdomen. Garlic is also helpful because it has powerful antibacterial effects.

Put your mind to work. Some studies have shown that visualization exercises, in which you form clear mental images of the healing powers of your body, can increase immunoglobulins and possibly help STIs heal more quickly.

Here's how it works. Twice a day, find a quiet place and relax by taking slow, deep breaths. Create a mental image of your reproductive organs, but with a slight blur over them; the blur represents the infection. Form a picture in your mind of thousands of white blood cells pouring into your organs. As they work, they'll flush out inflammation and clear away the blur, revealing healthy tissue underneath.

Medical Options

Get prescribed antibiotics immediately. If you're treated for an STI early enough, a single course of oral antibiotics will cure it for good. PID requires long-term therapy with multiple antibiotics.

Finish the prescription. Often a woman with PID who takes antibiotics starts feeling better within 2 days. But the antibiotics haven't finished working. You'll need to finish the full prescription – 1 to 2 weeks' worth – to eliminate all the bacteria from your body. Women who give up on antibiotics too soon may see the infection come straight back, says Dr Jacobs.

Stay in touch with your doctor. You'll need to make an appointment for 2 to 3 days after you begin treatment with antibiotics to ensure that the drugs are working. Make another appointment for when the treatment is finished. Your doctor will make sure that the infection is gone and that you don't need an additional round of antibiotics.

when to see a doctor

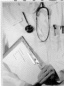

If you have a foul-smelling vaginal discharge, along with a dull ache in the lower abdomen or back, or fever and chills accompanying either of the above: see your doctor straight away. These are early signs of PID.

If you develop symptoms after having unprotected sex: you could have chlamydia, gonorrhoea or another sexually transmitted disease, which can increase your risk for PID.

If you have flulike symptoms or a heavy vaginal discharge or bleeding, along with pelvic pain, go to casualty. If you have PID, the infection may have reached a serious stage. It's not uncommon for PID to be misdiagnosed as endometriosis, so you may want to ask the doctor about getting your white blood cell count checked and having a pelvic ultrasound; these tests will help differentiate between the two conditions.

CHAPTER
21

Perimenopause

You may notice typical patterns as your body begins the 4- to 10-year transition out of its reproductive phase and into the perimenopause – which ends with the permanent liberation from tampons, period alerts and PMS.

Starting in your early forties, expect your periods to gradually become lighter and your cycles to lengthen or shorten. You can also expect to feel more sensitive to hot and cold temperature changes than you did in your twenties and thirties.

Women often become concerned about their health when they sense that they are nearing menopause. That can be a good thing because it can motivate them to make healthy lifestyle changes.

'Women often ask me what they should take for menopause,' says Dr Margery Gass, a professor of obstetrics and gynaecology. 'The good news is that they don't necessarily have to take anything to be healthy – that the transition to menopause is a perfectly natural process. The most important thing is a healthy lifestyle: nutritious food, normal weight, adequate calcium and vitamin D, exercise and no smoking.'

Coping with Change

If your hormone shifts are causing discomfort, remind yourself that the perimenopause doesn't last for ever. For example, you may experience premenstrual symptoms – such as irritability or monthly bloating – for the first time in your life, but the symptoms will disappear as your hormonal fluctuations settle down. Even hot flushes, if you get them at all, might occur only for a month or two. More typically, they come and go for 2 to 3 years.

Other changes, such as a thinning, less moist vaginal lining, are permanent, but may or may not cause any complications, such as uncomfortable sex or more frequent infections.

If you've fallen behind on healthy habits, your first step to avoiding difficulties is to get back on track by eating well, exercising regularly and practising sensible self-care. It's a good idea to cut back on caffeine and alcohol during perimenopause. That's because during this time women often become more sensitive to stimulants, which can disrupt sleep cycles or mood. Additionally, caffeine and alcohol relax the capillaries and promote hot flushes.

How or when to take further action depends

entirely on how severely you experience certain changes and to what extent these changes affect your overall quality of life.

MANAGING MENSTRUAL DIFFICULTIES

When you approach the perimenopause, you are coming to the end of a lifetime's supply of approximately 400,000 eggs. You won't ovulate as regularly as you used to. Although your ovaries are working their way out of the oestrogen production business, oestrogen sometimes peaks rather than plummets during the transition – sometimes as high as pregnancy levels. Then there's progesterone, which comes and goes according to whether you ovulate. Normal hormone shifts are enough to stimulate premenstrual discomfort, but the dramatic fluctuations that occur during perimenopause explain why some women experience menstrual or premenstrual discomfort for the first time in their lives – and why women who have always had PMS have it more severely.

Menstrual irregularities are also common. Even if your periods were always regular, you may find that they're coming more often, sometimes even twice a month, and then disappearing altogether for a few months. Many women experience unusually heavy menstrual flows as well. To manage menstrual difficulties, here are some strategies you may want to try.

Medical Options

Look into short-term hormone replacement therapy (HRT). Deciding whether or not to take hormones long term is a serious decision, and you must consider all the pros and cons. But in the mean time, your doctor may advise you to undergo HRT on a trial basis. It will quickly ease hormone-related changes while you decide whether or not to continue the therapy once you reach the menopause, says Dr Mary Jane Minkin, clinical professor of obstetrics and gynaecology at Yale University School of Medicine.

Supplemental oestrogen and progesterone provide immediate relief from symptoms such as menstrual difficulties, hot flushes, insomnia, vaginal dryness or urinary frequency, says Dr Minkin. 'Plus, when you are just taking hormones short term, you don't need to be as concerned about increasing your risk for breast cancer.'

Consider contraceptive pills. Oral contraceptives aren't for everyone. They contain higher amounts of hormones than those used in HRT, which means even greater concerns about stroke, heart attack and oestrogen-sensitive cancers. But as long as you don't smoke or have a history of blood clotting, birth control pills are a reasonable way to resolve menstrual irregularities.

Of course, birth control pills also offer solid protection against a pregnancy that might prove particularly difficult at this stage in life.

Start with progesterone alone. Although the root of irregular cycles at menopause is often hormonal, you don't necessarily have to undergo fully-fledged HRT for just this one issue. A small dose of premenstrual progesterone 10 to 12 days before your period might be enough to regulate your cycle and prevent heavy periods due to inconsistent ovulation, says Dr Gass.

In addition, progesterone can protect your endometrium, the lining of the uterus, from being overstimulated by oestrogen, which is a real concern when ovulation is hit-or-miss. Your doctor can prescribe a progesterone tablet.

Ask your doctor if hormone treatment is causing bleeding. Healthy women who don't smoke may take oral contraceptives for cycle control and get the added benefits of contraception and treatment of hot flushes. Women can use oral contraceptives or HRT if they are having hot flushes along with their irregular bleeding. But a side effect may be even more erratic periods.

Your doctor may advise you to take a 'cyclic dose' of hormones – rather than a 'continuous' dose – to allow a more 'scheduled' time for bleeding. 'HRT is a much lower dose of hormones than oral contraceptives. Sometimes HRT is just not strong enough to control a woman's irregular cycles in perimenopause,' says Dr Gass. Once you are a couple of years beyond the menopause, you may decide to switch to 'continuous dose' hormones, which shut down the cyclic bleeding completely.

Alternative Therapies

Try black cohosh. A herb, black cohosh appears to interact with the pituitary gland and reduce the production of luteinizing hormone – the hormone that often triggers the aggravating symptoms of menopause. Women who take black cohosh often maintain more stable levels of hormones, which keeps the menstrual cycle on track. There also may be a reduction in menstrual pain.

In a study of 80 menopausal women, researchers found that black cohosh was as effective as HRT at lessening the severity of hot flushes, memory loss, depression and mood swings, as well as improving the thickness of vaginal tissues. Black cohosh is used instead of – not with – conventional HRT. The recommended dose is usually 20 drops of 1:1 tincture three times daily, for no more than 6 months. (For more information on black cohosh, see the chart on page 61.)

Try this sexy herb. The herb Agnus castus (vitex), also known as chasteberry, is well recognized for regulating levels of progesterone and prolactin. The progesterone boost can smooth out your periods, whether they're infrequent, abnormally long, abnormally short, or unusually heavy or light. The prolactin boost from Agnus castus reduces bloating, improves sex drive and increases vaginal tone.

The recommended dose of Agnus castus (vitex) is 60 drops of 1:5 tincture twice daily, or tablets containing 250 milligrams of 4:1 extract twice daily.

If you are taking birth control pills, be aware that Agnus castus may counteract their effectiveness. When using Agnus castus, be patient: it often takes several months to bestow the full effects.

OUTWIT HOT FLUSHES

When the ovaries are changing over to their less active status at the time of the perimenopause, more than 70 per cent of women experience what are technically known as 'vasomotor symptoms'

– nervous system reactions by the part of your brain that regulates body temperature.

A full-out hot flush is unmistakable. Following a feeling of pressure in the head, your pulse quickens, and the skin on your chest, neck and head feels warm and sweaty as blood rushes to the surface. After approximately 4 minutes, the flushed feeling dissipates, and you feel cold and clammy. For some women, it feels as if their heart is racing, or they experience vertigo, weakness or shortness of breath. For others still, the feeling is more a sensitivity to heat than actual sweaty incidents.

Every woman has individual triggers that provoke hot flushes. As you get more experience, you may find yourself recruiting a family member to take things out of the oven or using only the low setting on the hair dryer. Even so, steadying your hormone levels is the only established method to actually treat hot flushes, and even then you may have some symptoms.

Fortunately, there are plenty of time-tested methods to reduce the discomfort.

Home Remedies

Reduce the heat in your diet. Don't order spicy chicken wings unless you're willing to suffer the consequences. The spices used in Indian, Mexican and Eastern cuisines can trigger hot flushes. In the kitchen, you may want to cut back on salsa, curry concoctions, hot-pepper sauce and black pepper.

Breathe away heat. Several studies have shown that women who practise a relaxing breathing technique can reduce hot flushes. While sitting in a comfortable chair, close your eyes and relax your muscles as much as possible. Slowly inhale and exhale until you can slow your breathing down to as little as seven or eight breaths a minute. Work to increase the depth of your belly breathing and decrease the depth of your chest breathing. If you practise this technique daily for 10 to 20 minutes, you may find that you're having fewer hot flushes than you did before.

THREE THINGS I TELL EVERY FEMALE PATIENT

DR MONA SHANGOLD, a gynaecologist, offers this special advice for women approaching the perimenopause.

1

EXERCISE REGULARLY. All women should get 20 minutes of aerobic exercise daily, combined with strength training 2 to 3 days a week.

2

MAINTAIN A HEALTHY WEIGHT. You'll have more energy and will be healthier overall than if you allow that extra weight to accumulate.

3

USE EXERCISE TO CONTROL MOODINESS. Whether mood changes are caused by sleep deprivation, night sweats or changes in brain chemicals associated with ageing, they can often be prevented with exercise.

Dress to keep cool. When you're venturing out for the day, think 'layers'. If you find yourself getting hot, you can start peeling off layers one at a time. 'Lots of perimenopausal women find that they are no longer comfortable in polonecks and clothes that hug the body,' Dr Gass adds. You may be more comfortable wearing breathable, loose fabrics, such as linen and cotton.

Treat your feet. Research confirms that if you keep your feet cool, you'll have fewer night sweats. Don't wear socks at night. If you do get a hot flush, put your feet in a cold bowl of water – it will help cool your whole body.

Nutritional Treatments

 Take sweat-stopping nutrients. Research suggests that combining vitamin C and bioflavonoid supplements may strengthen and stabilize capillaries and other small blood vessels, which can prevent hot flushes from occurring. You can find supplements that combine vitamin C with bioflavonoids at most health food stores. Look for a supplement that combines 500 to 1,000 milligrams of vitamin C with 200 to 500 milligrams of bioflavonoids per capsule.

Try vitamin E. Many women report that taking 400 IU of vitamin E daily helps prevent hot flushes. It doesn't work straight away, however. You may have to take vitamin E for at least 6 weeks before noticing any effects.

Alternative Therapies

Try essential oils. In addition to smelling great, essential oils such as rose, geranium and peppermint have cooling properties, says Dr Jane Buckle, an expert in holistic nursing. Put 6 to 8 drops of an essential oil in a water-filled small spray bottle. Keep the bottle by the bedside or in your bag, and spray it on your neck, chest and shoulders when you feel a sweat coming on.

Medical Options

Ask your doctor about medical treatments. Oestrogen is the best approach for hot flushes, but some women can't take oestrogen for medical reasons. A number of other medications may be helpful, says Dr Gass. A low-dose progesterone acts on the part of the central nervous system that controls body temperature. Some women get relief from clonidine tablets (Catapres).

when to see a doctor

If you have abnormally heavy bleeding or spotting between periods: make an appointment to see your doctor. These symptoms are often normal at the time of perimenopause, but they can also be caused by endometriosis, fibroids or even cancer.

If you experience hot flushes, vaginal dryness or other perimenopausal symptoms prior to the age of 40: about one in 100 women between the ages of 15 and 40 will experience premature ovarian failure, also known as 'early menopause'. You may need medical treatment to protect your bones and maintain fertility.

Yet another approach is to take antidepressants. Studies have shown that paroxetine (Seroxat), fluoxetine (Prozac) and venlafaxine (Effexor) may reduce the severity and duration of hot flushes.

OVERCOMING VAGINAL AND SEXUAL PROBLEMS

Just as your reproductive organs have a developmental stage at puberty, they also go through changes as you exit your childbearing phase. Your uterus, cervix and urinary tract slightly decrease in size, and the skin lining your reproductive organs begins to thin.

Declines in oestrogen affect the amount of blood flow to the pelvic area, as well as mucus production in the vagina. It's not uncommon for perimenopausal women to need lubrication, often for the first time, during sex. They also tend to get more vaginal or urinary tract infections.

None of this, however, means that you're going to enjoy sex less over the years. In fact menopause and beyond often bring the best lovemaking because couples grow in intimacy and confidence.

If you find that sex is compromised – either due to discomfort from physical changes or due to a lower libido – hormone therapy is one of the most powerful remedies. Here are some additional ways to deal with the changes.

Home Remedies

Switch to showers. Taking long baths removes lubricating oils from the skin. Quick showers, on the other hand, will help keep your skin soft and supple.

Use a water-soluble moisturizer. The most effective products you can buy for long-term management of vaginal dryness are labelled as vaginal moisturizers. They act directly on the tissue to make it less dry. Plus, they maintain a healthy acid balance in the vagina, which can help prevent infections. Some examples are Replens-MD and K-Y.

Use commercial lubricants. Vaginal lubricants such as Astroglide, Lubrin and Durex Sensilube will help prepare mucous membranes for intercourse. Apply the lubricant to your vaginal opening and to your partner's penis. Avoid lotions and oils that aren't marketed specifically for genital health, such as petroleum jelly or cocoa butter. They can actually increase friction and promote infection.

Revive your relationship. It's not uncommon for women to blame their hormones for a decline in libido, when what's really happening is a problem in the relationship. If the sex itself is a problem, you need to really talk about what will make you more comfortable or aroused. If you're growing apart emotionally, make an effort to invest more time with your partner in order to recapture the fun and intimacy that you shared earlier in the relationship.

Medical Options

Change contraceptives. If you are already using oral contraceptives at perimenopause, your remedy for a diminished libido may be as simple as switching to a different progestogen formula. Certain progestogens have 'androgenic' effects that boost sex drive; others can depress libido.

Ask your doctor about products that contain androgenic progestogens, such as levonorgestrel (Mirena – the coil or Logynon – a pill) or norithesterone (Norimin). Nonandrogenic formulations have norgestimate (Cilest) or desogestrel (Marvelon) as the key ingredient.

Consider topical oestrogen. Applying oestrogen cream, available by prescription, to the vaginal area will help improve tone and comfort. Some products are inserted outside the vagina; others are designed to treat vaginal dryness and

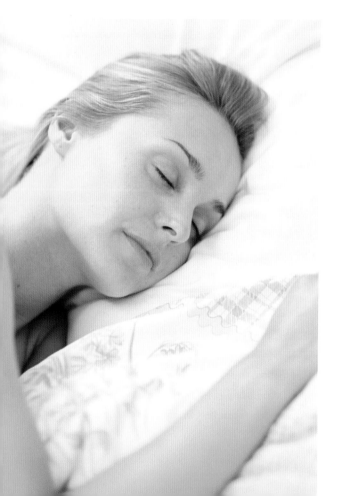

sensitivity – they come in the form of a ring, which is inserted in front of the cervix.

FEEL VITAL AGAIN

Some women have no specific physical complaints during the time of the perimenopause but may feel a general plummet in their energy or mood. 'Women at midlife tend to have a lot of irons in the fire,' says Dr Gass. 'They're caring for ageing parents or taking care of children and grandchildren. I advise women to take a step back and try to see how much stress they're experiencing.'

A minority of women may experience depression or anxiety due to hormone shifts, but it's more likely that multiple perimenopausal changes are having a snowball effect on your overall quality of life. Hot flushes, night sweats and menstrual discomfort, for example, can start a pattern of poor sleeping habits, which in turn can lead to malaise and moodiness, especially if you're too tired to keep up with regular exercise and other healthy lifestyle behaviours.

Before your mood or overall sense of vitality starts going downhill, it's essential to tackle individual symptoms as soon as they appear, says Dr Sadja Greenwood, an assistant clinical professor of obstetrics and gynaecology.

Home Remedies

Maintain regular sleep patterns. If night sweats or other perimenopausal complaints are keeping you up at night, you may experience disruptions in your natural sleep cycle. You may find yourself trying to compensate by snoozing late at weekends – but that can make it even harder to get back on track. It's important to go to bed and wake up at the same time every day. Maintaining a regular sleep/wake cycle helps minimize hormonal fluctuations, and you'll also feel more rested overall.

If you find that your sleep cycles have been disrupted, you may have to make a few changes. For example, dim the lights after sunset. It will help give your body the signal that it's time to unwind and begin preparing for sleep.

Make sure you're getting enough iron. Symptoms of iron deficiency include weakness, fatigue and low energy. Women who don't eat meat, or those who are experiencing heavy menstrual bleeding, are prime candidates for iron deficiency anaemia. Prevent this energy-draining situation by making sure that your daily supplement contains 100 per cent of the recommended daily allowance of 14.8 milligrams of iron.

In addition, ask your doctor to test your iron levels. If you're bleeding heavily each month, your doctor may recommend that you take even more iron than the recommended daily amount. You don't want to take extra iron unnecessarily, however. Excessive iron can cause just as many problems as too little.

Keep a worry book. Every day, take a few moments to write down frustrations and concerns that may be keeping you from getting all the rest you need. Just jotting them down may relieve some of the emotional pressure. So will outlining possible solutions – such as 'get organized tomorrow'.

Take a progesterone supplement. The body's production of progesterone declines as a woman approaches the perimenopause. This can be a problem because progesterone has a calming effect. When levels decline, women may experience irritability or insomnia. In fact, natural forms of progesterone were used as sedatives in the 1930s. Unfortunately, the synthetic progestogens in HRT and contraceptives might have the opposite effect and trigger anxiety and mood swings. One solution is to take a natural progesterone supplement, available in health food shops and pharmacies. Follow the instructions carefully and make sure that you purchase a product that contains pharmaceutical-grade progesterone. Your doctor can also prescribe a natural progesterone-containing gel called Crinone.

Medical Options

Have your thyroid tested. Low levels of thyroid hormones can drain your energy and lead to depression, while an overactive thyroid can produce feelings of anxiety and panic. Since thyroid hormones and oestrogen affect one another, it's likely that you'll need to have your thyroid medication (if you take it) adjusted at perimenopause, especially if you're undergoing HRT.

CHAPTER
22

Menopause

We think of oestrogen as affecting mainly the ovaries and uterus. But our bodies are really soaked in this reproductive hormone.

Blood vessels throughout the body contain oestrogen receptors, molecular docking sites that allow oestrogen to be delivered to the various tissues. Oestrogen helps regulate cholesterol levels, blood pressure, even the metabolism of certain nutrients. Oestrogen and other sex hormones play a role in the part of brain chemistry responsible for cognitive function, the sleep/wake cycle and moods. And oestrogen – or the lack of it – determines whether bones are strong or weak.

At the menopause, reproductive hormone levels plummet. We have less than half of the oestrogen that we had in our reproductive years, and the progesterone that once was released from the ovaries is nearly phased out. How can a woman survive without oestrogen and progesterone when nearly every tissue and organ in the body is affected by reproductive hormones?

Actually, women do very well. Even those who undergo hormone replacement therapy (HRT) are not actually replacing all of their sex hormones. They're only supplementing a small fraction of what used to circulate in their premenopausal bodies.

Menopause is a natural transition in a woman's life, says Dr Margery Gass, a professor of obstetrics and gynaecology. The reason the ovaries stop putting out massive quantities of oestrogen and progesterone is that the hormones are no longer needed for reproductive functions. After all, progesterone's main purpose is to service the uterus – either to stimulate a monthly period or to nurture a growing baby. If there aren't any more eggs, it's logical for progesterone levels to diminish. After menopause, oestrogen and other sex hormones continue to affect parts of the body that aren't involved with reproduction. That's why the ovaries and adrenal glands continue to produce maintenance levels of sex hormones – between 10 and 50 per cent of the amounts that were produced in reproductive years.

If the body needs additional oestrogen, it can produce extra amounts by recycling other hormones. Fat cells produce 'backup' oestrogen as well.

Of course, if illness or surgery has disabled your ovaries or adrenal glands, you will need to take supplemental hormones to maintain bone mass, healthy cholesterol levels and so on. For everyone else, it is a personal decision if you want to give your hormones a little help.

The decision to take supplemental hormones isn't a small one. Nor are the various questions surrounding the use of HRT easy to sort out. In the following pages, we'll take a look at the issues involved with hormone management. And since more than just hormonal changes occur at menopause, we'll guide you towards maximizing your personal fulfilment and all-around wellness.

Making the Mental Shift

There are good reasons why the body is programmed to reduce the production of hormones at the end of ovulation. In anthropological terms, menopause is of profound value to society, says Dr Sadja Greenwood, an assistant clinical professor of obstetrics and gynaecology.

In primitive cultures, such as the Hadza tribe of Northern Tanzania, postmenopausal women bring in 70 to 80 per cent of the food for the tribe while their daughters are busy nursing babies and rearing children. 'Even women in their sixties and seventies are doing hard labour, digging up tubers and carrying water for miles,' Dr Greenwood says.

Similarly, Western women are busier than ever at the menopause. Apart from grandmothering their children's children, they're often caring for older parents. This is also a time when careers and creativity are often at their peaks.

'One of the reasons why women make such valuable contributions to society after menopause is that they develop a sense that there's more to life than the daily grind,' says Dr Greenwood. 'They want to connect with nature and other people in a more profound way than ever.'

Here are a few ways to make the most of this exciting time.

Rise above ego. Statistically, many middle-aged men are interested in dating 20- and 30-something women. Some women find that they become invisible to men around the time of menopause.

This is no reflection of your own attractiveness or value. Instead of working harder to look younger, allow your self-worth to flow from within. You will find yourself needing less validation from others, and you'll be more satisfied on a spiritual level when you pay attention to your heart's longings and inner guidance. This is the time to join the trend of women going back to college at midlife, start the business that you always talked about or discover an entirely new personal passion.

Strengthen and renew female bonds. Girlfriends make every rite of passage more meaningful. When physical or emotional difficulties arrive, women have a special way of forming a circle of safety and love. If you catch yourself deprived of quality girlfriend time, you're never too old to organize a slumber party or sign up for a women's retreat where you stay up late, singing, drumming and telling stories of your life.

Volunteer. You don't need grandchildren to experience the life-affirming gift of sharing decades' worth of wisdom and talents. Not only does volunteering make life meaningful, but research shows that people who have a lot of human connections live twice as long as those who don't. Whether you're interested in comforting shelter animals, reading to primary school pupils or offering history tours of your town, you'll find plenty of volunteer opportunities. Look in your local newspaper. Or look at www.do-it.org.uk, the home of volunteering on the Web. Or try Australian Volunteer Search: www.volunteersearch.gov.au; in New Zealand: www.volunteeringnz.org.nz.

Focus on good posture. Due to the natural loss of muscle tone that happens with age, your abdomen *will* protrude more than it did in younger years, even if you exercise diligently, says Dr Gass. Hormone shifts and a downshifting of metabolism also encourage fat storage.

Yes, you need to watch how much you eat, and regular exercise is important, but you also need to accept that your figure is designed to change with age.

In fact, some postmenopausal women find it life affirming to decorate their homes with artwork that reflects the human figure in all shapes and sizes.

when to see a doctor

If you've started HRT and are experiencing breast pain, nausea, bloating or other side effects: call your doctor right away. Lowering the dose or switching to a different hormone may be all that's needed to resolve the problem.

If you're having breakthrough bleeding: it's common when women start HRT that combines oestrogen and progesterone – but it can also be caused by endometriosis or uterine cancer. You'll need a comprehensive examination by your doctor to make sure that you're healthy.

Whatever figure you have, good posture will make you look and feel more youthful. Make an effort to keep your head level, pull your shoulders back and walk tall. Rounded shoulders and a stooped back call attention to stomach imperfections and steal vitality.

Rethink Your Hormone Status Annually

If you were taking oral contraceptives during the perimenopause to manage premenstrual discomfort or erratic menstrual bleeding, once you hit the menopause the birth control pill is no longer necessary to shut off your system. Rather than oral contraceptives, you may wish to switch to lower doses of hormones in HRT. It will prevent problems that don't go away after menopause, such as vaginal dryness.

Whether you have any bothersome symptoms or not, the menopause is a call for every woman to evaluate her hormone management plan, says Dr Steven Petak, an associate professor of reproductive medicine and endocrinology.

'When your doctor first confirms that you are menopausal – and every annual period-free anniversary after that – you're going to want to decide if hormones help you meet your current health goals, especially the key areas like bone density and heart protection,' he says.

Between a fifth and a third of menopausal women choose HRT as an integral part of their long-term health goals. Another group decide that HRT is not necessary and conflicts with their health goals. The remaining group haven't really thought about supplement hormones and forgo treatment with HRT.

'Whatever you choose to do in the area of hormone management, be as informed as possible, and be specific about your needs. If you do that, you and your doctor are more likely to make the best decision for you,' says Dr Gass. The following steps are essential for making educated decisions about managing your hormones.

Review your current health status with your doctor. You have to determine your most pressing long-term health concerns. You can then match your goals with the current data on what hormones offer. In order to be specific, you'll need to complete the following:

- A complete physical checkup

- Personal and family health history, particularly concerning cancer and cardiovascular disease

- Baseline bone mineral density scan

- Complete lipid profile – total cholesterol, HDL (high-density lipoprotein), LDL (low-density lipoprotein) and triglycerides

- Smear or Pap test

- Mammogram

- Test for thyroid-stimulating hormone (TSH)

Rule out risks. The next specific question to ask is whether hormones are any kind of a threat, either because of a family history of certain illnesses or because of red flags in your current health reports. You need to abstain from taking HRT, or be closely monitored, if you have the following conditions.

- Breast and endometrial cancers, gallbladder disease, or other illnesses commonly triggered or aggravated by oestrogen

- A blood-clotting disorder

- Bleeding from the uterus that hasn't been evaluated

HORMONE REPLACEMENT STRATEGIES

If you are considering hormone replacement therapy (HRT), keep in mind that it can take some trial and error to find the regime that works best for you.

Dr Brian W. Walsh, an assistant professor of obstetrics and gynaecology at Harvard Medical School, offers the following advice.

Give it a short-term trial. Even though HRT is meant to be taken long term, there's nothing wrong with trying it for about 3 months to see if side effects will be an issue, says Dr Walsh. In addition, if new health information changes your thinking about HRT, you can stop at any time.

If you stop, stop gradually. Women who abruptly discontinue HRT may be faced with hot flushes, excessive menstrual bleeding, vaginal dryness or difficulties sleeping.

If you decide to phase out HRT, work with your doctor to reduce the dosage gradually.

- Hypertension
- Migraine and other headaches that are aggravated by hormones
- Smoking

Compare forms and dosages. When researching the pros and cons of taking hormones, keep in mind that generalizations about the effects of oestrogen and progesterone are often meaningless. Every formulation of hormones has different effects; how the hormones are taken makes a difference; and the dosage can have a significant impact. (To compare the subtle differences among hormone formulations, see the chart on page 209.)

'If you are leaning towards taking HRT, then it's necessary to be flexible and adopt the spirit of experimentation while you sample different forms and see what affects you best,' says Dr Petak.

For example, 'natural hormones' – those designed to more closely approximate the body's own chemistry – are reportedly less symptomatic in terms of mood changes, menstrual discomfort and headaches than the more synthetic brands and formulations that most doctors use. (Don't be confused by the terms 'natural' and 'synthetic': both types are created in laboratories.)

Doctors don't always recommend natural hormones, also known as custom formulations, because they haven't been as well-studied as other products and they tend to cost more. For some women, however, they're the only way to go. Other women actually fare better on synthetic versions – perhaps because the dosages and formulations may be more consistent than the natural formulations.

Weigh the Pros and Cons

Taking hormones isn't a guaranteed insurance package for your health. Whether or not you should take hormones, and the types of hormones that you take, will always be an educated guess on the part of you and your doctor. But the more educated you are, the less guessing you'll have to do. Hormone management requires well-rounded, careful research. The following review takes an in-depth look at what we currently know about what hormones can and cannot offer.

HORMONES AND CANCER RISKS

Excessive stimulation of an organ by hormones can result in tumour formation, and oestrogen is particularly active in breast tissue and the uterus.

In fact, oestrogen stimulates the lining of the uterus to grow so actively that it can increase the risk of endometrial cancer threefold. However, if you take progesterone along with oestrogen, you don't have this to worry about. By helping the uterine lining to thin out, progesterone actually has the opposite effect.

The risk of colon cancer is reduced when you take HRT. Research shows that taking oestrogen lowers your risk by as much as 40 per cent.

On the other hand, the risk of breast cancer is a very real concern. A large-scale study monitored women's breast cancer rates over a 10-year period. Women who stayed on HRT the whole time had almost double the rate of breast cancer as those who stayed on HRT for a shorter time.

In an analysis of more than 50 medical studies, the risk of breast cancer increased by 2.3 per cent each year in women using HRT. This review is one of several that have led experts to make the general conclusion that oestrogen causes a 'moderate' increase in breast cancer risk – essentially changing the risk from 10 women out of 10,000 per year to 13 women out of 10,000 per year.

Another landmark study was abruptly halted when its results revealed the breast cancer risk to be higher than previously estimated – for every 10,000 women, there were 8 more cases of breast cancer among those on HRT than among those who took placebos.

Each study is worth considering, but experts try to base recommendations on the pool of data as a whole. To put the risk in perspective, remember that the majority of women who get breast cancer are not taking hormones. Not taking oestrogen is no assurance that you aren't going to get cancer, says Dr Petak. Breast cancer has genetic causes and all sorts of other triggers besides oestrogen.

The kind of breast cancer that is associated with HRT tends to be the most treatable kind. In addition, research shows a correlation between the length of time on HRT and breast cancer risk. You have some control over your risk by limiting the number of years that you take HRT.

'You'll see all kinds of numbers, but we have enough to go on for general recommendations,' says Dr Petak. To balance your hormones and also protect against breast cancer, here's what doctors advise.

Limit HRT. The 'moderate' risk for breast cancer that appeared in the studies didn't clearly show up until women had been taking hormone replacement therapy for 10 years or longer, says

Dr Mary Jane Minkin, clinical professor of obstetrics and gynaecology at Yale University School of Medicine. If you want the benefits of HRT, such as strengthening bones, but want to minimize your risk for breast cancer, giving yourself a limited time on HRT is a reasonable compromise.

Don't focus only on breast cancer. While long-term HRT increases the risk for breast cancer, it can reduce the risk for other serious conditions.

When you're considering whether or not to

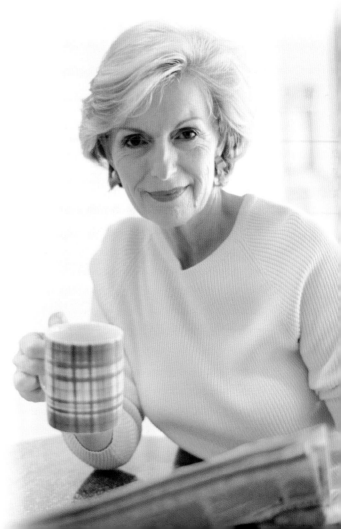

take HRT, it may be helpful to list all of the benefits – such as bone protection, fewer hot flushes, better sexual health, and possibly the prevention of colon cancer and Alzheimer's disease – on one side of a sheet of paper. On the other side, list the potential risks. If a moderately increased risk of breast cancer is the only downside, you may decide that the potential benefits of HRT make it worth doing.

Look deeper into family history. It's true that if you have the genetic mutation for breast cancer, your risk for getting the disease rises 50 per cent, even without taking oestrogen. But don't assume that your risk for cancer is unusually high just because your female relatives got it. What really matters is when they were diagnosed.

Women who develop breast cancer before menopause are more likely to have a genetic predisposition to the disease. If the women in your family developed breast cancer at an early age, that might be an argument to forego HRT.

Reduce progestogen. While the progestogen component of HRT has a protective effect against cancer of the uterus, recent evidence indicates that combined oestrogen–progestogen therapy may raise the possible risk for breast cancer more than taking oestrogen alone. To get the uterus-protecting benefits of progestogen while preventing the double risk factor of oestrogen plus progestogen, ask your doctor about taking progestogen less frequently, says Dr Minkin. With 'intermittent cyclical dosing', you may be advised to take progestogen every other month – or even every 3 months – while taking oestrogen daily.

Watch your alcohol intake. In a large study, researchers noted that the women who took hormones and consumed 'substantial' amounts of alcohol had an elevated risk for breast cancer. 'Substantial' is defined as 5 grams or more of alcohol daily – equivalent to 60 to 80 millilitres (2 to 3 fluid ounces) of whisky or 80 millilitres (3 fluid ounces) of wine. Whether or not you're on HRT, experts advise limiting alcohol intake to two to three drinks weekly.

Step up your breast screenings. The slightly elevated breast cancer risk that occurs when taking HRT is an important reason to keep up with breast self-examination, as well as with regular mammography (starting at 50). Keep in mind that HRT sometimes makes the breasts feel lumpier. HRT can also make it difficult to get an accurate mammogram reading; the treatment contributes to a denser concentration of cells in some women's breasts. Make sure that all of your doctors (and mammography radiographers) know that you're taking HRT.

HOW HORMONES AFFECT YOUR HEART

Protecting the heart has been a major justification for taking supplemental hormones after the menopause. However, the latest recommendation is that women at risk for heart disease should take one of the cholesterol-lowering drugs known as statins rather than HRT for heart protection after menopause. And several recent studies support the view that HRT won't help all female hearts.

'It's not that HRT isn't valuable,' says Dr Margo A. Denke, an associate professor of internal medicine. 'It eases menopausal symptoms and can protect bones during and shortly after menopause. But it just doesn't appear to prevent heart disease as well as we had hoped.' On the other hand, a significant body of research shows that statin drugs do cut cholesterol and prevent heart attacks.

If you're already taking HRT, should you switch to a statin? Here's how to tell.

- Stick with HRT if you want relief from menopausal symptoms, if your cholesterol is normal and if you're concerned about bone health.

- Add a statin if you fit the description above but you have high cholesterol that hasn't responded to dietary changes. Adding a statin drug will get your cholesterol under control.

- Switch to a statin if you have high cholesterol, if you're postmenopausal and if you're taking HRT just for heart protection.

HOW HORMONES AFFECT YOUR BONES

One in three women over 50 in the UK has osteoporosis. Worldwide, the lifetime risk of an osteoporotic fracture for a woman is 30 to 40 per cent, while for men the figure drops to about 13 per cent. It's no coincidence. Oestrogen has a tremendous effect on the strength of the skeleton. It helps the intestines absorb calcium, and it helps the kidneys hoard this important mineral. It also stimulates the production of vitamin D, which helps the bones take up calcium.

Oestrogen also plays a key role in bone remodelling – the process by which the bones rebuild themselves over time. When oestrogen levels decline at menopause, the bones begin to lose density and mass at an accelerated rate. By the age of 60, women can lose 15 to 30 per cent of peak bone mass. This decline starts at around the age of 30 but becomes much more aggressive at menopause. Women can lose 3 to 5 per cent of their bone mass annually.

The diet and exercise recommendations in chapter 27 are essential for bone protection.

If you already have osteoporosis or have a high risk for developing it, your doctor may advise treatments other than hormone replacement therapy. But for most women, HRT may offer valuable benefits for bone protection. Other steps to protect your bones include:

Get the best tests. There are several ways to measure bone mineral density. Those heel or wrist scans that may be offered at your local health club are a good place to start – but keep in mind that the most serious injuries are hip and spinal fractures. If you have high risk factors for osteoporosis, you'll need to ask for tests that measure bone density at the hip, spine and wrist. An X-ray test called DEXA (dual energy X-ray absorptiometry), which can detect bone loss at an early stage, is your best choice.

Consider adding testosterone to HRT. Oestrogen may not be the only sex hormone that helps protect the bones. Higher levels of testosterone in the body have been linked to higher levels of bone density. One study that compared the use of estradiol (a kind of oestrogen) with estradiol plus testosterone found significantly greater increases in bone density in those using the combined therapy.

'We're not certain if the testosterone itself is benefiting the bones, or if testosterone is converting to oestrogen,' says Dr Petak. Experts don't recommend adding testosterone to HRT just for bone health.

Because long-term safety hasn't been proved, testosterone isn't recommended for routine use. But if you have other health issues, such as depressed libido, the addition of testosterone to HRT may boost testosterone levels to a more normal female range.

Take ipriflavone as a fallback. This is a laboratory-derived version of isoflavones, bone-protecting compounds that are found in soya foods. Ipriflavone can strengthen bones without exerting hormonelike effects on the breasts and uterus.

Some small studies point to ipriflavone's ability to prevent bone breakdown and increase bone density. 'The benefit is probably equivalent to taking a very small dose of oestrogen,' says Dr Bruce Ettinger, an ipriflavone researcher.

The recommended dose is 600 milligrams daily, combined with 1,000 milligrams of calcium. It's safe, though you may experience bloating, diarrhoea or stomach irritation. Ipriflavone supplements are available at health food shops and some pharmacies.

Keep up with exercise. In a 5-year study, women who did high-impact, weight-bearing exercise three times weekly gained or maintained bone density while also building muscle and improving balance. Women in the same study who didn't follow the exercise recommendations lost bone density.

Feeling Good Overall

The potential benefits of HRT are wide-ranging. It may play a role in boosting libido, preventing middle-age weight gain, maintaining memory and improving overall vitality, says Dr Gass.

Hormones are hardly a fountain of youth, she adds. While some women experience an extra 'glow' when taking supplemental hormones, not everyone does.

So far, HRT has been proven to do only three things: improve hot flushes, relieve vaginal dryness and improve bone density. While hormones may provide other benefits, women always have to weigh the potential downsides, such as the increased risk of blood clots or breast cancer.

As long as the potential benefits of HRT add up to a happier, healthier life, it's certainly worth considering. But it's not a panacea, and there are times when it's not the best choice. For example:

- If your main health concern is improving cholesterol, other medication, such as the statins, should be your first choice.

- If you already have osteoporosis, you should take alendronate, risedronate, raloxifene or calcitonin, not hormones. HRT should not be used as the first line of treatment for osteoporosis.

- If you already have heart disease, don't turn to HRT.

Your Guide to Menopause Management Options

There are dozens of types of HRT. So if one doesn't suit you, another might. This at-a-glance guide can help you sort through your options with your doctor.

Oral Oestrogens

Product	Main Roles	Unique Benefits	Potential Disadvantages
Estradiol (e.g. Progynova, FemTab, Elleste-Solo, Zumenon) **Estropipate** (Harmogen) **Conjugated equine oestrogens** (e.g.Premarin)	Relieve hot flushes Relieve vaginal dryness Relieve urinary complaints Increase bone mass	Raise beneficial HDL cholesterol and lower LDL Some studies suggest lower risk for Alzheimer's disease and diabetes Might prevent gum disease and improve skin tone	Side effects include bloating, breast tenderness, headaches, nausea and irregular bleeding Risk of blood clots Risk of breast and uterine cancers Raise triglyceride level

Oestrogen Nasal Sprays

Product	Main Roles	Unique Benefits	Potential Disadvantages
Estradiol (e.g. Aerodiol)	Same as oral formulations	Same as oral formulations	Can cause nosebleeds in some people

Oestrogen Injections

Product	Main Roles	Unique Benefits	Potential Disadvantages
Custom formulations	Same as oral formulations	Same as oral formulations	Erratic hormone levels make them unpopular form of HRT

Transdermal Oestrogen Patches

Product	Main Roles	Unique Benefits	Potential Disadvantages
Estradiol (e.g Fematrix, Estraderm, Menorest, Evorel, Elleste-Solo MX)	Relieve hot flushes Relieve vaginal dryness Relieve urinary complaints Increase bone mass	May help control blood pressure and blood vessel constriction More even hormone levels than oral forms Less frequent reported side effects such as headache, nausea and mood swings Shown to reduce depression in clinically depressed, post-menopausal women	Most common side effects include bloating, breast tenderness, headaches, irregular bleeding (blood clot risk not as high as with oral forms) Can irritate skin at site of application Patch can fall off

continued

Topical Oestrogen Formulations

Product	Main Roles	Unique Benefits	Potential Disadvantages
OESTROGEN CREAMS: **Estradiol** (e.g. Oestrogel, Sandrena) **Estropipate** (e.g. Hormogen) **Conjugated equine oestrogens** (e.g. Premarin)	Relieve vaginal dryness and vaginal atrophy	Faster vaginal symptom relief than with oral and patch oestrogens Less breast and uterus cell proliferation than with oral and patch forms Estradiol products may also protect against urinary infections	Can be messy Not approved for hot flush relief or for bone and heart protection benefits
OESTROGEN RING: **Estradiol** (e.g. Menoring 50)	Relieves vaginal dryness and vaginal atrophy Prevents and treats urinary infections	Low-fuss method that doesn't require daily routine of oral and vaginal methods Doesn't have to be used with progesterone	Isn't approved for hot flush relief

Custom Oestrogen Formulations

Product	Main Roles	Unique Benefits	Potential Disadvantages
Estriol/estrone/17-beta estradiol combination (e.g. Hormonin) **Estriol cream** (e.g. Ovestin)	Same as other oral and transdermal oestrogens	Often recommended by natural health care practitioners for having fewer side effects and health risks Estriol cream doesn't need to be accompanied by progesterone to protect the uterus	Custom formulations lack thorough testing and assurance of reliability Prescription can be made up only at pharmacy specializing in compounding

Synthetic Progestogens

Product	Main Roles	Unique Benefits	Potential Disadvantages
Medroxyprogesterone acetate (e.g. Provera) **Norethisterone** (e.g. Micronor HRT) **Norethisterone acetate** (e.g. Evorel) **Norgestrel** (e.g. Cyclo Progynova) **Levonorgestrel IUD** (e.g. Mirena) **Dydrogesterone** (e.g. Duphaston)	Protect uterus from overstimulation from oestrogen Relieve oestrogen-dominated conditions, including fibrocystic breasts, endometriosis, ovarian cysts and uterine fibroids	Norgestrel and norethisterone can help reduce breakthrough bleeding	Associated with mood changes, depression and anxiety Side effects include fluid retention, headaches, breast tenderness Counteract beneficial cholesterol effects of oestrogen replacement therapy

'Natural' Progesterone

Product	Main Roles	Unique Benefits	Potential Disadvantages
Progesterone vaginal gel (e.g. Crinone)	Relieves hot flushes Normalizes menstrual cycle Relieves PMS complaints in perimenopausal women	Sufficient progesterone to protect uterus from oestrogen stimulation Reports of 'emotional boost' benefit Decrease in headaches, depression and mood swings when compared with synthetic progestogens Doesn't produce messy discharge	Can cause drowsiness

Combination Oestrogen/Progesterone Products

Product	Main Roles	Unique Benefits	Potential Disadvantages
Estradiol/ norethisterone acetate (e.g. Adgyn Combi, Novofem, Kliovance) **Conjugated equine oestrogen/ medroxyprogesterone** (e.g. Premique, Prempak-C, Tridestra) **Estradiol/levongestrel** (e.g. Nuvelle, FemSeven Conti, FemSeven Sequi)	Relieve hot flushes Relieve vaginal dryness Relieve urinary complaints Increase bone mass Protect uterus	Simpler regime than with separate products	Most common side effects include bloating, breast tenderness, headaches, mood changes and nausea Breakthrough bleeding more common in combined products
Tribolone (e.g. Livial)	Combines oestrogenic and progestogenic activity with weak androgenic activity	Good for hot flushes Can help protect against osteoporosis (but not as first line treatment).	Can cause weight gain and increased facial hair May encourage breakthrough bleeding

continued

Androgens ('Male Hormones')

Product	Main Roles	Unique Benefits	Potential Disadvantages
Mesterolone (e.g. Pro-Viron) **Testosterone undeconate pills** (e.g. Restandol) **Testosterone injections** (e.g. Sustanton, Virormone) **Testosterone implants** (e.g. Testosterone Organon) **Transdermal matrix testosterone patch** (e.g. Andropatch, Testogel)	Androgen-containing products for treatment of hot flushes in women who aren't helped by oestrogen alone Increased sexual desire, arousal and general sexual enjoyment	Offer some protection against bone loss May also increase energy, improve mood and help manage weight Helpful for maintaining lean muscle mass after menopause	Inappropriate doses can lead to male features (body hair, lower voice, muscle weight gain), acne and feelings of aggression, agitation or depression Can severely disrupt cholesterol levels

Osteoporosis Drugs

Product	Main Roles	Unique Benefits	Potential Disadvantages
SELECTIVE OESTROGEN RECEPTOR MODULATORS: **Raloxifene** (e.g. Evista)	Spine fracture preventive Treatment for osteoporosis Act as oestrogens in some tissues and anti-oestrogens in others	Produce favourable changes in blood lipids that protect against cardiovascular disease; don't stimulate the breasts and the uterus (common with oestrogens); may reduce breast cancer risk; don't need to be accompanied by use of progestogens	Increased risk of blood clots (also common with oestrogens) Generally not beneficial for treating hot flushes and other symptoms that oestrogen relieves
BISPHOSPHO-NATES: **Alendronate** (e.g. Fosamax) **Risedronate** (e.g. Actonel) **Disodium Etidronate** (e.g. Didronel)	Proven to reduce risk of spine and hip fracture Treatment for osteoporosis	The only drugs proven to specifically reduce hip fracture risk	No effect on hot flushes or other symptoms
SPRAY OR INJECTION: **Calcitonin** (e.g. Forcalcitonin Miacalcic)	Slows bone loss, increases spinal bone density and relieves pain associated with hip fractures	Favoured for women 5 or more years past menopause, particularly women who want to reduce spinal fracture risk	Injection of calcitonin can cause allergic reaction, flushing of face and hands, urinary frequency, nausea and skin rash; calcitonin spray can cause runny nose No effect on hot flushes or other symptoms or hormone-related health risks

Over-the-counter Hormone-regulating Products

Product	Main Roles	Unique Benefits	Potential Disadvantages
Black cohosh (Remifemin and various other herbal product brands)	Hot flush relief, vaginal dryness treatment, hormone-related mood swing relief and menstrual cycle regulation	Not associated with risks of oestrogen-sensitive cancer May protect against age-related memory decline May enhance sex life	Recommended only for 6-month intervals and without the use of HRT; potency and reliability not regulated; may produce gastrointestinal side effects
Phyto-oestrogen/ isoflavone supplements (Promensil, Estroven and various other brands)	Recommended to lower cholesterol and reduce risk of cardiovascular disease May help relieve hot flushes and vaginal dryness	Act similar to body's own oestrogen and may provide protection against bone loss, heart disease and breast cancer	Not proven safe to use in conjunction with HRT Effectiveness and long-term safety not established Over-consumption may stimulate breast and uterus; similar cancer risks to HRT
Soya foods (soya nuts, soya milk, tofu, various brands)	Recommended to lower cholesterol and reduce risk of cardiovascular disease; may help relieve hot flushes and vaginal dryness	Act similar to body's own oestrogen and may provide protection against bone loss, heart disease and breast cancer	Effectiveness and long-term safety not established Over-consumption can stimulate breast and uterus, creating similar cancer risks to HRT
7-isopropoxy-isoflavone ('Natural Ipriflavone', various brands)	Mild bone loss prevention and bone density increase	May lower cholesterol and offer cancer protection; does not appear to have hormone-like effects on the breasts and uterus	Bone protection milder than prescription options
Progesterone (wild yam or soya cream, various brands)	Hot flush relief; regulates menstrual cycles; protects uterus when oestrogen is used	None	Potencies and reliability not regulated
Agnus castus (vitex or chasteberry)	Relieves vaginal dryness, improves libido in women with elevated prolactin levels and curbs PMS in perimenopausal women	Can enhance progesterone while reducing prolactin hormone	Potency and reliability not regulated
DHEA	Converted by body to testosterone to improve libido, general vitality	None	Same risk as with prescription androgens Efficacy and ability of body to absorb DHEA unclear

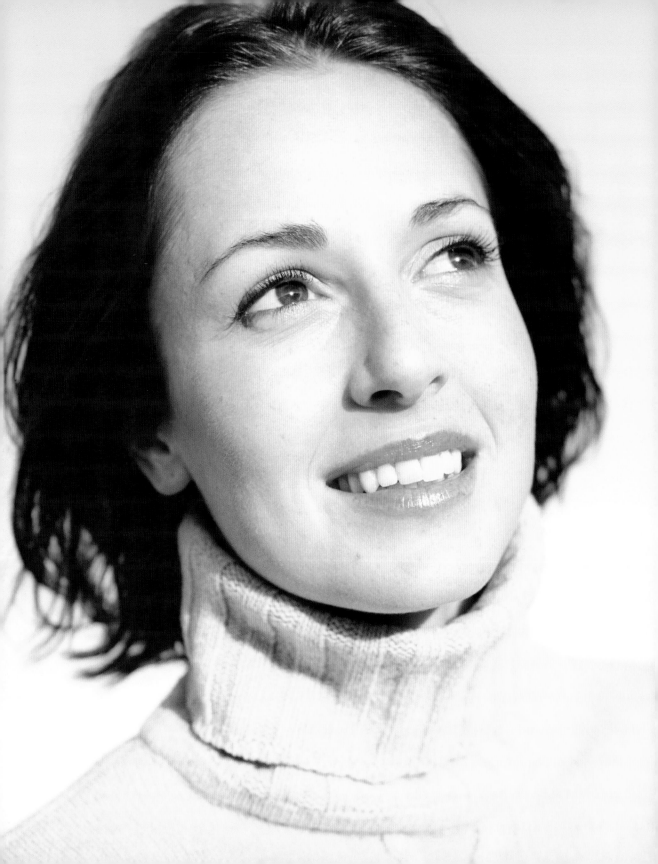

PART 4

Primary care: essential protection against major health threats

CHAPTER
23

Heart Disease

If cancer tops your list of health worries, you're not alone. Studies have shown that women tend to overestimate their chances of getting cancer and they fail to think enough about another serious health threat: heart disease.

Deaths from stroke, heart attack or other forms of cardiovascular disease are second only to deaths from cancer.

The good news is that heart disease is nearly always preventable. Studies have shown that women who follow a healthy lifestyle – refraining from smoking, exercising regularly, eating healthy foods and so on – can slash their risk of heart disease by 82 per cent.

Even if you're premenopausal, don't put off taking care of your heart. Around one-quarter of deaths from heart disease are in people under 65.

It's true that a woman's risk of heart disease increases as she gets older. After the menopause, when the body's production of oestrogen declines, there's an increase in atherosclerosis – the accumulation of fatty deposits in the arteries that can reduce blood flow and increase the risk of heart-damaging clots. But atherosclerosis actually starts much earlier, even in the teenage years.

Many women have the sense that they don't need to worry about heart disease until after the menopause. But they may be ignoring risk factors that could be treated, such as high blood pressure or high cholesterol, because they don't think they have to worry about them yet.

Here's what leading cardiologists say women should be doing, right now, to protect their hearts.

Lifestyle Strategies

Maintain a healthy weight. Many of us put on a little weight over time, but those extra pounds can substantially boost your risk for developing heart disease. Women who are overweight are much more likely to develop diabetes – and diabetes is one of the main risk factors for heart disease. Obesity also increases cholesterol and puts more strain on the heart.

Most women who are overweight know it. However, while the *amount* of extra weight is important, the way it's distributed on your frame also makes a difference. Doctors often use a guide called body mass index (BMI) to determine how close you are to your ideal weight. You'll find a detailed guide to calculating BMI on page 83. For now, just remember that your BMI should fall

216

somewhere between 18.5 and 24.9, and your waist should measure less than 35 inches. If your waistline is larger than that and if your BMI is above 25, it's time to get serious about losing weight.

If you follow the guidelines in chapter 5, you'll find that losing weight doesn't have to be an all-consuming chore – and the more you lose, the healthier your heart will be.

Get serious about exercise. Every woman knows that exercise is important for health, but people don't always realize just how damaging a sedentary lifestyle can be. Women who are sedentary have about twice the risk of heart disease as those who are physically active. Put another way, not getting regular exercise is potentially as harmful as smoking or having high cholesterol.

Obviously, vigorous activity is great for your heart – but what if you're not a serious athlete? Studies have shown that even modest levels of activity can make a real difference. Women who walk, ride a bike or exercise at the gym for 30 minutes most days of the week can achieve nearly the same health benefits as those who go all out.

In fact, you don't even have to get the exercise all at once. While one longer daily walk of 30 minutes is preferable, women who exercise three times daily for 10 minutes each time will get measurable cardiovascular benefits, too.

You don't even have to do 'formal' exercise to protect your heart. Vacuuming can be exercise if you do it vigorously. So can gardening, doing dishes or making the beds. Look for opportunities to exercise throughout the day. This might involve

ANGINA: HEED THIS WARNING SIGN

About 2 million people in the UK suffer from angina, a condition that may cause chest pain or other symptoms that occur when narrowed blood vessels prevent the heart from getting all the blood and oxygen that it needs. Women are nearly twice as likely as men to get angina. In a way, angina may be a good thing because it's often a clue that a woman is developing heart disease.

'Often there's not actually a sensation you would call "pain" with angina, but rather a deep discomfort or tightness under the breastbone that can radiate up to the shoulder or jaw,' says Dr Rose Marie Robertson, a cardiologist. The lack of sufficient blood flow to the heart, which causes angina symptoms, can also result in fatigue or shortness of breath. It usually comes on when women are doing something physical and subsides when they're at rest. 'Hopefully, angina will lead a woman to seek medical attention before

things become worse,' she notes. If you experience any of the pain or other symptoms associated with angina and they last for more than 5 minutes, call an ambulance – you could be having a heart attack and need medical attention right away.

Angina doesn't always mean that surgery or angioplasty is needed. It can often be treated with medication, but some women may need surgery to improve blood flow to the heart.

walking around the perimeter of your office building in your lunch hour, taking stairs instead of lifts and walking to the corner shop instead of hopping in the car and driving. Taking a dog for a walk is great, too.

If you smoke, do your best to stop. The risk of heart disease in smokers is two to four times higher than in non-smokers. As every ex-smoker knows, quitting is hard – it may be the hardest thing you've ever done. But the payoff is dramatic. If you haven't been able to quit smoking on your own, talk to your doctor about starting a stop-smoking programme. (For more information on getting cigarettes out of your life, see chapter 7.)

Consider aspirin. Studies have shown that this over-the-counter painkiller 'thins' the blood and reduces the risk of heart-damaging blood clots. In a recent study, Italian researchers looked at nearly 4,500 men and women. Those who took 100 milligrams of aspirin daily were 44 per cent less likely to die of heart disease.

The one problem with aspirin is that it may cause stomach upset and increase the risk of bleeding. Researchers have found that enteric aspirin – coated to protect the digestive tract – dissolves in the small intestine instead of in the stomach and is less likely to cause side effects than normal aspirin.

While the dosage of aspirin used in the Italian study may be different from the dosages that are

GOOD NEWS FOR CHOCOLATE LOVERS

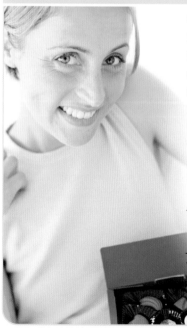

Who says heart-healthy eating has to be dull? Researchers have found that chocolate contains chemical compounds called antioxidants, which prevent harmful oxygen molecules in the body from damaging cholesterol – the process that makes it more likely to stick to artery walls.

Chocolate is so effective, in fact, that it blocks free radicals better than green tea, grape juice or blueberries – all of which are potent antioxidants. As a bonus, the active compounds in chocolate, called flavonoids, make the blood 'thinner' and may reduce the risk of harmful clots in the arteries.

Of course, chocolate is high in calories as well as fat. While it may have some benefits for women, it's hardly as nutritious as fresh vegetables, legumes or other wholesome foods.

The key is moderation. For the average person who's physically fit, having an occasional cup of cocoa or a bar of chocolate can be part of a healthy diet.

commonly available in other countries, doctors often recommend taking a 75-milligram dose – the amount found in low-dose aspirin – once daily, particularly if you have already experienced a heart attack or have other risk factors. Of course, consult with your doctor before beginning any aspirin regime.

Nutritional Treatments

Eat lots of fruit and vegetables every day. Women who follow this simple advice can dramatically reduce their risk for heart disease. What makes fruit and vegetables so powerful? They're packed with antioxidants – powerful plant chemicals that block the effects of free radicals, harmful oxygen molecules in the body that make cholesterol more likely to stick to artery walls. Fresh fruit and vegetables are high in fibre, which helps remove cholesterol from the body. They're also filling, which means that women will be less likely to fill up on other, less healthy foods.

According to the Department of Health, women should eat at least five servings each of fruit and vegetables daily. 'It's so simple, it's unbelievable,' says Dr Mosca.

Cut back on fat. This includes cooking oils, butter and lard, as well as fatty foods such as red meats, fast foods and rich desserts and snacks.

WHAT WORKS FOR ME

DR LORI J. MOSCA, an associate professor of medicine and director of preventive cardiology, has seen too many women suffering, unnecessarily, from heart disease. In her own life, she does everything possible to keep her heart and arteries healthy.

I definitely practise what I preach in terms of heart health. No matter how busy the family gets, we have a couple of priorities. We sit down every night and eat well together – and we exercise together, too.

We always cook meals that are heart healthy. The meals might include salad, soup and a main course – something like a stir-fry made with garlic, olives, capers, broccoli and chicken, served on pasta.

One trick I've learned is to do a lot of cooking on Sundays. I make things like soup or pasta sauce and store them in plastic containers. That way, if we're stretched for time during the week, we don't have to cook hamburgers. We can take something out of the freezer, make a quick salad and have a nutritious meal.

I always find time to exercise. I work out in the mornings before I wake my two boys. As a competitive triathlete, I do 20 minutes of swimming, 20 minutes of cycling, and 30 to 40 minutes on the treadmill. One day a week, I do strength training, and another day I take a stretching class. I also swim with my kids regularly, and I ride a bike with my husband.

Exercise helps me unwind, too. Sometimes I run through the park near our home and listen to the birds. It's so serene. I love the feeling of the sun on my back and the wind through my hair.

The fats in foods – especially saturated fats and trans fatty acids – raise your blood cholesterol levels and increase the risk of heart disease.

Women should limit total fat intake to 25 per cent of total calories – 20 per cent is even better. In addition, do everything you can to restrict your intake of saturated fat – the kind found in red meat, full fat milk and other animal foods – to no more than 7 per cent of total calories.

Study after study has shown that women who limit their consumption of animal foods and fill up on fruit and vegetables can dramatically lower the risk of heart disease.

Follow the Mediterranean example. Even though people in Italy, Greece and other Mediterranean countries consume more fat than other Westerners, their rates of heart disease are a fraction of what they are in those countries. What are they doing differently?

For one thing, they consume very little saturated fat. They enjoy meat, but they have much smaller portions than we do. Much of the fat in their diets comes from olive oil, which contains heart-healthy monounsaturated fats. They also eat large amounts of whole grains, fresh fruit and vegetables and other plant foods. As a result, the

Mediterranean diet is among the healthiest in the world.

Sip a little wine with meals. Or pour a glass of grape juice. They contain chemical compounds called flavonoids, which have been shown to reduce fatty buildups in the arteries and reduce the risk of heart disease.

Sprinkle some flaxseed (linseed) on your cereal. This nutty-tasting grain is rich in alpha linolenic acid, which helps to prevent blood-blocking buildups in the arteries. Women are advised to have at least 2 tablespoons of ground flaxseed daily.

Eat more fish. It's among the most powerful strategies for preventing heart disease. One study found that men who ate mackerel, herring, wild salmon or other fish several times a week were 34 per cent less likely to die from heart disease than those who ate less. The results are assumed to apply to women as well.

Experts recommend that women eat fish twice a week. If you don't like fish, it's fine to take fish oil supplements. Look for products that contain docosahexaenoic acid, or DHA. The recommended dose is 300 milligrams daily.

Take heart-healthy nutrients. Women who eat a nutritious diet will get most of the nutrients that they need for long-term heart health – but supplements can provide extra insurance. Women are advised to take the following:

- **Vitamin E.** Take 200 IU daily. If you have a high risk for heart disease – you're a smoker, for example, or have a family history of heart disease – take 400 IU. Vitamin E helps prevent cholesterol from sticking to artery walls.

- **Vitamin C.** Take 500 milligrams daily. Like vitamin E, it helps prevent fatty accumulations in the arteries. It also lowers levels of Lp(a), a type of blood fat that's harmful for the heart. If you are on cholesterol-lowering medication, check with your doctor before taking vitamin C supplements.

- **B vitamins.** They help lower levels of homocysteine, an amino acid that increases the risk of high cholesterol and artery disease. The advice is to take 800 micrograms of folic acid daily; 10 micrograms of vitamin B_{12}; and 10 milligrams of vitamin B_6.

- **Coenzyme Q_{10}.** It boosts the heart's pumping ability – but a number of medications, including antidepressants and cholesterol-lowering drugs, can deplete coenzyme Q_{10} from the body. Whether or not you're using other medication, it's a good idea to take 100 milligrams of coenzyme Q_{10} daily.

Mind-body Techniques

Keep stress under control. Studies have shown that women with high levels of stress in their lives may have a higher risk of heart disease.

THE COUPLES CONNECTION

Marriage is about sharing – everything from tackling the daily chores and caring for the children to paying the mortgage.

Now there's some evidence that sharing may go further than anyone imagined. If your husband has heart disease, there's a good chance that your risk for getting it is also high.

In one study, researchers surveyed 177 couples 2 months after the husband had either had a heart attack or undergone open-heart surgery. They found that even though wives didn't share the same physical risk factors as their husbands – they were unlikely to have high cholesterol or elevated blood pressure, for example – they often shared unhealthy lifestyle habits, such as smoking or being overweight.

In some cases, the wives had even greater risks than their husbands after the initial hospitalization because they didn't always join their husbands in adopting heart-healthy habits. After the hospitalizations, in fact, the women were twice as likely as the men to continue smoking.

Of course, just as couples may share bad habits, they can also work together as a team to reverse them. It may not be easy to change these kinds of risky behaviours, but when couples work together, it's probably easier to do.

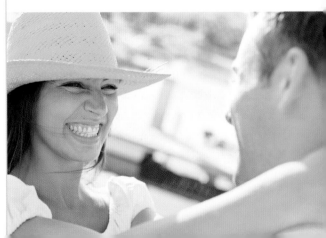

You can't eliminate stress, of course, but you can take steps to keep it under control – by exercising, practising yoga or meditation, or simply taking some deep breaths at the end of the day.

Accept what you can't change. Stress itself doesn't necessarily increase the risk of heart disease – it's how you respond to stress. Many of the things we get stressed out about just aren't that important. You have to step back and ask yourself, 'Am I going to let this bother me or not?'

Take a holiday. A recent study showed that men who took annual holidays were less likely to die of heart disease than those who kept their noses to the grindstone. The same applies to women. It makes sense because few things reduce stress more quickly than taking a holiday. In addition, holidays are a good time to spend quality time with family and friends, and studies have shown that maintaining social connections is an important strategy for keeping the heart healthy.

Let go of anger. The same goes for hostility and irritability. If you're always on edge and ready to snap at people or overreact to difficult situations, your heart may be paying the price.

Studies show that the less angry and hostile you are, the less your blood pressure responds when you're provoked. Having a positive, optimistic view of the world is clearly good for you.

Get in touch with your spiritual side. Research has shown that people who are spiritual have a lower risk of heart disease than those who don't practise a religion or cultivate spiritual beliefs.

Spirituality provides important support in many ways. It allows you to take a bad event and put it in a different perspective. It allows you to have less fear and anxiety, and it provides solace. Going to church also performs an important social function by providing a sense of community.

Medical Options

Many of the things that increase the risk of heart disease, such as smoking, putting on weight or not getting enough exercise, are easy for women to recognize – and reverse – on their own. But other types of risk factors are 'silent' – you won't know you have them unless you work with your doctor.

The first step in taking action against heart disease is to identify all your risk factors, but it is clear that many women have nowhere near the awareness that they need.

Some risk factors you can't change, of course. If you have a family history of heart disease, there's not much you can do about it. But other risk factors can be controlled – if you know you have them. That's why it's important to discuss your concerns about heart disease with your doctor.

Don't wait for your doctor to bring it up either. Many doctors aren't aware that women, including premenopausal women, can have a high risk for heart disease. Ask your doctor what your risk factors are and what you can do about them.

Women are often amazed to learn that they have heart disease, but it can often be predicted years or even decades before it occurs. But if you don't know you have high cholesterol or high blood pressure, you'll have missed the opportunity to prevent future problems.

Get regular blood pressure checks. High blood pressure has been called a 'silent' disease because it doesn't cause symptoms at first. By the time it does cause symptoms, damage to the arteries has already occurred. It's essential to get your blood pressure checked regularly because high blood pressure boosts the heart's workload and greatly increases the risk of heart disease and other cardiovascular problems.

You want your blood pressure to be ideally under 140/85.

If your blood pressure has climbed to 160/90 or higher, it's essential to take action – by exercising,

VITAMIN ALERT!

If you take a statin and niacin, don't also take antioxidants over and above the amount in your multivitamin. (Antioxidants prevent harmful oxygen molecules in the body from damaging artery walls.)

In a new study, taking high-dose antioxidants reduced to zero the benefits of taking the cholesterol drugs simvastatin and niacin for raising the type of HDL that actually clears your arteries, called HDL2. But subjects taking the same drugs without antioxidants showed a healthy gain in levels of beneficial HDL2 of 42 per cent. High doses of antioxidants in this study were 1,000 milligrams of vitamin C, 800 IU of vitamin E, 100 micrograms of selenium and 25 milligrams of beta-carotene.

limiting salt intake, losing weight if you need to or taking medication – and see your doctor.

Keep an eye on cholesterol. If you were to do only a few things to protect your heart, maintaining healthy levels of cholesterol would certainly be near the top of the list.

Cholesterol, also known as lipids, enters the bloodstream every time you eat. Over time, the fatty molecules are taken up into artery walls, where they restrict blood flow, promote the development of blood clots, and greatly increase the risk of heart attack and other cardiovascular conditions.

According to the latest guidelines, here's what you should strive for.

- **Total cholesterol:** Keep it under 5 mmol/litre. Keep in mind, though, that a total cholesterol reading over 5 mmol/litre may not be a bad thing if your HDLs are high (for more on this, see below).

- **LDL:** It stands for low-density lipoprotein, the 'bad' cholesterol. Ideally, your LDL should be below 3 mmol/litre. Note that not all labs currently test for LDL and HDL separately.

- **HDL:** Aim for more than 1.15 mmol/litre.

- **Triglycerides:** Keep them under 1.5 mmol/litre.

Many doctors believe that the ratio of total cholesterol to HDL is more accurate than total cholesterol alone as a marker for heart disease. To determine your ratio, divide your total cholesterol reading by your HDL number. The Framingham Cardiovascular Institute recommends a total cholesterol/HDL ratio below 4.

Keep in mind that these guidelines are variable, depending on other risk factors you may have. If your doctor says your risk for heart disease is low to moderate, for example, it may be acceptable to have a higher LDL reading. If you have multiple risk factors for heart disease, on the other hand, you'll want to keep LDL lower.

These days, there's no reason for most people to have high cholesterol. Apart from lifestyle changes, such as lowering your intake of saturated fat, there are a number of very effective cholesterol-lowering drugs that can bring the numbers down to a healthy level.

Think twice about hormone replacement therapy (HRT). 'In healthy women, we don't recommend HRT solely for the purpose of preventing heart disease, but there are many other

when to see a doctor

If you experience chest pain, or if you have fullness or tightness in your chest, are suddenly dizzy, fatigued or nauseated, or if you're having trouble breathing or are cold and clammy: call 999 immediately. These are the most common signs of a heart attack in men and women. Women are more likely than men to have less typical symptoms, such as fatigue or shortness of breath alone.

reasons to take it,' Dr Mosca says. Supplemental hormones can reduce the risk of osteoporosis, the bone-thinning condition that's the leading cause of fractures in older women.

Hormone therapy also can prevent hot flushes and other types of menopausal discomfort. It's best to discuss the pros and cons of HRT with your doctor.

24

High Blood Pressure and Stroke

The frightening thing about high blood pressure, or hypertension, is that it doesn't cause any symptoms in the early stages. Even when the numbers reach potentially dangerous levels, you probably won't feel different than you did before.

But even in the absence of symptoms, the force of blood roiling through the arteries will be doing serious damage.

Unless high blood pressure is diagnosed and treated in the early stages, it can lead to a host of cardiovascular conditions, including stroke and heart disease, says Dr Debra R. Judelson, a cardiologist.

About one-third of adults in Britain and Australia are now classified as having high blood pressure, and up to half of these people are not taking medication for it.

Statistics show that more women than men die from strokes. Women often enjoy healthy blood pressure levels until they reach the menopause. Then, when their oestrogen levels decline, blood pressure starts creeping upwards – and the women won't even suspect there's a problem.

Understanding the Numbers

Blood pressure measures the force with which blood travels through blood vessels. The numbers typically start to rise when artery walls thicken, constrict or lose their elasticity, which makes it harder for blood to push through them. In the majority of cases, the change in blood vessels occurs long before actual changes in blood pressure can be detected. There's usually no known cause; only about 10 per cent (or fewer) of cases of high blood pressure can be attributed to specific conditions, such as kidney or blood vessel abnormalities. You don't want your blood pressure to be *too* low because that can result in dizziness or fatigue. But for most women, the lower the blood pressure, the healthier they'll be.

When you have your blood pressure taken, there are two numbers to consider. The first, higher number measures systolic pressure – the pressure that's generated when the heart is actually pumping blood. The second, lower number measures diastolic pressure – the pressure when your heart rests between beats.

Here's what the readings mean.

- Ideally, blood pressure should be below 140/85 milligrams per decilitre.

- If your systolic pressure is 160 or over, and the diastolic pressure is 85 to 89, you're heading into risky territory, especially if you have other risk factors for stroke or heart disease, such as obesity or a family history of high blood pressure, or if you're post-menopausal or African-Caribbean.

- A reading of 160/90 or higher means that it's time to take action. Even if only one of the numbers is high, you may need medical treatment.

BRINGING THE NUMBER DOWN

Many people require medication to control high blood pressure, but this isn't always necessary.

'With a healthy lifestyle, many women can prevent hypertension from developing – or at least reduce its severity,' says Dr Samuel J. Mann, an associate professor of clinical medicine and expert in hypertension. Here's what doctors advise.

Lifestyle Strategies

Maintain a healthy weight. 'Excess weight is the biggest risk factor for high blood pressure,' says Dr Matthew Gillman, associate professor of ambulatory care and prevention at Harvard Medical School. Studies have shown, in fact, that men or women who lose as little as 4.5 kilograms (10 pounds) can send their blood pressure plummeting.

The only way to lose weight is to consume fewer calories than you burn. You can do this by eating

---

WHAT WORKS FOR ME

DR DEBRA R. JUDELSON is a cardiologist who specializes in treating women with cardiovascular problems. Here's what she does to make sure that her risks for high blood pressure and stroke are as low as they can possibly be.

I eat fewer processed foods these days, and I also go for a brisk walk every morning before I shower. This is my thinking time. By the time I'm dressed and ready to leave the house, my day is already planned.

I've also worked to reduce the stress in my life – and not just by using relaxation techniques. I've changed my entire life.

I used to be a type A personality. I was working incredibly hard – always in a hurry. Then, just before I reached 45, I began wondering why I was working so hard. I realized that I was trying to make a lot of money to pay for a big house and exotic holidays or other things I really didn't need. But I wasn't necessarily reaching my goal of happiness. I stopped the 80-hour weeks. I now keep my office time limited. Sometimes I go in at 9 o'clock – it allows me to spend time with the kids in the morning. I don't rush very much any more. I have a degree of peace and comfort throughout the day that sustains me.

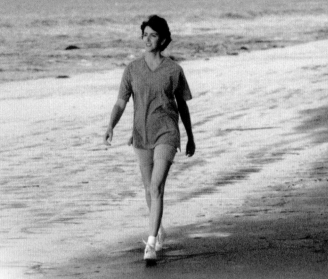

smaller servings, consuming fewer high-fat foods (fat contains more calories than protein or carbohydrates) and avoiding snack foods. Portion size is important, and be aware that manufacturers of processed low-fat foods tend to replace the fat in those foods with sugars, which also contribute to weight gain.

At the same time, you'll need to exercise regularly to burn off the calories you consume. 'Concentrate on increased physical activity,' Dr Gillman recommends. (For more information on healthy weight loss, see chapter 5.)

Keep your body moving. Even if you're at a healthy weight, regular exercise is among the best ways to prevent – or reverse – high blood pressure. Studies have shown, in fact, that men and women who are sedentary are 20 to 50 per cent more likely to develop high blood pressure than those who are physically active. How much exercise do you need? A total of at least 30 minutes a day of gardening, walking, jogging, cycling, weight lifting or other types of exercise is probably enough to keep blood pressure in check. (For more information on exercise, see chapter 4.)

If you smoke, try to quit. Every time you light up, your blood pressure climbs – and it stays up for an hour or more afterwards. (For information on how to quit smoking, see chapter 7.)

Nutritional Treatments

Follow the DASH diet. It stands for 'dietary approaches to stop hypertension', and it's considered one of the most effective ways to keep blood pressure in a healthy range. The diet suggests you have:

- Eight to 10 daily servings of fruit and vegetables (each about 115 grams/4 ounces)

- Seven to eight daily servings of whole grains (one slice of bread)

- Two to three daily servings of low-fat or fat-free dairy foods (45 grams/1½ ounces)

- Two or fewer servings of meat (each about 90 grams/3 ounces)

The DASH diet is so effective that one study found that men and women who followed the eating plan were able to lower their blood pressure as much as they would have had they taken prescription drugs.

Cut right back on salt. Dietary guidelines call for limiting salt consumption to 2,400 milligrams daily (1 teaspoon). However, several recent studies suggest that this number may be too high. When men and women without high blood pressure lowered their salt intake by about a third of the recommended limit – to ⅔ teaspoon, or 1,500 milligrams – their systolic pressure fell by 7 millimetres; in those with high blood pressure, the drop was 11.5 millimetres. People who lowered salt intake and followed the DASH diet had even better improvement.

Westerners eat huge amounts of salt because of all the processed foods. When buying soups or other processed foods, look for the words 'low sodium' or 'sodium free' on the label. Avoid ultrasalty foods such as crisps, pickles and soy sauce, and use the salt cellar sparingly.

Eat fish two or three times a week. It's rich in omega-3 fatty acids, which have been shown to help lower blood pressure. Fatty fish has the largest amounts of omega-3s. This includes wild salmon, tuna and sardines.

If you're not a fish eater, you can get the same beneficial fats by eating flaxseed (linseed) or walnuts or using oils made with flaxseed, rapeseed or walnuts.

Imbibe moderately. Moderate drinking (one glass of wine or beer for women, no more than twice that for men) won't affect blood pressure and has been shown in several studies to be good for your heart and arteries.

Drinking to excess, however, can cause long-term rises in blood pressure, and more than a drink a day increases the risk of breast cancer. So if you do drink, limit yourself to about 45 millilitres (1½ fluid ounces) of spirits, 150 millilitres (¼ pint) of wine or 300 millilitres (½ pint) of beer a day. It's also a good idea to limit your coffee intake. Those who consume too much caffeine –

in the form of coffee, tea or caffeinated fizzy drinks – may experience rises in blood pressure of as much as 10 points. Limit yourself to about two servings of coffee, tea or colas daily.

Keep cholesterol in check. It makes the arteries less elastic, and it also leads to accumulations of fatty material, called plaque, on the artery walls – the cause of heart attacks. As the arteries narrow, blood moves through them with greater force.

The best way to control cholesterol is to avoid saturated fats in the diet and increase your consumption of whole grains, pulses and other fibre-rich foods. (For more information on controlling cholesterol, see chapter 23.)

Alternative Therapies

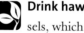 **Drink hawthorn tea.** It dilates blood vessels, which can result in modest drops in blood pressure.

To make a tea, steep 1 to 2 teaspoons of crushed herb in a cup of boiling water for 10 minutes. You can drink the tea several times daily.

Get in touch with 'hidden' emotions. Folklore to the contrary, daily anxiety and stress don't play much of a sustained role in high blood pressure, even though they may affect blood pressure in the moment. However, emotions that are held deep inside may send blood pressure soaring, at least in some women.

'One-quarter to one-third of the hypertension cases I see are related to repressed or, so to speak, hidden emotions,' says Dr Mann. 'These are people who have had childhood traumas or who cope with emotional stress by not dealing with it.

WHEN BAD THINGS HAPPEN TO HEALTHY WOMEN

Job Stress Raised Her Blood Pressure

In retrospect, Barbara Smith isn't surprised that her blood pressure rose to 140/90. When she was in her early thirties, she suffered the death of her mother. She also had put on weight, and she had a family history of hypertension. At the time, however, she was very shocked to realize that her blood pressure had risen so high.

'You don't really pay attention to your risks until it happens to you,' she says.

Her doctor immediately put her on hypertension medication, but she didn't work very hard at making basic lifestyle changes until she left her high-stress job a few years later.

'I started walking every day,' she says. 'I got involved in my community, and I read books about health and spirituality. I also meditated every day and became a vegetarian. It took time, but my blood pressure went down even further.'

But the changes didn't last. When she started a new job the following year, her health routine fell apart. Her blood pressure rose higher than it had ever been. In fact, she ended up in hospital after a test revealed that her blood pressure had risen to an alarming 170/100.

Barbara, now 51, admits that she struggles to find a balance between career demands and healthy living. 'I keep saying a mantra to myself: "I'm not going to let my job keep me from eating properly and exercising."'

She continues to take medication, but she also eases daily stress by visiting friends and doing things she enjoys, like flower arranging and going to the theatre.

'I know I don't have to do everything, that it's OK to let some things go,' she says. 'I write little notes to myself about the priorities in my life. I read them whenever I feel things getting out of control.'

They're the ones who are even-keeled – who never complain – and are actually less likely than most to feel depressed.'

People whose hypertension is related to hidden emotions tend to achieve less success with blood pressure-lowering medication.

'For some women, shifting attention to what has been hidden away can rapidly lower blood pressure,' says Dr Mann. 'Some can heal themselves, and others can benefit from consulting with a psychotherapist.'

Medical Options

Ask your doctor to check your blood pressure twice. Nearly one in four people, including women, suffers from 'white-coat hypertension'. In other words, their blood pressure is usually normal, but it jumps when they visit the doctor, often because of simple anxiety. They could end up being treated for hypertension that they don't have.

The opposite can also happen. It's normal for

blood pressure to rise and fall periodically. It's possible for a woman to have normal blood pressure in the doctor's surgery, but soaring blood pressure at home.

'Always make sure that you really have hypertension before getting treated,' advises Dr Mann. The way to do this is to ask your doctor to take more than one blood pressure reading during your visit. Another option is to buy a blood pressure cuff and periodically check your own pressure at home.

Consider medication. If you aren't able to control your blood pressure with lifestyle changes, your doctor will probably advise you to take pressure-lowering medication. There are many classes of drugs to choose from. Some of the main ones are:

- **Diuretics.** Also called 'water pills', they cause the body to eliminate water, which causes blood pressure to fall.

- **Beta-blockers.** They block the action of a body chemical called epinephrine, thereby slowing the heart rate and causing a drop in blood pressure.

- **ACE inhibitors.** They cause blood vessels to stay dilated, allowing blood to flow with less force.

Blood pressure drugs are safe for most women, but they can cause a variety of side effects, including dizziness, dehydration, decreased levels of potassium or sedation. They can even cause blood pressure to drop too low in some cases. Doctors usually resort to medication when lifestyle measures aren't effective.

REDUCE YOUR RISK OF STROKE

Heart disease and cancer get all the headlines, but stroke is the third leading cause of death in both men and women in the West. Overall, women are three times more likely to die of a stroke than they are of breast cancer. About 25 per cent of those who suffer from strokes are younger than 65, and more than half are women. Doctors have done a good job of educating women about breast cancer, but stroke is much more common.

There are two main types of stroke: ischaemic strokes, which occur when a blood clot blocks the flow of blood through an artery in the brain, and haemorrhagic strokes, which occur when brain blood vessels leak or burst.

The same strategies that lower blood pressure – such as cutting back on salt and eating a low-fat diet – also reduce the risk of stroke. It makes sense because high blood pressure damages arteries throughout the body, including those in the brain.

Home Remedies

Give up smoking immediately. It's bad for blood pressure, and it's even worse for stroke. Studies have shown, in fact, that compared with non-smokers, smokers have double the risk of having a stroke. If you give up, within 5 years your risk will be the same as that of a non-smoker.

Take aspirin daily. It reduces the tendency of blood to form clots in the arteries, which can help prevent strokes. Aspirin is usually advised for those who have already had a stroke or who have a high risk for having one. Even if your risk for stroke is low, you may want to take a daily low-dose aspirin, which contains 75 milligrams. Of course, check with your doctor to make sure daily aspirin is right for you.

Nutritional Treatments

 Take vitamin E. It is thought to be healthy for blood vessels and may reduce the risk of heart attack or stroke. Experts recommend a dose of 100 to 400 IU daily.

Take extra B vitamins. They lower levels of a chemical in the body called homocysteine. 'High homocysteine levels may be as risky as high cholesterol,' explains Dr Wayne M. Clark, a neurologist.

Leafy green vegetables and beans are among the best dietary sources of folate (folic acid) and vitamins B_6 and B_{12}. You may want to take supplements as well. Look for a multivitamin that contains 1 milligram of folic acid, 25 milligrams of vitamin B_6 and 250 micrograms of vitamin B_{12}.

Medical Options

Don't go in for a second round. In an international study that followed 6,105 stroke survivors for 4 years, those who took the blood pressure drug perindopril (Coversyl/Aceon) plus the diuretic indapamide had 43 per cent fewer second strokes than those who took placebos.

Throughout the world 20 per cent of stroke survivors will have another one within 5 years – and second strokes are often more disabling, or deadly. 'Now, we're finally seeing evidence that secondary strokes can be prevented,' says Dr Stanley Rockson, a cardiologist. Discuss this with your doctor if you've had a stroke.

when to see a doctor

If you experience migraine headaches that are preceded by difficulty talking or partial paralysis on one side of your body: contact your doctor straight away. These types of migraines mean you may have a slightly higher risk of stroke.

If you experience sudden numbness or weakness in the face, arms or legs, or if you're having trouble speaking, walking or maintaining your balance: get to a casualty department. You may have experienced a 'mini-stroke' or stroke warning called a transient ischaemic attack, which could potentially be followed by a full-fledged stroke.

If you're suddenly suffering from depression, and you haven't had depression in the past: this is sometimes caused by a 'symptomless' stroke, especially in those aged 50 and older.

If you notice that your pulse is irregular: this is sometimes caused by atrial fibrillation, an irregular heartbeat that increases the risk that blood clots will travel to the brain.

CHAPTER

25

Diabetes

A few decades ago, a diagnosis of diabetes meant a lifelong sentence of dietary austerity – and a vastly increased risk of blindness, nerve damage and other serious symptoms.

Things have improved dramatically since then. Diabetes is still a serious illness, but it can almost always be controlled – and one type may even be prevented and possibly reversed in some people through a combination of medication and important lifestyle changes.

'Diabetes is a very manageable disease – but it does take some work,' says Dr Karen E. Friday, an endocrinologist.

Diabetes occurs either when the pancreas doesn't make enough insulin or when the insulin that is produced isn't efficiently used by the body's cells. Insulin is a hormone that transports energy-giving glucose, the sugar found in foods, into the cells. When insulin is in short supply, the cells don't get all the glucose they need. Instead, the glucose accumulates in the blood. Small amounts of glucose are essential for health, but at high levels it literally becomes toxic. Uncontrolled high blood sugar can lead to kidney failure, blindness, stroke, nerve damage and heart disease.

There are two main forms of diabetes. Type 1 – formerly called juvenile-onset or insulin-dependent diabetes – occurs when the immune system destroys beta cells, insulin-producing cells in the pancreas. Type 1 diabetes accounts for 5 to 10 per cent of all diagnosed diabetes cases and is thought to be caused by genetic and environmental factors. People with type 1 diabetes need daily insulin injections or insulin delivered by a pump to manage their blood sugar.

The second form of diabetes, which accounts for 90 to 95 per cent of all diabetes cases, is type 2, previously known as non-insulin-dependent or adult-onset diabetes. Those with type 2 have a condition called insulin resistance in which their bodies do not respond efficiently to insulin. Blame this one on lifestyle factors. People who are genetically susceptible and are overweight, eat a lot of processed foods and don't exercise regularly have the highest risk of developing it. 'It's mostly associated with obesity and sedentary lifestyles,' says Dr Mitchell A. Lazar, an expert in the treatment of diabetes. Other risk factors for type 2 diabetes include a family history of the disease, age and ethnicity: African-Caribbeans are more likely than Caucasians to get type 2 diabetes. Women with a history of gestational diabetes – a type of diabetes that occurs during pregnancy and then disappears – and those who have had a baby with a birth weight exceeding 4 kilograms (9 pounds) are also at an increased risk for later developing type 2 diabetes.

If you have diabetes, one of the most important things you can do, apart from controlling it, is to keep an eye on your heart health. People with diabetes have a very high risk of heart disease, as well as stroke.

Almost before anything else, doctors advise people with diabetes to get their other risk factors under control. These include:

■ **Elevated blood pressure.** Be sure to keep it under 140/85.

■ **High cholesterol.** It is recommended that people with diabetes keep cholesterol levels below 5.

■ **Pregnancy.** About one in 20 pregnant women will develop gestational diabetes. Your doctor can screen for gestational diabetes around the sixth month of pregnancy. If you have it, you'll have to be especially vigilant about taking care of yourself later on.

SPICE UP YOUR METABOLISM

Cinnamon is more than a flavoursome kitchen spice. There's good evidence that it can help prevent or at least delay the onset of type 2 diabetes.

In studies, leading scientist Dr Richard A. Anderson has tested more than 50 spices and herbs – including cinnamon, allspice, catmint and turmeric – to see which ones make fat cells more responsive to insulin. The research is important because insulin-resistant cells can't take in enough energy-giving glucose from the blood, which can lead to diabetes.

'Cinnamon is the champ,' says Dr Anderson. It contains a substance called methylhydroxy chalcone polymer, or MHCP, which in laboratory studies increased glucose metabolism up to twentyfold.

In the future, the compound may be available in supplement form. For now, Dr Anderson recommends eating ¼ to 1 teaspoon of cinnamon daily, particularly if you have high blood sugar, insulin resistance or type 1 or type 2 diabetes. Sprinkle cinnamon on your porridge or stir it into foods, such as yoghurt, throughout the day. 'We've heard from people with diabetes who have begun adding cinnamon to their diets,' he says. 'They say it's the best thing they've tried since sliced bread.'

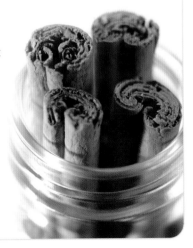

MUST-HAVE MONITORING

If you have diabetes, you will need a variety of checkups regularly. If your doctor's surgery has a diabetes nurse, he or she can help teach you how to do blood sugar self-monitoring (daily).

In addition, your surgery or hospital clinic will check the following things at least once a year:

- Blood test for glycosylated haemoglobin
- Foot check for sores or ulcers
- Eye screening for retinopathy, a condition that can lead to blindness
- Lipids (total cholesterol, HDL, LDL and triglycerides) to check heart disease risk

Catch It Early, Treat It Well

The goal of treating type 2 diabetes is straightforward: to keep blood sugar levels as normal as possible with a combination of lifestyle changes, or with lifestyle changes plus medication, possibly including insulin. Women with type 1 diabetes need to maintain a healthy lifestyle, too, and take insulin. If you have either type of diabetes, you will also be instructed by your doctor on how to monitor your blood sugar levels at home. Your doctor also can check for kidney problems by measuring protein in the urine. This is important because diabetics have a higher risk of kidney disease. You should also go for yearly eye checkups to check for early, treatable changes in the eyes.

The sooner diabetes is diagnosed, the better your chances of managing it effectively. With type 1 diabetes, people may be able to come off insulin early in the disease with the help of lifestyle changes and certain medication. And an early diagnosis for type 2 diabetes is important because if it continues uncontrolled for years, the high glucose and insulin levels eventually destroy the pancreas so it can't produce a sufficient amount of insulin. Once the pancreas is no longer producing insulin, there may be no going back – you might require medication for the rest of your life.

'But type 2 diabetes may possibly be reversed in some people, up to a point, if they lose weight and exercise,' says Dr Katherine D. Sherif, an assistant professor of medicine. In some cases, in fact, people are able to give up taking medication once they make fundamental changes in their diets and exercise habits, she adds.

It's important to recognize the early signs of type 2 diabetes because it's during the initial stages of the disease that reversing it may still be an option. Women need to be especially alert because they have a higher risk than men for developing heart disease if they have diabetes.

Your first clues, if you have type 2 diabetes, may be frequent trips to the lavatory and excessive thirst. Extremely high blood sugar may also be accompanied by fatigue and visual blurring. The main symptoms of type 1 diabetes are unexplained weight loss and hunger, sometimes called 'starvation in the midst of plenty.' But if you are at risk for either form of diabetes, see your doctor regularly for checkups, even if you don't have any symptoms.

Preventing diabetes, of course, is a lot better than treating it later. Long before people actually develop the disease, the body's cells may be

WHEN BAD THINGS HAPPEN TO HEALTHY WOMEN

She Traded In Her Chocolate Bars for a Treadmill

Fifty-two year old Sylvia Charity wasn't surprised when she first noticed the telltale signs: frequent lavatory trips, a raging thirst and light-headedness. Both type 1 and type 2 diabetes run in her family, and her mother recently died of complications from the disease.

Sylvia quickly had her blood sugar level tested. The test was positive. 'My worst fear was confirmed – I had type 2 diabetes. I was heartbroken at first, then became very angry because I felt responsible for allowing my fear to become a reality,' she says. 'You really don't want to admit that this is happening to you.'

Like many women her age, Sylvia had put on some weight over the years. She had slacked off on exercise, and she spent most of her days confined to a desk at work.

'After always being able to do whatever I wanted, like eating a piece of cake or having a banana split, I finally realized I was going to have to adjust my life,' she says. 'At first it felt like the end of the world, but now I know I can live with this.'

Sylvia, who describes herself as a 'chocoholic', stopped buying chocolate bars. She cut back on high-carbohydrate meals, and she always balanced the carbohydrates with small portions of meat and vegetables. She got her doctor's approval and started working out on a treadmill three or four times a week. She's now up to 25 minutes a session. 'I've lost more than 9 kilograms (20 pounds), and my blood sugar stays pretty much in control.

'This is not an overnight thing,' she says. 'Temptation is all around you. But I've got six grandchildren that I want to be around to see. I know I need to get my priorities straight and to be in control of my life again.'

---

becoming increasingly resistant to insulin, mainly because of poor lifestyle habits.

'If we could get people to restrict calories, exercise and eat properly, in theory we could prevent type 2 diabetes,' says Dr Francine Ratner Kaufman, an expert in endocrinology and metabolism.

Lifestyle Strategies

If you don't have diabetes, the following lifestyle tips will help ensure that you never get it. Even if you've already been diagnosed with diabetes, you can use this guide to help control your glucose levels, reduce symptoms and generally keep the disease at a manageable level.

Control your weight. It's easier to talk about losing weight than actually doing it. There's a good reason for this: human beings have a genetic tendency to overindulge and hold on to every last calorie. 'Our genes aren't that different from those in our caveman ancestors,' says Dr Kaufman. 'If a bison came along only once a week, those genes enabled us to survive by storing calories incredibly efficiently. Now, with fast food everywhere, we're still storing those calories efficiently, but it leads to obesity.'

The problem with obesity is that it increases the risk of insulin resistance. This means that it's more difficult for glucose to enter the body's cells. The glucose sits in the blood and starts to poison the blood vessels, nerves and pancreas. Insulin resistance is more likely to occur when body fat is stored in the abdomen rather than in the hips or buttocks – but any fat accumulation may be a factor. As little as 9 extra kilograms (20 pounds) of fat can make you insulin resistant.

The best way to lose weight is to follow our weight-loss guidelines, which are discussed in detail in chapter 5. But one point is worth mentioning here: diets that promise dramatic weight loss in a short period of time almost never succeed. Traditional diets, which involve a combination of physical activity and sensible eating, may be slower, but they've been proven to work.

'I always try to be realistic when I advise a woman about weight loss. For example, I might say to aim for losing 10 per cent of her weight over 6 months,' says Dr Sherif.

Do you have to keep losing weight to control diabetes? There are plenty of good reasons to reach and maintain your ideal weight, but there's a good chance that you'll notice significant improvements in blood sugar control in the meantime. If the diabetes is at an early stage, and your body's cells and insulin levels are close to normal, losing as little as 4.5 kilograms (10 pounds) may be enough to keep your blood sugar from getting into the diabetic range.

THE BLUES–BLOOD SUGAR CONNECTION

Doctors have known for a long time that depression and diabetes seem to go hand in hand. But which comes first: the depression or the diabetes?

Scientists looked at dates from the medical records of 1,680 people with newly diagnosed type 2 diabetes and compared them with records for the same number of people without the disease. They found that those with diabetes had suffered significantly more bouts of depression prior to their

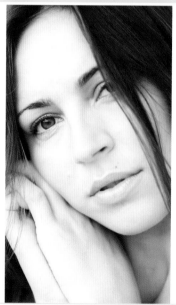

diagnoses. In fact, in those who had been diagnosed with diabetes and depression, the depression came first three-quarters of the time.

It is not possible to say that depression causes diabetes, but it is possible that both depression and diabetes are linked to a common factor – one that hasn't yet been identified.

If you have a family history of diabetes or if you have other risk factors for the disease, it's worth paying attention to your moods.

It's not always easy to tell at a glance if you're truly overweight or how much weight you might need to lose. Doctors recommend a tool called the body mass index, or BMI. We discuss this is more detail in chapter 5, but here's how it works. To find your BMI, multiply your weight in pounds by 703 and divide that number by your height in inches. Divide that number again by your height in inches, and you have your BMI. A BMI of 25 to 29.9 means that you're overweight. Anything above 30 is considered obese.

To make the calculations easier, check out the online BMI calculator at www.bbc.co.uk/health/ yourweight/bmi.shtml. A metric version is also available.

Take regular exercise. It's among the best strategies for treating both types of diabetes, and evidence suggests it may also help prevent type 2 diabetes. 'Exercise has two beneficial effects. It alters muscle cells to improve their resistance to insulin, and it also allows sugar to get out of the blood into the skeletal muscle in the absence of insulin,' says Dr Lazar. If you exercise regularly, your cells will be less resistant to insulin and will take in more glucose, which in turn keeps blood sugar levels in a healthy range.

Taking regular exercise will also help you maintain a healthy weight, control your cholesterol and keep your blood pressure numbers normal. It can dramatically reduce your risk of heart disease, which is important because women with diabetes are two to four times as likely to die from heart disease as those without diabetes.

For a complete guide to exercise, see chapter 4. Keep in mind, however, that even if aerobics classes or weight lifting aren't for you, simply walking for 40 minutes a day can reduce your risk of diabetes by an impressive 40 per cent. If you walk for a full hour at a good pace, you can cut the risk in half.

Talk to your doctor before starting an exercise routine, particularly if you already have diabetes or if you haven't put on your walking shoes for a while. Your doctor might recommend that you have a stress test, just to make sure that your heart can handle the workouts.

'There's no reason to go from being sedentary to running a marathon,' says Dr Lazar. 'Increase your pace gradually. Start by walking ½ kilometre (¼ mile), then slowly increase the distance,' he advises.

Nutritional Treatments

Eat natural foods. Humans didn't evolve to eat fast food and high-sugar, high-fat snacks. The ideal diet today is the same one that fuelled our ancient ancestors: fibre-rich whole grains, fresh fruit and vegetables and pulses – and the 'good' fats, such as olive and flaxseed (linseed) oils and the omega-3 fats.

In the past, people with diabetes were advised to avoid desserts and other sugary foods. Nutritionists still worry about this, but research has shown that the key to controlling diabetes is to eat a balanced diet. Keep your overall diet healthy and have only small portions of cake, biscuits and sweets very occasionally.

According to experts, the optimal diet includes 10 to 20 per cent of daily calories from protein; 30

per cent (or less) of total calories from fats with less than 10 per cent coming from saturated fats; and the rest from complex carbohydrates, which are mainly found in fruit, vegetables, beans and grains. If your LDL cholesterol reading is 100 or more, you need to take extra care to make sure your saturated fat intake is less than 7 per cent.

Include more fibre in your diet. A study found that people who increased their fibre intake from 24 to 50 grams daily had dramatic improvements in blood sugar levels. In fact, the high-fibre diet was as effective as some diabetes medications.

Rather than trying to work out how much fibre is in different foods, you can simply try to get a total of 13 daily servings of a mixture of fruit, vegetables, beans, brown rice and whole grain pastas, cereals and breads. For optimal glucose control, try to get an equal mix of soluble fibre (found in oranges, grapefruit, prunes, cantaloupe melon, raisins, oat bran and muesli) and insoluble fibre (found in some greens, vegetables, pulses and whole grains).

Avoid sugary drinks. There's nothing wrong with having fruit squashes or fizzy drinks on occasion, but they're brimming with sugar and little else. When you take in a lot of calories from sugar, you'll be less likely to get enough calories from wholesome, nutrient-packed foods.

People with diabetes should drink mainly water. When you do fancy a fizzy drink or squash, look for products that are sugar-free – and drink them in moderation, no more than one a day.

Consider supplements. In the past few years, researchers have found that a number of essential nutrients can play a powerful role in controlling

diabetes. You can't get enough of these nutrients from foods, however, so you'll need to get extra amounts in supplement form.

- **Vitamin E.** It strengthens immunity and plays a key role in preventing infections. This is important because people with diabetes are much more likely to get infections than those without the disease. Vitamin E also helps prevent heart disease, a common consequence of diabetes. People with risk factors for diabetes are advised to take 400 IU vitamin E daily. For those who already have the disease, the recommended dose is 400 to 600 IU daily.

- **Vitamin C.** It lowers blood glucose levels and helps insulin work more efficiently. Take 500 milligrams of vitamin C daily.

- **Alpha lipoic acid.** This is a co-factor for the enzyme that converts the broken-down glucose in the body's cells to a form that will be used to produce energy. It also helps prevent cells from becoming resistant to insulin. Some experts advise people with type 2 diabetes to take 400 to 600 milligrams of alpha lipoic acid daily. For prevention, take 100 milligrams daily. Important: if you're already taking medication for diabetes, talk to your doctor before supplementing your diet with alpha lipoic acid.

- **B-complex vitamins.** Take them if you're using alpha lipoic acid, which depletes B vitamins from the body. Look for a supplement that contains 100 per cent of

MORE VEGETABLES, LESS MEAT

The mantra of diabetes experts is 'low fat, high fibre'. But what about meat? According to one study, people with diabetes might want to give up all meat, including fish and chicken, and fill their plates with vegetables instead.

Researchers divided people with type 2 diabetes into two groups. One group was given a low-fat vegan diet (consisting of whole grains, vegetables, pulses and fruit, and no animal products), while the second group was given a low-fat diet that included fish and poultry. Both groups stayed on the diets for 12 weeks.

In the vegan group, fasting blood sugar levels dropped by 28 per cent – more than twice the amount of those in the fish-and-poultry group. People in the vegan group also lost an average of nearly 7.5 kilograms (16 pounds), compared with a 3.5-kilogram (8-pound) loss in the meat-eating group.

Even better, some of the people in the vegan group were able to discontinue or reduce their levels of blood sugar medication. None of the meat eaters could. As this study indicates, unlike the complex carbohydrates in a plant-based diet, refined foods, especially the sugars and fats, and calorie-dense foods, such as meat and dairy products, are absorbed rapidly. This prompts blood sugar spikes that lead to increased insulin requirements and the accumulation of fat.

Most people with type 2 diabetes are overweight, reflecting their intake of these refined foods, and have an increased risk for insulin resistance.

The heavier you get, the more insulin resistant your cells become. The sugar that is in your blood because it can't get into the cells damages the nerves, pancreas and arteries.

Unrefined plant foods may interfere with carbohydrate and glucose absorption, resulting in lower blood sugar and lower insulin requirements.

They are also sources of protective antioxidant nutrients, which are vital to the prevention and reversal of the arterial damage that is associated with diabetes. They are some of the most powerful tools we have against obesity and diabetes.

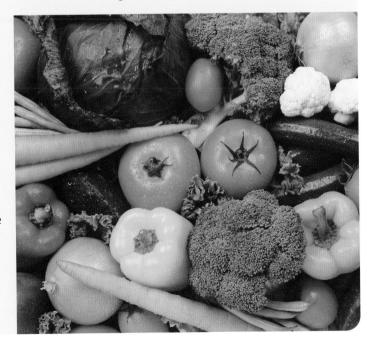

the recommended daily allowance for all the B vitamins.

- **Multimineral supplements.** Look for a product that contains chromium, magnesium, zinc and selenium. Chromium and magnesium improve insulin efficiency, zinc improves insulin production in the body and selenium helps protect the kidneys from damage. The recommended dose for people with diabetes is 400 micrograms of chromium (where a deficiency has been diagnosed). Otherwise, people with diabetes can keep their chromium levels at their optimum by consuming food sources such as lean meat, offal (especially liver) and oysters, whole grains, brewers yeast, nuts and seeds, and vegetables and pulses.

Alternative Therapies

Until recently, most doctors dismissed alternative healing techniques for serious conditions such as diabetes. But recent studies

PROTECT YOUR ORAL HEALTH

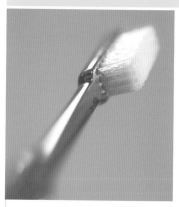

Gum disease may threaten more than your teeth and gums. Although not proven scientifically, it is thought that gum disease may be a trigger for the clinical onset of diabetes in individuals already predisposed to the disease. There is also evidence that gum disease can worsen the degree of control of diabetes.

In one study, researchers found that among overweight adults with the highest insulin resistance levels, one in two also suffered from severe gum disease.

It's possible that gum disease, which is caused by chronic bacterial infections that affect the whole body, may somehow trigger insulin resistance. The process is believed to be due to inflammatory substances produced in response to the infection. Molecules of these substances prevent insulin from docking on its receptors on the cells' surface. This reduces the uptake of glucose by the cells and results in insulin resistance.

'Oral health is far more important than we previously thought,' says Dr Sara G. Grossi, an assistant professor of oral biology. 'Gum disease may affect other conditions in the body, such as heart disease, stroke, respiratory diseases and diabetes. Periodontal disease in people with diabetes constitutes a significant health risk since it could lead to difficulty in controlling blood sugar and therefore worsen diabetic status.'

The best way to prevent gum disease is to brush and floss your teeth twice daily, eat a balanced diet rich in antioxidants – and visit your dentist regularly for checkups and teeth cleanings.

have shown that remedies outside mainstream medicine, such as medicinal herbs and mind–body techniques, may play an important role in keeping diabetes under control.

Let go and relax. Simply taking a deep breath and relaxing your muscles may result in significant dips in blood sugar. A study of 18 people with diabetes found that relaxation exercises were able to reduce blood sugar levels by 9 to 12 per cent.

When you're under stress, the brain secretes hormones that make you more susceptible to all diseases, including diabetes.

There are many relaxation techniques to choose from. One of the easiest is called progressive relaxation. Begin by breathing deeply for a minute or two. Spend the next 10 to 15 minutes progressively relaxing all the muscles in your body, starting at your toes and working upwards to your head. In your mind, imagine that the muscles are getting heavy, warm and loose. By the time you're finished, you'll notice that stress and tension have slipped away. If you do this every day, you may find that your blood sugar levels have dropped into a safer zone. (For more relaxation techniques, see chapter 6.)

Battle depression. Studies have shown that people with diabetes are twice as likely to suffer from depression than non-diabetics. Depression is a real problem because it makes people less likely to focus on the lifestyle changes that are needed to keep blood sugar under control.

If you've been feeling depressed or anxious, your doctor may recommend that you talk to a therapist or get a prescription for antidepressant medication. On the home front, really push yourself to take more exercise and to spend time with friends. They're among the best ways to ease depression.

Try milk thistle. It contains a compound called silymarin, which appears to improve insulin resistance and glucose control. Take 140 to 210 milligrams of silymarin from standardized milk thistle extract daily. The supplement label will tell you how much silymarin the milk thistle product contains.

Syndrome X: The Beginning of Diabetes

Long before people suffer from diabetes, their bodies have begun laying the groundwork for future problems. They may have what doctors refer to as insulin resistance or syndrome X, which leads to other problems, including high cholesterol and triglyceride levels, high blood pressure and accumulations of fat. These conditions can increase the risk of diabetes as well as heart disease.

'People who are diabetic may have been insulin resistant for years,' says Dr Sherif. 'One day, the pancreas just can't crank out enough insulin any more. Blood sugar builds up, which leads to diabetes. And by that time, half of them also have developed coronary artery disease.'

Researchers have found that insulin resistance and syndrome X have a common cause: the fat that accumulates through years of munching refined carbohydrates, which are generally found in snacks and other processed foods.

The problem with refined carbohydrates, and possibly with refined fats and excess protein, is that they're quickly turned into glucose in the body. The cells get overloaded with glucose, so the body stores it in the form of fat.

That fat does more than cling to just the abdomen – or the hips, buttocks, thighs and everywhere else. It promotes the production of a hormone called resistin, which essentially orders cells to ignore instructions from insulin to gobble up glucose that's circulating in the blood. In other words, it makes the cells resistant to insulin, one hallmark of type 2 diabetes. Although this mechanism is not proven, researchers think that resistin may be the link between obesity and type 2 diabetes.

We're all at risk from syndrome X, which is caused by poor diets and lifestyles. But you can reverse it, and sometimes type 2 diabetes as well, by eating a proper diet, taking nutritional supplements, getting regular exercise and reducing stress. If you have a family history of diabetes, or if you have high cholesterol, high blood pressure or abdominal obesity, it may be helpful to see your doctor for an oral glucose tolerance test. 'It tells how your body handles sugars after eating,' says Dr Sherif. 'If sugar levels don't drop after a couple of hours, it means that your body isn't handling glucose and you're probably insulin resistant.' The test may be helpful for women with a condition called poly-cystic ovary syndrome (PCOS), which causes symptoms such as irregular periods, unexpected weight gain and acne outbreaks. Most women with PCOS are insulin resistant and have a very high risk of developing type 2 diabetes. If they're not treated, many do go on to develop the disease. (For more information on PCOS, see chapter 17.)

DOES TELEVISION CAUSE DIABETES?

For years, doctors have known that an active lifestyle protects against diabetes and all its life-threatening complications. But American researchers wanted to find out if the reverse was true: would long stretches of TV watching – the sedentary activity that consumes 40 per cent of our leisure time – increase the odds?

They analysed the viewing habits of nearly 38,000 men, aged 40 to 75, for more than 10 years. After adjusting for age, physical activity levels, alcohol use and smoking, those who watched TV more than 4 hours a day doubled their odds of getting diabetes, compared with those who watched less than 2 hours weekly. Those who viewed 40 hours a week tripled their risk.

And if TV watching keeps you up late, you may face a second risk. Another study suggests that getting less than 6½ hours of sleep nightly raises the odds of insulin resistance, a diabetes precursor.

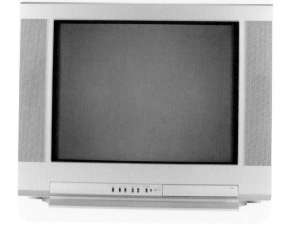

CHAPTER

26

Cancer

Almost every week, another cancer myth makes the Internet rounds. You've probably seen cancer alerts about deodorant, shampoo and even electrical appliances. It's enough to make women swear off consumer products for ever. Your best bet is to ignore those warnings – and empower yourself with facts. Doctors know what causes cancer, and those lists of 'carcinogenic' goods looping through cyberspace usually have very little basis in truth. What does count is how you live. If every woman ate well, exercised, didn't smoke and safeguarded herself against infectious diseases, particularly the sexually transmitted kind, nearly three-quarters of cancer deaths among women would never happen.

'The majority of cancer risk can be attributed to lifestyle,' says Dr Therese Bevers, an expert in clinical cancer prevention. Diet and smoking make up most of the risk pie, she explains, with inherited cancers accounting for between 5 and 10 per cent of cases. 'But even then, lifestyle or environmental factors may actually trigger it,' she says.

Does that mean you'll stay cancer-free if you follow the rules of good health? Not necessarily, says cancer expert Dr Mitchell L. Gaynor. But you greatly improve your odds.

Many Diseases, Similar Strategies

Cancer may sound like one disease, but it's actually dozens of diseases that attack different organs and spring from different causes. What all cancers share, though, is the uncontrolled growth and spread of abnormal cells – cells that eventually destroy the body if they aren't stopped.

Your immune system is uniquely equipped to recognize and destroy deviant cells before they become cancerous. Your detoxification system, which is controlled by the liver, rids your body of cancer-causing toxins. But sometimes this arsenal of defences fails, due to poor diet, illness, lack of exercise or stress. That's when cancerous cells may slowly begin accumulating. 'A tumour is the manifestation of a process that may have taken decades to happen,' says Dr Gaynor.

That's why keeping your body, mind and spirit in potent fighting shape is the key to preventing cancer and to living with cancer once you have it.

'If you get cancer, the healthier you are, the less likely you'll be to have other medical conditions that might interfere with treatment, and the better you'll be able to get through it,' says Dr Marilyn Leitch, a surgical oncologist. 'You don't have to die from cancer.'

Here's how to lower your general cancer risk, plus ward off the most common women's cancers.

YOUR CANCER PREVENTION PLAN

Some day, you may be able to have an injection that would protect you against cancer the same way as you get a jab against tetanus. In fact, it's one of the hottest areas of medical research today. Until a breakthrough occurs, however, your best bet is to do everything you can to lower your risk – starting with dietary changes.

Nutritional Treatments

Eat wholesome foods. Like so many lifestyle diseases, cancer risk can be reduced by good eating. Experts recommend having five or more servings of fruit and vegetables daily, plus plenty of other plant-based foods, such as wholegrain breads, rice, pasta and beans. Prepare low-fat meals, and limit your consumption of meat, particularly high-fat red meats.

Women who try to overhaul their diets all at once often get frustrated and fail. Dr Leitch

TURNING OUT THE LIGHTS MAY HELP TURN OFF CANCER

The hormone melatonin – which is secreted by the pineal gland at night when it's dark, and is curtailed by light – has been lauded as everything from a promising sleep aid to the fountain of youth. But its greatest potential may lie in its potency against breast cancer.

In a recent laboratory study, Dr Steven M. Hill, professor in the department of structural and cellular biology at Tulane University, gave female rats a preparation to induce breast cancer. Then he treated them with a combination of melatonin and 9-cis-retinoic acid, a derivative of vitamin A. The animals given the

treatment developed significantly fewer tumours than those that didn't get the treatment. In addition, the onset of tumours was delayed from 5 to 7 weeks.

The vitamin A derivative is a known cancer fighter, and adding melatonin to the mix appeared to make it even more effective.

Besides its ability to prevent or delay breast cancer, melatonin may aid in the treatment of existing breast tumours by altering oestrogen receptors and by starving tumour cells of the hormone they need for growth. Dr Hill isn't suggesting that women

take melatonin supplements to prevent or treat breast cancer. But it might make sense to encourage the pineal gland to produce as much of this healing hormone as possible by turning out the lights when the sun goes down and going to sleep early.

'By getting up at 5 every morning and staying up until 11 or 12 every night, with artificial lights on, you're giving your pineal gland only a short period in which to make melatonin,' says Dr Hill. He suspects, in fact, that melatonin deprivation may explain why some reproductive cancers are on the rise.

advises making the changes slowly. For example, substitute fruit or vegetables for chips one day; on another, replace red meat with fish, whole grains or pulses. 'You can't go on a grape-fruit diet for the rest of your life, nor would you want to,' she says. 'But if you have a more comprehensive plan that lets you eat enough to feel satisfied, then you're more likely to stick with it over time.'

Increase your odds with superfoods. 'I think the most exciting advance in the next decade will be predicting who's at risk for cancer, and preventing it largely through nutrition,' says Dr Gaynor. Scientists have found that many foods contain protective antioxidants and phytonutrients, which boost your body's natural defences against carcinogens. Some of the best include:

- **Tomatoes and fresh tomato sauce.** They contain lycopene, a plant pigment that blocks the harmful effects of naturally occurring molecules called free radicals. Lycopene has been linked to reductions in lung, breast, colon, cervical and other cancers.

- **Fish and flaxseed (linseed).** They contain omega-3 fatty acids, which fight cancer by inhibiting the body's production of prostaglandins, chemicals that promote tumour growth and inhibit the ability of the immune system to detect cancers. Oily fish such as tuna, wild salmon, mackerel, cod and halibut contain the most omega-3s. Or you can take 2 tablespoons of flaxseed oil daily.

- **Cruciferous vegetables.** Cabbage, broccoli, cauliflower, Brussels sprouts and kale contain formidable cancer fighters, including sulforaphane and indole-3-carbinol. Dr Gaynor recommends having six servings of cruciferous vegetables weekly.

- **Mushrooms.** They're packed with compounds called polysaccharides, large, chainlike molecules that have both anti-tumour and immune-stimulating properties. Enoki and maitake mushrooms contain the largest numbers of these molecules.

- **Olive oil.** It contains anthocyanins, flavonoids and phenols, which are known cancer combatants. They're not bad for your heart, either.

- **Green tea.** Studies have shown that people who drink about 4 cups of green tea daily have a lower risk of cancer than those who don't drink tea.

- **Garlic.** Along with spring onions, leeks and onions, it contains sulphur compounds, which have anti-cancer properties.

Use vitamins as needed. If you're eating at least six to eight servings of fruits and vegetables daily, you're probably getting enough immune-boosting, cancer-fighting nutrients. But if your diet needs a little help, you may want to consider taking a multivitamin that contains 100 per cent of the RNI (or recommended daily allowance) for most nutrients (including B vitamins), as well as separate daily supplements of the following: 1,500 micrograms of vitamin A; 10 micrograms of vitamin D;

500 milligrams of vitamin C; 70 to 270 milligrams of vitamin E; plus calcium (500 milligrams a day for women under 50; 1,000 milligrams for women over 50) if you don't consume three daily servings of dairy products.

Lifestyle Strategies

Get physical. Regular exercise can reduce your risk of a variety of cancers, including colon, breast, endometrial and ovarian cancers.

'You should take at least 30 minutes of moderate-to-heavy physical activity a day,' says Dr Leitch. (For a complete guide to fitness, see chapter 4.)

Live lean. Excess weight gain has been associated with increased breast cancer risk.

Every woman knows just from looking in the mirror if her weight is close to what it should be. In scientific terms, a body mass index (BMI) of 25 to 29.9 is considered overweight, and anything over 30 is obese. To calculate your BMI, take your weight in kilograms and divide that number by your height in metres. Divide that number again by your height in metres, and you'll have your BMI. (For more information on weight control, see chapter 5.)

Take a stress break. When you experience stress in your life, the body produces higher amounts of stress hormones, which suppress

DO LOW-CALORIE DIETS PREVENT CANCER?

Before you sit down to your next big meal or raid the refrigerator for a midnight snack, consider this: eating much less than you usually do could potentially add years to your life and prevent or delay the development of cancer or other diseases.

For more than 10 years, a group of scientists has been studying two groups of 60 male and 60 female rhesus monkeys. Animals in one group are allowed to eat as much as they want, while those in the second group consume about a third less calories. Preliminary results suggest a dramatic difference between the groups. Of the 60 well-fed monkeys, six have developed cancer. In the restricted-calorie group, only two have developed cancer. Other animal studies have shown similar effects.

It's possible that calorie restriction significantly slows cell division in the body, which reduces the likelihood of diseases that rely on cell proliferation, such as cancer and endometriosis according to Dr Mark Lane, principle investigator of the primate calorie restriction and ageing project at the US research body the National Institute on Aging.

Animals who eat less also have lower incidences of heart disease, cataracts and ulcers. They live longer, too. In human terms, you'd see an average increase in life span from 80 to 100, and the maximum age limit would rise from 120 years to 140 years, the scientists say.

Should you reduce your calorie intake by one-third? Probably not. It's just not realistic.

immunity and increase the likelihood of cancer. Soothing stress with relaxation strategies, such as yoga or meditation, not only appears to prevent some cancers but also helps prevent relapses in those who have already had cancer.

'Get in touch with your essence,' says Dr Gaynor. 'Make a list of things in your life that serve you and things that don't – and try to get rid of those things not serving you. Play music that you find relaxing. Try yoga, deep breathing, guided imagery – anything that relaxes you.' (For a stress-reduction action plan, see chapter 6.)

Medical Options

Get a complete checkup. If you've never had a formal cancer risk assessment, you could arrange for a health screen at a private hospital or clinic.

BREAST CANCER

It's true that breast cancer strikes more women than any other kind of cancer. But your overall risk is probably much lower than you think, and there are ways to make it lower still.

Statistics show that about one in eight women will develop breast cancer during her lifetime. Hereditary factors, such as carrying the BRCA1 or BRCA2 breast cancer gene, account for 5 to 10 per cent of all breast cancers. The rest are mainly due to lifestyle factors, such as what you eat and how you live.

Here's an anti-breast-cancer plan that will tilt the odds in your favour.

Nutritional Treatments

Consume 10 daily servings of fruit and vegetables. In one recent study, women at high risk for breast cancer increased their daily intake of fruits and vegetables from 5.8 servings to 10 or more servings. After 2 weeks, researchers found that free radical damage to the DNA in the women's white blood cells had dropped by 21.5 per cent.

When choosing fruit and vegetables, look for those that contain a variety of phytochemicals, says Dr Caroline L. Apovian, an expert in nutrition and weight management. Some of the best ones to include in your diet are citrus fruits and berries, cruciferous vegetables (such as broccoli and cabbage), leafy green vegetables, tomatoes, and yellow and orange vegetables.

Get more fibre in your diet. Dietary fibre helps reduce the amount of oestrogen that circulates in the blood, and it reduces oestrogen's impact at the cellular level, says Dr Apovian. Over a woman's lifetime, this can reduce the risk of breast cancer. Fibre also makes the stools bulkier, which can allow the body to excrete oestrogen more efficiently.

All plant foods contain fibre. When you plan your menus, be sure to include plenty of fruit, vegetables, whole grains, pulses and nuts. We recommend 25 to 35 grams of fibre per day for general good nutrition.

Get 'good' fats in your diet. Diets that are high in animal fats and high in foods, such as margarine, that contain trans fatty acids have been linked to higher breast cancer rates. Replace these with monounsaturated fats, such as those in olive and rapeseed oils, or with omega-3 fatty acids, such as those in fish and flaxseed (linseed).

Drink moderately or not at all. Research suggests that women who have two drinks a day may increase their risk of breast cancer by 25 per cent. If your overall breast cancer risk is average, it's probably safe to have a drink or two on occasion, but you should steer clear if you have a history of breast cancer in your family or have been diagnosed. 'One drink a day may be too much for women who already have breast cancer or for those at high risk,' says Dr Apovian.

Lifestyle Strategies

Get up and go. Don't underestimate the power of physical activity to safeguard you against breast cancer.

Even a little bit of exercise can help – but the harder you exercise, the greater your protection. Brisk walking for 3 or more hours a week can lower your breast cancer risk by 30 per cent.

'I recommend exercising for at least half an hour, 3 or 4 days a week,' says Dr Julie R. Gralow, an assistant professor of medical oncology at a leading medical school. 'Then augment that with

WHAT WORKS FOR ME

DR JULIE R. GRALOW is an assistant professor of medical oncology at a leading medical school. Here's what she does to reduce her own risk of cancer.

I try to practise what I preach on cancer prevention, but I'm the first to admit I'm not perfect. I don't smoke, but I do drink a glass or two of wine a week. A little bit is enjoyable, and it relaxes me.

I travel around the world a lot for work, and I try to be reasonable about my diet. I don't eat much meat, but I do eat fish. But I'm always struggling to get enough fruit and vegetables. In hotels, if I'm ordering room service, I have some control. During business meetings, I often order the vegetarian dish. Airport lounges now offer fruit, so I buy some. It's a little more work to get what you need, but it can be done.

Of course, there are days I look back and am mortified by what I've eaten, so I take a

multivitamin with extra calcium just to make sure I'm getting everything I need.

I definitely believe in exercise. When I'm staying overnight anywhere, I always carry my trainers, bathing suit and exercise clothes and try to fit in exercise, even if it's only at the hotel gym or around the local area. I've actually jogged around the Kremlin and through Shanghai.

At home, I run a couple of times a week, and my husband and I try to plan an event every weekend, such as a bike ride or walk. Occasionally we've cycled 50 miles a day. Every August I participate in a sprint triathlon (swimming, cycling, running) with a group of female cancer survivors who I work with.

To reduce stress, I make sure to schedule in some quiet time. I love novels, and I read a couple of nights a week and at weekends. I'm also a big fan of massages, and I try to get them whenever I can, especially when I'm travelling in Asia.

a bike ride or something else you enjoy doing at weekends or other days.'

Stay slim. One reason exercise is so crucial is that it controls fat, a tissue that produces large amounts of oestrogen – and oestrogen, as we've seen, increases the risk of breast cancer. Fat is even riskier after a woman reaches the menopause, when the incidence of breast cancer rises.

'If you weigh 70 kilograms (11 stone) and you put on just 7 kilograms (1 stone 1 pound) at menopause, your risk of breast cancer increases,' says Dr Gralow.

Medical Options

Use hormone replacement therapy (HRT) for a limited time. Women who have reached menopause may be advised to take HRT in order to reduce the risk of osteoporosis; supplemental oestrogen also reduces hot flushes and other types of menopausal discomfort. However, there's some evidence that women who use hormone replacement therapy for an extended time may have a higher risk of breast cancer.

Studies indicate that limiting HRT to less than 5 years – just long enough to get through the

WOMEN BLAME STRESS FOR BREAST CANCER

Science has found strong links between cancer and diet, genes and lifestyle. But cancer survivors tend to pinpoint something else: stress. Do patients' beliefs – even when not scientifically proven – help them survive?

To find out, Dr Donna Stewart, a professor at the University of Toronto, surveyed nearly 400 breast cancer survivors who had been disease-free for at least 2 years.

They were asked what they felt was the cause of their cancers, and why the cancers hadn't recurred.

Stress was overwhelmingly named as the leading culprit, cited by 42 per cent of the respondents. Known scientific risk factors – such as genetics (26.7 per cent), environment (25.5 per cent), hormones (23.9 per cent) and diet (15 per cent) – trailed considerably.

'We know that stress alters immune function, and these women may in fact be partly right that stress contributed to their cancers,' says Dr Stewart. 'But the evidence isn't very clear.'

When the women were asked why their cancers hadn't returned, 60 per cent credited

their positive attitude. This was followed by diet (50 per cent), healthy lifestyle (40.3 per cent), exercise (39.4 per cent), stress reduction (27.9 per cent) and tamoxifen (3.9 per cent).

Dr Stewart and her colleagues concluded that patients' personal beliefs about the cause of their cancers – even when their opinions were at odds with scientific evidence – were important in helping them cope with and manage the disease and that these beliefs should be worked with and not be discounted by doctors and health professionals.

period of hot flushes and menopausal mood swings – won't elevate the odds of getting breast cancer and will still probably protect against osteoporosis to some extent.

See your doctor regularly. You'll need to have regular mammograms, starting at the age of 50. If you have a high risk for breast cancer, your doctor may recommend starting mammograms earlier. You should also practise self-examination on your breasts throughout your life.

Some women, including those with dense breast tissue, may benefit from having a yearly MRI. Women who have a very high risk for breast cancer may be advised to undergo a procedure called ductal lavage, which can detect malignant cells years before a tumour shows up on a mammogram.

Consider chemo-prevention. If you have a strong family history of breast cancer or you've had it yourself, talk to your doctor about taking tamoxifen, a selective oestrogen receptor modulator that can reduce a woman's risk of developing the disease by almost 50 per cent. Preliminary studies suggest that another drug, raloxifene, may be similarly beneficial.

LUNG CANCER

Preventing lung cancer can be summed up in two words: don't smoke. If we all heeded this advice, lung cancer cases among men and women alike would drop by 80 per cent.

Your chances of getting breast cancer are greater, but lung cancer is more likely to kill you if you get it. In fact, it's now the number-one cancer killer of women, mainly because more women are starting to smoke at an earlier age, when their lungs are most vulnerable. 'Mutational changes in the lungs start to develop immediately, so it's worth quitting earlier rather than later,' says Dr Anne L. Davis a pulmonologist. 'Giving up smoking is the most important thing a woman can do.'

If you've smoked for years, and you've smoked a lot, your risk of lung cancer is naturally greater than if you never smoked.

But the risk drops dramatically once you quit and your lungs start repairing the smoke damage. In just 10 years, your risk may be up to half that of a smoker. Even if you wait until middle age to give up smoking, you can reduce your risk considerably.

For tips on giving up the habit, see chapter 7.

Nutritional Treatments

Eat your way to lung health. The chemical compounds in fruits and vegetables can protect the lungs from cancerous changes. In one study, women who ate more than six daily servings of fruits and vegetables were able to reduce their lung cancer risk by 21 to 32 per cent.

Some of the best choices include cruciferous vegetables (such as cabbage and broccoli), citrus fruits and vegetables high in carotenoids (such as tomatoes, squashes and carrots). Apples and onions are also good choices because they contain a compound called quercetin, which has been shown to reduce lung cancer rates.

Cook curry. It contains curcumin, a compound that appears to detoxify smoking-related carcinogens in lung tissue.

Lifestyle Strategies

Exercise early or late. 'Exercise is good for your lungs, but my only warning is to avoid exercise outside in highly polluted areas,' says Dr Davis. If you can't avoid the fumes from urban traffic or industry, at least take your exercise in the early morning or later in the evening, when traffic is lighter.

Check for radon. After smoking, radon is the main cause of lung cancer. It's formed during the natural breakdown of radium in rocks and soil, and it gets trapped in cellars and other air-tight spaces. If you live in a high-radon area, or if you just want to make sure that your house doesn't have elevated levels of this odourless, radioactive gas, look in your phone book for a testing service.

Medical Options

Get tested straight away. One reason lung cancer is so deadly is that the most common diagnostic test, a chest X-ray, isn't sensitive enough to detect tumours when they're small enough to be cured. If you are a heavy smoker or former smoker, and are worried about a persistent cough or coughing up blood, talk to your doctor about referral to a chest clinic.

COLORECTAL CANCER

For some reason, people often think that cancers of the colon or rectum (colorectal cancers) are more likely to strike men than women. The opposite is true: slightly more women now die from colorectal cancer each year than do men. However, this is one type of cancer that can almost always be prevented. Experts say that if you get tested and have a reasonable diet, you shouldn't get colorectal cancer.

Most colorectal cancers begin as a polyp, a tissue growth inside the colon or rectum. Over many years, they may gradually change to cancer.

'Usually there's adequate time to prevent cancer by removing polyps before they turn cancerous,' says Dr Mary Elizabeth Roth, an oncologist. Even a malignant polyp, if caught before the cancer spreads, can be removed almost all the time for full recovery.

Medical Options

Be aware. If you have a high risk of colorectal cancer – because you have a family history of colon cancer, for example, or if you have inflammatory bowel disease – you may be advised to have regular colonoscopies. Recent research has found that colonoscopy is the most effective method of screening for colon cancer. During a colonoscopy, a slender, flexible lighted tube is inserted through the rectum. It allows the doctor to see any abnormalities throughout the large intestine.

If you have any rectal bleeding, go and see your doctor who may arrange for you to have a flexible sigmoidoscopy. During this test, the doctor gently inserts a soft, bendable tube about the thickness of the index finger into the anus (rectal opening) to examine the rectum and lower colon.

Talk to your doctor about hormone replacement. 'Women who have been on oestrogen replacement therapy – even those who have been on it for just 1 year, starting at the age of 60 or 70 – have a lower incidence of colon cancer,' says Dr Roth. 'The lowest rate is among those who've been on it since the menopause.'

Nutritional Treatments

Eat plenty of fibre. Cereals and breads contain fibre, but most of it is too refined to protect your colon from carcinogens. 'The best sources of fibre are raw vegetables and fruit,' says Dr Roth. 'Fibre literally cleans away potential carcinogens from your intestine.'

One study found that people who ate more than six daily servings of fibre-rich fruit and vegetables had a 40 per cent lower risk of colorectal cancer than those who only ate two daily servings.

Cut right back on fat. The saturated fat in meats, butter and other animal foods may cause cellular changes in the intestine that can lead to cancer.

Eat barbecued foods sparingly. Meat that's charred on the barbecue (or grilled) produces cancer-causing compounds that can increase the risk of colon cancer, says Dr Roth. She recommends barbecuing only on occasion. When you do barbecue, don't let the flames touch the meat, which increases the production of cancer-causing compounds.

Take folic acid. Studies have shown that taking 400 micrograms of folic acid (the synthetic form of folate) daily may reduce the risk for colon cancer.

Get extra calcium. This essential nutrient is believed to bind to toxic bile acids released from the liver. This is important because bile acids may trigger cancer when they come into contact with the colon wall.

The best dietary sources of calcium include low-fat milk and cheese, fortified cereals or soya milk, and vegetables such as broccoli and turnips. You also may want to take a calcium supplement. Experts recommend taking 700 milligrams daily if you're postmenopausal and you aren't undergoing hormone replacement therapy. Younger women can take 500 milligrams daily.

Home Remedies

Keep regular bowel habits. If you exercise regularly, drink plenty of fluids and get enough fibre in your diet, your bowel movements will naturally stay regular.

This is important because constipation may increase the risk for colon cancer by allowing harmful substances to linger in the intestine, says Dr Roth.

UTERINE OR ENDOMETRIAL CANCER

A woman's body produces oestrogen, which offers significant protection to your heart and bones. But too much oestrogen can boost the risk of uterine and other reproductive cancers, which usually strike after the menopause. In fact, high exposure to oestrogen over many years may be your single biggest risk factor for uterine cancer.

If you started menstruating before the age of 12, entered the menopause after 50, never gave birth and have a history of infertility, you've been exposed to relatively large amounts of oestrogen over time – and your chances of getting uterine cancer are elevated.

You can't change your menstrual or reproductive history, but there are other ways to reduce your lifelong exposure to oestrogen. Here's what doctors recommend.

Lifestyle Strategies

Maintain a healthy weight. Fat tissue does more than hug your thighs and hips. It converts certain hormones into oestrogen. Women who are obese are two to five times more likely to develop endometrial cancer than are slimmer women. (For more information on achieving – and maintaining – a healthy weight, see chapter 5.)

Nutritional Treatments

Follow a low-fat diet. Foods that are high in fats, particularly animal fats, can raise your risk of uterine cancer in two ways. Fatty foods lead to weight gain – and fat tissue itself, as we've seen, increases the risk of cancer. High-fat foods also appear to boost the body's production of oestrogen.

Research has shown that women who consume diets low in fat and high in complex carbohydrates have a reduced risk for developing endometrial cancer.

Medical Options

Consider birth control pills. Taking oral contraceptives for up to 5 years defends against endometrial cancer – not only while you're using them but for years afterwards. Most contraceptive pills contain progesterone, which helps reduce the body's exposure to oestrogen. It's the same reason that pregnancy – which shifts the hormonal balance towards greater levels of progesterone – also safeguards the uterus.

RYE PROTECTS AGAINST COLON CANCER

The next time you eat a sandwich made with rye bread, you might be enjoying powerful protection. A recent study in Finland looked at 17 people who ate either about four slices of whole grain rye or the same amount of refined bread, every day for 4 weeks. Researchers found that the wholegrain rye reduced levels of bile acids – digestive fluids that are thought to promote colon cancer – by an average of 26 per cent.

Unfortunately, a lot of rye bread is made from refined flour. To get the benefits from rye, check the labels and look for the term 'whole rye flour' or 'whole rye meal'.

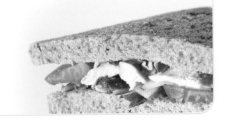

Add progesterone to hormone replacement therapy. The use of supplemental oestrogen after the menopause has given new meaning to the term 'golden years'. But taking oestrogen without balancing it with progesterone may increase the risk for endometrial cancer. 'It's pretty clear that a lot of uterine cancer is preventable with the use of progesterone during oestrogen replacement,' says Dr Joanna M. Cain, a gynaecologist.

Be wary of tamoxifen. Used to prevent breast cancer, it acts like oestrogen in the uterus, sometimes encouraging growth of the uterine lining and slightly raising the risk of endometrial cancer. If you're taking tamoxifen, have a yearly gynaecological examination – and make sure you report any abnormal bleeding to your doctor.

Report unusual bleeding to your doctor. A number of conditions, many of them harmless, can cause abnormal menstrual bleeding. With endometrial cancer, however, abnormal bleeding is almost a given.

If you're bleeding abnormally, especially after menopause, contact your doctor who will organize an endometrial biopsy – a test that looks for cancerous changes in the tissue lining the uterus.

Have regular smears. You should have regular smear/Pap tests. The smear/Pap test is most effective at detecting cervical cancer, but it may detect endometrial cancers as well. If you have the hereditary form of colon cancer, your chance of developing uterine cancer is also higher.

OVARIAN CANCER

'The most significant factor related to ovarian cancer is the number of ovulations that you have over a lifetime,' says Dr Cain. 'Things that suppress ovulation – such as contraceptive pills, having children, breastfeeding, later menstruation or early menopause – will all decrease your risk.'

About 10 per cent of ovarian cancers are genetic. If your mother, sister or daughter has had ovarian cancer or breast cancer, particularly at a young age, or if you've had breast cancer yourself, your chances of getting ovarian cancer are greater.

Whatever your initial risk, following the general anti-cancer plan that we discussed at the beginning of this chapter will go a long way towards providing lifetime protection. In addition, here are some other strategies that you'll want to follow.

Medical Options

Get tested if you have a strong family history. If more than one member of your close family has had ovarian cancer, ask your doctor to refer you to a genetic counsellor or gynaecologist to find out if you carry the BRCA1 or BRCA2 gene. These genes increase the risk for both ovarian and breast cancers.

'You'll want to discuss what you're going to do if you have the gene,' says Dr Cain. 'Doctors recommend removing the ovaries after a woman has finished having children. If someone's not at that point yet, we can test with transvaginal ultrasound (with a small instrument inserted into the vagina) and a CA-125 screen every 6 months.' CA-125 is a blood protein that's sometimes elevated in women with ovarian cancer. These tests are recommended only for women with a higher-than-average risk of ovarian cancer, Dr Cain adds.

Report symptoms immediately. Many women have subtle symptoms, such as mild nausea, a little diarrhoea that doesn't get better or a slight pain in the pelvic region, about 6 months to a year before they're diagnosed with ovarian cancer. Other symptoms of ovarian cancer include long-term swelling of the abdomen, unusual vaginal bleeding, pelvic pain or pressure, back pain, leg pain or digestive disorders, such as flatulence, indigestion or stomach pain.

Chances are, the symptoms will turn out to be nothing to worry about, but having prompt check-ups can ease your mind and also aid your chances of recovery if it turns out to be ovarian cancer.

Review reproductive options with your doctor. Having one or more pregnancies is one way to reduce the risk for ovarian cancer, especially if your first baby arrives before you're 30. If you breast-feed for a year or more, you'll improve your odds further.

This doesn't mean that women should rush into having children before they're ready. The goal is to reduce your body's long-term exposure to ovulation, and this can be achieved with the use of birth control pills. Women who take birth control pills for more than 5 years are 60 per cent less likely to get ovarian cancer than women who have never used them.

CERVICAL CANCER

Your mother and grandmother probably worried more about cervical cancer than you do. Thanks

---

SPEAK UP TO RELIEVE CANCER PAIN

About 90 per cent of people with cancer have at least moderate pain at some point in their illness, but half don't find relief.

New research shows that a frank talk with your doctor could make all the difference. Researchers studied 67 people with cancer pain. Counsellors met with half of the group to set pain relief goals and rehearse what to say at future doctor visits. The other half received standard pain control advice.

Two weeks later, after all the patients had seen their doctors, those who had received coaching felt 20 per cent less pain. Those who'd reported severe pain now described it as moderate.

'Cancer patients should know that their doctors are just as concerned about symptoms such as pain as they are about treating their cancer directly,' say the researchers.

'Don't be afraid to tell your family doctor.'

To help ease cancer pain, take these steps.

Ditch these myths. Cancer patients worry that treating pain may keep their doctors from treating their cancer aggressively or that they'll become addicted to painkillers. Neither is true.

Set goals. For example, you may hope to sleep through the night without pain. Rehearse. Have a run-through with a friend or relative before your doctor visit so that you feel more confident.

to the development of Pap/smear tests, which allow for early detection, deaths from cervical cancer plummeted by nearly three-quarters between 1955 and 1992.

But don't let vigilance blip off your radar screen. Your risk may be higher than you think, particularly if you or your partner has been sexually active outside the relationship, or at other times in your lives.

The leading cause of cervical cancer is infection with HPV – the sexually transmitted, and often symptomless, human papillomavirus. The more sexual partners you and your partner have had, the greater your likelihood of HPV infection.

All women may be at higher risk for HPV than they believe. Even if you've had few sexual partners in your life, your partner may unwittingly harbour the infection.

WHEN BAD THINGS HAPPEN TO HEALTHY WOMEN

She Survived Both Breast and Ovarian Cancers

Corinne Greene considers herself blessed. Not just because she's still alive and active after a devastating diagnosis of breast cancer in 1988 and a more recent diagnosis of ovarian cancer. Rather, she says, she treasures what she's learned on her path to wellness.

'I value every day, and I try to stay cognizant of the miracles that happen all the time,' she says. 'Most days everything works right in our bodies. That's a miracle.'

Corinne was 35 years old when she first noticed a lump in her breast 14 years ago, while she was rocking her 3-year-old son to sleep. She had a lumpectomy, chemotherapy and radiation, and the tumour disappeared.

Then, in 1998, she noticed pain and severe bloating in her abdomen. After seeing her doctor for 4 months with these symptoms, her doctor organized a sonogram. At that point, she was quickly diagnosed with advanced ovarian cancer, and she underwent a total hysterectomy. She still receives chemotherapy. 'I'm trying to keep the cancer under control until

a treatment comes along that works; my doctor calls it "co-existing" with the disease,' she says. 'I put myself in God's hands, and I focus on my children and husband. My goal is not to give the cancer any more than I've already given it.'

In addition to healthy living, including not eating red meat, Corinne incorporates a few complementary approaches into her healing strategy, such as yoga and visualization. 'When I have chemotherapy, for instance, I visualize it as white light going through my body, instead of poison,' she says.

More important, she says, are the profound relationships that have been made richer and stronger through adversity – relationships with other cancer survivors, as well as with her children and husband.

'We're a very close, tight-knit family, and we don't take each other for granted,' she says. 'My kids have developed a different level of awareness about what's important. My husband and I are still very passionate about each other. I think that's what's kept me going.'

So far, there isn't a sure way to prevent HPV. The use of condoms can help, but it's possible for HPV to be transmitted during skin-to-skin contact with an infected area, such as skin of the genital area not covered by the condom, even if symptoms aren't apparent. Doctors are currently working on an experimental vaccine, and within a few years it could be available. If successful, it may pretty much wipe out cervical cancer.

Here are some other important strategies.

Medical Options

Have an annual Pap/smear test. One of the most important things you can do is have a Pap/smear test every year, beginning at 18 or when you first start having intercourse, whichever comes first. Pap/smear tests can detect the signs of cervical cancer long before it becomes a real threat.

Cervical cancer is almost completely preventable with regular Pap/smear tests. It can also be successfully treated when abnormalities are detected early.

It's not uncommon for mild dysplasias (precancerous cell abnormalities) to show up during Pap/smear tests. These abnormalities don't always become cancerous. They may even disappear by themselves. If you have a positive test, don't be surprised if your doctor doesn't seem too concerned. He or she might schedule a follow-up test to keep track of changes.

If the dysplasia is more advanced, your doctor will refer you to a colposcopy clinic to have the abnormal cells treated. It's a simple procedure that can be done in the clinic, either with the use of liquid nitrogen (cryosurgery), electro-cautery or with a cone biopsy.

Lifestyle Strategies

Don't light up. If you smoke, do everything possible to give up right away. Doctors believe that tobacco smoke creates chemicals that damage DNA in cervical cells. If you smoke, you're twice as likely to get cervical cancer as a non-smoker.

Nutritional Treatments

Consume retinoids. Found in a wide variety of fruits and vegetables, retinoids such as vitamin A and beta-carotene appear to slow the growth of epithelial cells in the cervix, which is where most cancerous and precancerous abnormalities occur.

SKIN CANCER

We all like that sun-kissed look, but our love affair with the sun is a prime health hazard. Skin cancer is the most common of all cancers.

'Heredity plays a role, and the more irregular moles you have, the more likely it is that you may develop melanoma,' says Dr Diane Berson, a leading dermatologist. 'But protecting yourself from the sun is the most important thing you can do.' Fortunately, most skin cancers are highly curable, especially non-melanomas, such as basal cell and squamous cell carcinomas, which account for the majority of cases.

Malignant melanomas are less common, but they're also less curable. Catching them early is your best chance of making a complete recovery.

Wearing sunscreen is essential, of course. It's especially important to start using it early because 80 per cent of sun exposure occurs before you turn 18.

We recommend wearing, at all times, a water-proof, sweat-proof sunscreen with at least 15 SPF and full ultraviolet A (UVA) and ultraviolet B (UVB) protection. Apply it 20 minutes before exposure and reapply every 2 hours. You should also avoid the sun as much as possible between 10 a.m. and 4 p.m. (For a complete guide to skin care, see chapter 8.) Practising healthy habits, such as refraining from smoking and eating a low-fat diet, will contribute to the overall health of your skin, including reducing cancer risk and having fewer wrinkles.

It's important to check your skin. When looking at moles, remember the letters A (asymmetry), B (border irregularity), C (changes in colour) and D (changes in diameter). If you notice any one of these changes, you could have a higher risk for developing melanoma.

Non-melanomas often start as pale or pink, waxlike, pearly nodules, or as red, scaly patches. Report to your doctor any skin changes, including scaling, oozing or bleeding from bumps or moles. Skin cancer is the one cancer that shouldn't be missed, because it's visible.

It's also worth drinking a few cups of green tea daily or using skin-care products that contain green tea extract. Green tea is rich in antioxidants, which have been shown to prevent skin cancer in laboratory mice. Some researchers believe green tea is probably just as effective in humans.

Osteoporosis

One of the scary things about osteoporosis, a bone-thinning condition that primarily affects women after menopause, is that it develops over decades without causing overt symptoms. It doesn't hurt. You won't see any visible signs. But year after year, the bones get progressively weaker. You won't suspect there's a problem until you actually fracture a wrist, hip or spinal bone or notice a substantial decrease in your height.

Osteoporosis is incredibly common. Your risk of developing it rises with age, especially in the first 5 to 7 years after menopause, when drops in oestrogen may result in a 20 per cent loss of bone mass. For women aged 50 years and older, the risk of suffering an osteoporosis-related bone fracture at some point is about 50 per cent.

The good news? Even if you have risk factors for osteoporosis – such as a family history of the disease, a thin or small-framed body, a history of irregular or skipped periods, smoking or drinking excessive amounts of alcohol, not getting enough calcium, being inactive or having taken steroids or other bone-thinning medications – the odds for preventing it can be very much in your favour.

'Osteoporosis is a disease of heredity and lifestyle,' says Dr Bess Dawson-Hughes, director of the calcium and bone metabolism laboratory at the US Department of Agriculture. 'You can't do much about heredity, but you can prevent much of it with lifestyle modifications.'

Nutritional Treatments

Throughout your life, bone cells called osteoblasts are continually adding new bone to your skeleton while cells called osteoclasts demolish old bone in order to supply the rest of your body with much-needed calcium.

The prime bone-building years are between childhood and early adulthood. In other words, at that time new bone is added to your skeleton faster than old bone is destroyed. By the age of 30, your bones are as dense and strong as they'll get. After that, bone loss gradually begins to outpace bone construction. Everyone – male or female – needs an adequate level of oestrogen to build bone during their youth. Oestrogen deficiency in pre-menopausal women is a significant risk factor for bone loss, and once a woman reaches the menopause, declines in the body's oestrogen cause the bones to lose calcium and break down at an accelerated rate.

'Whether you get enough calcium and build adequate bone mass early in life or not, your body will start reabsorbing bone from your skeleton during your perimenopausal and post-menopausal years, which can lead to osteoporosis,' says osteoporosis expert Dr Ethel Siris. 'If you enter menopause with a lower bone mass, obviously you'll be at a disadvantage,' Dr Siris notes.

The body uses the reabsorbed bone to keep your blood calcium at a healthy level to sustain life.

Get enough calcium. Calcium is important throughout your life, but your needs for this important mineral change over time.

If you're 50 years old or younger, you should be getting 700 milligrams of calcium daily through your food, plus a supplement if needed. If you're older than 50, you need 1,000 milligrams daily. That's a lot of calcium, but Mother Nature is generous – many delicious, wholesome foods are brimming with it, says Dr Robert R. Recker, a researcher in osteoporosis. Dairy products are your best bet, followed by calcium-fortified juices, breads and cereals.

How much calcium can you get in your diet? Consider this: just three daily servings of low-fat or fat-free milk, cheese or calcium-fortified soya milk or orange juice will provide more than 1,000 milligrams of calcium. When you add the calcium that you get from other foods, such as legumes or green salad vegetables, you'll get the calcium that your bones need to stay healthy – provided you eat all those foods day in and day out.

Consider supplements. Even women who eat healthy diets most of the time don't always get enough calcium. This is especially true of women who don't eat dairy foods – either because they don't like the taste or because they find them hard to digest. If you aren't getting enough calcium in your diet, it's fine to make up the difference with supplements, says Dr Siris.

She sometimes advises women to take chewable calcium supplements, such as Lamberts chewable calcium, as a portion of their daily calcium intake. You can also choose to take traditional calcium supplements. Supplements in any form are often overkill, Dr Siris notes, because your body is able to absorb only a certain amount of calcium at one time and then excretes the excess. Genetics play a role in determining how much calcium your body can actually use for optimal bone density. Your body never fully absorbs all of the calcium you ingest, but taking calcium in several servings or doses throughout the day will optimize absorption.

'You might think you're getting 900 milligrams of calcium at breakfast if you drink a glass of milk – which has about 300 milligrams – and take a 600-milligram supplement, but in reality you're only absorbing somewhat less,' she says.

One more point about supplements: those that contain calcium carbonate should be taken only with meals in order to prevent stomach upset. Supplements that contain calcium citrate, on the other hand, can be taken any time.

Be aware of the calcium robbers. Salt, caffeine and protein play a role in removing calcium from your body.

To safeguard your calcium stores, cut back on processed, tinned and fast foods, plus crisps, pickles and other items that are high in salt, says Dr Dawson-Hughes. The upper daily limit for salt is about 2,400 milligrams, assuming you consume 2,000 calories daily.

Dr Dawson-Hughes also advises drinking no more than two cups of coffee a day – although adding milk to coffee will replenish the calcium that's lost due to the caffeine.

It's also helpful to eat moderate amounts of protein. Women between the ages of 30 and 50 are advised to get about 10 to 15 per cent of their total caloric intake from protein each day.

Lifestyle Strategies

Get a little sun each day. Every time sunshine strikes your skin, the body produces vitamin D, which aids in the absorption of calcium. You get some vitamin D in fish oil, egg yolks and fortified milk, but few other foods contain this vital nutrient – so getting a little bit of sun makes good sense.

If you don't get much sun, you may want to take a multivitamin that contains vitamin D – or take a calcium supplement with vitamin D added. The recommended daily dose of vitamin D for over 65s is 400 IU.

Get plenty of exercise. Aerobic exercise is good for everyone, but for protecting the bones, you can't beat weight-bearing or resistance

WHAT WORKS FOR ME

DR FELICIA COSMAN, clinical director of the US National Osteoporosis Foundation, shares her secrets for keeping her bones strong.

My mother was diagnosed with osteoporosis in her early sixties. She suffered compression fractures of the spine, which resulted in height loss and back discomfort. That puts me at greater risk, so I've developed a personal strategy to prevent osteoporosis.

First, I make sure to get enough calcium each day. I don't drink milk, so I have around 150 millilitres (¼ pint) of calcium-fortified juice at breakfast – it provides about 200 milligrams of calcium. Reduced-fat dairy products offer as much calcium as full-fat dairy products, so at other meals I eat about 30–45

grams (1–1½ ounces) of low-fat cheese, which adds another 300 milligrams. I take one 500-milligram calcium chew, and I probably get another 200 milligrams from other foods in my diet, which includes about five servings of fruits and vegetables a day. I don't take vitamin D supplements, but I get outside in the sunshine most days during the week, and I wear sunscreen.

Exercise is a big part of my routine. I go to the gym at work three times a week – either during lunchtime or right after work. I jog on the treadmill for 25 to 30 minutes, and I do weight training for my back, upper body and legs.

I also plan to have a bone-density test as I approach the menopause in the next decade.

exercises, which are essential for increasing or maintaining bone mass.

What's the best exercise? You have plenty to choose from. Experts advise women to run, walk, ski or dance. In fact, any activity that gets you on your feet and moving against gravity for 30 minutes five times a week will keep or modestly increase your bone mass. (For details on starting an exercise programme and sticking to it, see chapter 4.) For additional benefits, add 15 minutes of muscle-strengthening exercises, such as lifting weights. (For a complete guide to bone-building exercises, see the photos and instructions on page 264.)

If you smoke, make every effort to give up. Cigarettes damage the bones in several ways. Smoking lowers levels of oestrogen, which hastens bone loss. In addition, women who smoke may absorb less of the calcium in their diets. (For details on how to give up, see chapter 7.)

Drink alcohol in moderation, if at all. Having more than a drink or two a day will interfere with the bones' ability to absorb calcium. Heavy drinking is even more detrimental because it often results in poor nutritional intake overall, which can increase the risk of osteoporosis and fractures.

Medical Options

As we've seen, the body's levels of oestrogen decline at menopause. Combined with the natural bone loss that occurs with age, this can vastly increase your risk for osteoporosis and related bone fractures. Women who have reached the menopause need to follow all of the bone-protection strategies that they depended on when they were younger – plus some that are unique to this stage of life.

'It's good to have an ongoing dialogue with your doctor about your bone status throughout your life,' says Dr Siris. 'Simply taking calcium and exercising won't stop osteoporosis. You need to discuss your risk factors and what you can do for protection.'

Get a bone test. Around the time you've reached the menopause and have one or more risk factors for osteoporosis, you'll probably want to undergo a test called central DEXA (dual energy X-ray absorptiometry), which measures bone density of the hip and spine. If you don't have any risk factors for osteoporosis, you can probably put off the test until you're between the ages of 60 and 65. We recommend that women have a baseline bone-density test at the first signs of menopause – or earlier if they have one or more of the risk factors for osteoporosis.

If you're still in your thirties or forties, there's no reason to have a bone-density test as long as you eat a nutritious diet, take regular exercise, have a healthy lifestyle and don't have any risk factors for osteoporosis.

Ask your doctor about taking oestrogen replacement. You may already be on oestrogen replacement therapy if you have been experiencing menopausal symptoms, such as hot flushes. If not, ask your doctor if you should be taking supplemental oestrogen for maintaining and increasing your bone mass. Oestrogen replacement therapy may be particularly important for those postmenopausal women who have low bone density. If you are uncomfortable with

WHEN BAD THINGS HAPPEN TO HEALTHY WOMEN

She Made Up for Lost Time – and Bone

About 12 years ago, Linda Harrigan, now 51 years old, felt a pain in her hip during aerobics class. The pain was bad enough to send her to her doctor. Even more shocking was the diagnosis: osteoporosis.

'My reaction was total surprise,' she recalls. 'I thought, "This is an old woman's disease."'

While the reasons for her condition weren't surprising (she had undergone a hysterectomy, which had halted her body's production of bone-building oestrogen), she could not understand why it was her doctor hadn't recommended supplemental oestrogen or extra calcium to offset the bone loss.

'I was angry,' Linda says. 'But I'm also a fighter. I never gave up, and I never stopped to be emotional.'

As soon as she got the news, Linda went on a bone-strengthening regime. She began taking 1,500 milligrams of calcium daily, from high-calcium foods and supplements, and she launched into an exercise plan that included walking, cycling, lifting weights and running on a treadmill. Because she has brittle bones, she stays away from pounding activities, such as horse riding or running on hard surfaces.

Linda also decided to begin low-dose oestrogen replacement therapy, and she gets a bone-density test every 2 years. Because she has a family history of breast cancer, however, she may discontinue the use of oestrogen and begin taking an osteoporosis-stopping drug.

'I've been told that my spine is what you'd find in a 90-year-old, so I worry sometimes that my body will start to crumble and fall apart. But I'm very upbeat about it. I just went for my yearly checkup, and I'm still the same height and my posture is excellent. I've been blessed.'

choosing oestrogen, there are alternatives you can discuss with your doctor.

Take medication to prevent bone loss. Most women can prevent osteoporosis by maintaining a healthy lifestyle – but if you already have it, your doctor may recommend medication that will prevent further bone loss.

In addition to oestrogen, there are a number of drugs for the prevention and treatment of osteoporosis. These include the selective oestrogen receptor modulators raloxifene (Evista), alendronate (Fosamax), calcitonin (Miacalcin nasal spray), and risedronate (Actonel). Each of these drugs reduces bone loss and also increases bone density.

If you're 65 or older and have osteoporosis, you'll probably want to take one of these drugs after you go off oestrogen replacement. If you don't have osteoporosis, you might not need drugs. Just continue your prevention programme.

strengthen your bones with exercise

If you do have osteoporosis, check with your doctor before starting an exercise plan. Physical activity is good for you, but you'll probably be advised to limit certain activities – such as those that require bending your back forwards, or high-impact exercises such as tennis or running.

There are two main types of exercises for building and strengthening bones: weight-bearing exercises, in which you move your body against gravity, and strength-training and resistance exercises, which are considerably more strenuous. Here are some of your choices.

Walking

This is among the best weight-bearing activities. When you walk, your legs are required to bear most of your weight, increasing stress on bones in the legs and hips. Researchers aren't sure why, but the stress felt by bones during exercise stimulates the bone-building cells, osteoblasts, to make new bone.

Walking is easier to do than many types of exercise, and it's an excellent way to retard bone loss as you age. Women who regularly walk throughout their lives have higher bone density than women who are sedentary. They also have a fracture rate that's 30 per cent lower.

Doctors advise taking a 30-minute walk 5 days a week. You don't have to do it all at once: two 15-minute walks will give the same benefits. To increase the intensity of your workout – and increase the bone benefits – walk faster, or choose an uphill route.

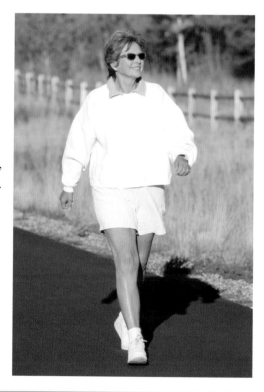

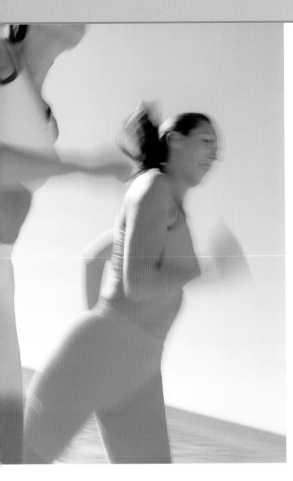

Running

This is a high-impact exercise. It stimulates more bone growth than walking – about three times more, according to recent studies. If your bones are already strong, high-impact activities (which include aerobics, dancing and tennis) are a good choice. If, however, you've already been diagnosed with osteoporosis, ask your doctor if your bones are strong enough for high-impact activities.

Many women incorporate high-impact activities into their regular walks – for example, by breaking into a run for a minute or two, then slowing back to walking speed. To give your body time to adjust to the vigorous exercise, start out by running for just 10 seconds. If it feels comfortable, gradually increase the time. Even a small amount of high-impact activity will prompt significant bone growth.

Gardening

You don't have to belong to a gym to get the bone-boosting benefits of resistance exercises. Activities such as mowing the lawn and gardening require a lot of digging, pulling and pushing. They're two of the best bone-preserving activities you can do.

Remember, though, to take it easy. If you haven't gardened for a while, rest frequently to prevent over-exertion – and drink plenty of water to prevent dehydration.

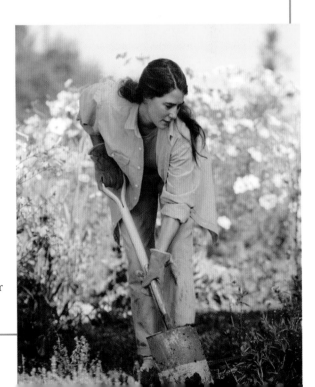

strengthen your bones
with exercise

Jumping Jack

If your bones are already strong and healthy, jumping is a good way to increase hip density. In fact, doing this type of exercise for 2 minutes daily can increase bone density in a matter of months.

Jumping jacks are good for beginning jumpers. Find a flat surface, either indoors or out. Avoid slippery spots or extremely hard surfaces, like concrete or tiles.

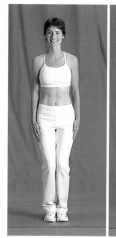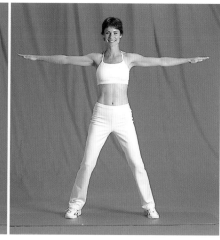

Stand with your feet together and arms at your sides (left). Bend your knees slightly, and jump while simultaneously moving your arms and feet out to the sides. Your feet should be approximately 1 metre (3 feet) apart. Your arms should be parallel to the floor (right). Land on the balls of your feet with your knees slightly bent.

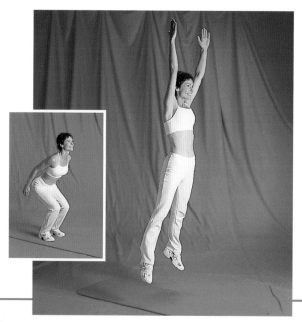

Power Jump

If you've been doing jumping jacks for at least 4 weeks, and you're sure you can jump and land safely, the 'power jump' is worth a try.

Stand with your feet hip-width apart and your elbows bent slightly at your sides (far left). Bend your knees 10 to 15 centimetres (4 to 6 inches), then jump straight up. As you jump, extend your arms up over your head, as if you were reaching towards the ceiling (near left). Land on the balls of your feet, keeping your knees slightly bent.

Seated Reverse Fly

This simple exercise will strengthen your shoulders and back.

Sit on a chair with your feet flat on the floor, hip-width apart. Hold a dumbbell in each hand, with the weights at chest level. Hold them about 30 centimetres (12 inches) from your body, with your palms facing each other as though you were holding a beach ball. Your elbows should be slightly bent (near right). Bend forward from your hips about 7 to 12 centimetres (3 to 5 inches).

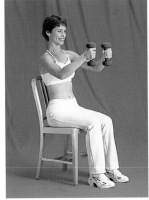 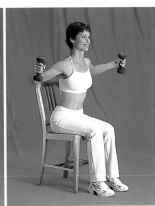

Keeping your back flat and your spine straight, slowly squeeze your shoulder blades together and pull your elbows as far back as possible (far right). Pause, then slowly return to the starting position. Repeat the exercise 8 to 12 times. Rest a moment, then do 8 more.

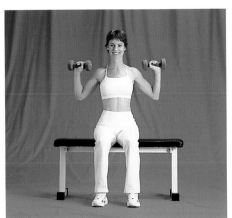

Overhead Press

This offers plenty of lifting and lowering – and lowering weights is what really counts when it comes to stimulating bone growth, according to researchers.

While sitting, hold a weight in each hand (top). Start with the weights at shoulder height; your palms should be facing forwards. Raise the weights above your head without bringing them together or locking your elbows (bottom), then bring them back down to your shoulders.

Important: don't try to lift weights that are too heavy. The weight should be challenging, but not overwhelming. If you find you can easily repeat the exercise more than 12 times, move to a heavier weight. If you can't do eight repetitions, the weight is too heavy. This advice on weight selection pertains to the military press exercise here, as well as the exercises requiring dumbbells, above and overleaf.

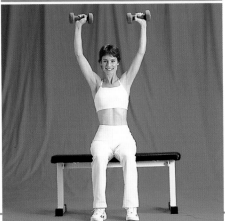

continued

strengthen your bones
with exercise

Squat

A type of resistance exercise, squats are an excellent way to strengthen the thighs – and new research suggests that the more muscle you have, and the less fat, the higher your bone density will be. Here's how to do them.

Stand with your feet shoulder-width apart (near right). Bend your knees and squat, as though you're sitting; hold your arms in front for balance. Slowly lower your buttocks until your thighs are almost parallel to the ground (far right). Don't let your knees extend beyond your toes. Hold the position for a second, then rise.

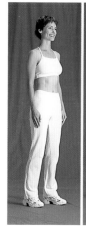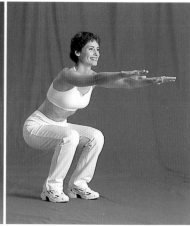

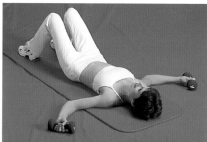

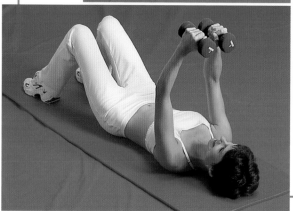

Chest Fly

This exercise improves chest and shoulder strength, as well as your posture.

Lie face-up on an exercise mat, with your knees bent, feet hip-width apart, and toes straight ahead.

Holding a dumbbell in each hand, extend your arms out to the sides, with your palms facing up and your hands at chest level (top). Bend your elbows at about a 45-degree angle.

Keeping your wrists straight and your lower back pressed into the floor, slowly lift both arms up and towards the centre of your body in a sweeping arc (bottom). Make sure not to lift the dumbbells directly over your head, and don't straighten your arms.

Stop just before the weights touch in mid-air over your chest. Pause, then slowly lower the weights. Repeat the exercise 8 to 12 times. Rest a moment, then do them again.

Wrist Flexion

Osteoporosis is often responsible for wrist fractures in women. This easy exercise will strengthen the wrists and protect against carpal tunnel pain, sprains and other injuries.

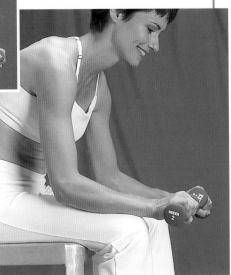

Sit in a chair, your feet hip-width apart. Holding a dumbbell in each hand, place your forearms on top of your thighs so your palms are facing up (left). Your hands will hang over your knees.

Slowly bend your wrists, curling the dumbbells up towards your arms (right). Your wrists and hands should be the only things moving. Bring your hands up as high as is comfortable. Hold, then slowly lower. Repeat the exercise 8 to 12 times. Rest, then repeat the exercise.

Wrist Extension

Like wrist flexions, this exercise will both strengthen and protect your wrists.

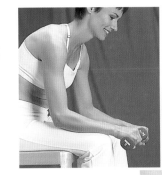

Sit in a chair with your feet hip-width apart. Holding a dumbbell in each hand, place your forearms on top of your thighs so that your palms are facing down (near right). Your hands will hang over your knees.

Slowly lift the dumbbells, bringing your knuckles up towards your arms (far right). Your wrists and hands should be the only things moving. Go as far as is comfortable. Hold, then slowly lower. Repeat the exercise 8 to 12 times. Rest, then repeat the exercise.

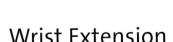

CHAPTER
28

Alzheimer's Disease

Occasional forgetfulness is one of the disconcerting signs of middle age. Maybe you occasionally misplace the car keys or find yourself racking your brain for a word that's just beyond reach. Deep down, you may worry that these flashes of forgetfulness are the beginnings of Alzheimer's disease or dementia.

The worry is understandable. Worldwide, dementia affects one person in 20 over the age of 65 and one person in five over the age of 80. Alzheimer's disease is the most common form of dementia, making up 55 per cent of all cases. Women are slightly more at risk of developing Alzheimer's than men. Medication can ease some of the symptoms for a time, but there isn't a cure, and scientists still aren't sure of what the underlying causes are. While researchers have found that people with Alzheimer's have abnormal tangles in and around nerve cells in the brain, which interrupt their normal connections and result in mental and physical deterioration, it isn't clear what triggers these changes in the first place.

Most memory problems, of course, are entirely normal – although research has shown that you can minimize the lapses with a little help. Even if you have a greater risk for developing Alzheimer's

disease – because it runs in your family, for example, or you've had a serious head injury in the past – you may be able to reduce that risk.

'There's no proven way yet to prevent Alzheimer's disease, but there are positive signs of progress,' says Dr Linda A. Hershey, a professor of neurology and pharmacology.

Most neurological problems take decades to develop. The earlier you start strengthening and protecting your brain, the better your chances of staying healthy throughout your life, says Dr Dharma Singh Khalsa, an expert On Alzheimer's disease. 'The brain is not a computer,' says Dr Khalsa. 'It's flesh and blood like any other organ – and it depends on the same things to keep it healthy.'

Nutritional Treatments

Eat wisely. The same foods that are healthy for the heart and arteries are also good for the brain, Dr Khalsa says. He advises people to eat an abundance of fresh fruits, green leafy vegetables, whole grains and soya foods. They're rich in protective phytochemicals, plant-based nutrients that may protect brain cells from future damage.

FOCUSING ON FISH MAY HELP TO FOCUS THE BRAIN

Our ability to bond with animals may be hardwired into our brains. Now researchers believe that they've found a way to harness the healing power of this inner circuitry to benefit those with Alzheimer's disease.

In one study, scientists placed glass tanks of brightly coloured fish in three nursing homes, then studied the effects on 60 men and women with Alzheimer's disease.

Researchers noted that two problems with Alzheimer's disease are that people often wander aimlessly or get lethargic – and it's hard to get them to eat. They observed that the fish tanks had a sedating, calming effect on wandering patients, so they'd sit down longer and eat. The tanks had the opposite effect on the lethargic patients – they were more likely to stay awake, which also made it easier for them to eat.

In fact, patients who watched the fish ate up to 21 per cent more than the non-fish watchers. Some patients who had previously been unresponsive were even prompted to talk.

It's not clear why watching fish had the effects it did. The researchers speculate that human beings may have an intrinsic need to bond with animals and that watching the fish fulfilled some deep-seated spiritual, emotional or even physical need.

Reduce the fat in your diet. Ideally, fewer than 20 per cent of your total calories should come from fat, especially if you have a family history of Alzheimer's disease. 'Fat plugs up arteries in the brain and reduces blood flow,' says Dr Khalsa. A high-fat diet also increases damage from free radicals, harmful oxygen molecules that damage tissues in the brain and other parts of the body.

Take a vitamin E supplement. High doses of vitamin E daily may delay mental declines in Alzheimer's patients. It's also possible that vitamin E may play a role in preventing the disease, says Dr Gary W. Small, an expert on age-related memory loss. For prevention, some experts advise taking 400 to 800 IU of vitamin E daily. Vitamin E is safe for most people, but it may increase the effects of blood-thinning medications, such as warfarin (Coumadin). If you're taking these medications, check with your doctor before supplementing your diet with vitamin E.

Take extra vitamin C. Like vitamin E, it's an antioxidant that blocks some of the effects of cell-damaging free radicals.

Consider an over-the-counter supplement. A product available in pharmacies and health food stores, phosphatidylserine (PS), is thought by some researchers to reverse certain types of age-related memory loss. One study has shown, in fact, that people who took PS had an improvement in their ability to remember names. Dr Khalsa advises taking 100 to 300 milligrams of PS daily.

Home Remedies

Take ibuprofen. Because brain inflammation appears to play a role in the development of Alzheimer's disease, taking ibuprofen (such as Nurofen) may delay its onset – or even prevent it entirely. Because ibuprofen may cause side effects, talk to your doctor before using it as part of an Alzheimer's prevention plan.

Stay physically active. In a 5-year study of people aged 65 and older, Canadian researchers

WHY EARLY DIAGNOSIS IS VITAL

Families often wait 3 to 4 years – dutifully fishing car keys out of sugar bowls and nodding at the same tale repeated over and over in a single conversation – before they seek professional help for a loved one exhibiting the early signs of dementia. Those 3 to 4 years could cost dearly. Here's why.

There are three stages of dementia. Stage 1, in which the patient begins to exhibit confusion, depression, irritability, anxiety, difficulty with everyday tasks and social withdrawal, but is still able to live on her own, lasts 2 to 4 years. Most families mistakenly attribute this stage to normal ageing. A doctor's opinion is frequently not sought until stage 2, which is often marked by troublesome behaviour such as agitation, paranoia or aggression and by more serious cognitive and physical slippage and a need for more care. By the time someone reaches stage 3, they often require around-the-clock care.

Families who receive an early diagnosis of Alzheimer's while their loved one is still at stage 1 may be able to slow down the progression of the symptoms by as much as a year or more with medications such as Aricept, Exelon and Reminyl, says Dr Steven Potkin, a neuropsychiatric researcher. 'Their loved one consequently gets to stay home longer and functions better than she otherwise would.'

New evidence suggests that if you miss that window of opportunity, the new drugs may not work as well. In a recent study, patients with mild to moderately severe Alzheimer's who received Exelon improved after 6 months; expectedly, those given a placebo didn't.

'But then the researchers gave the placebo group Exelon, and checked in with both groups over the next year and a half,' says Dr Potkin. 'Much to their surprise, while the original placebo group improved with Exelon, they never did as well as the people who had been given the drug from the beginning.'

found that those who exercised vigorously at least 3 days a week were up to 50 per cent less likely to develop Alzheimer's disease and 40 per cent less likely to suffer other symptoms of mental decline than their sedentary counterparts.

Even those who did only light activity such as easy walking had a much lower risk, says lead researcher Danielle Laurin. 'We need more research, but exercise may work by improving blood flow to the brain (hence providing more nutrients), which keeps brain cells healthy and alive.'

Exercise your brain. Reading the paper and discussing it, doing crossword puzzles or taking up a hobby – such as art, music or learning a foreign language – increases the connections between brain cells and decreases your chance of getting Alzheimer's.

Alternative Therapies

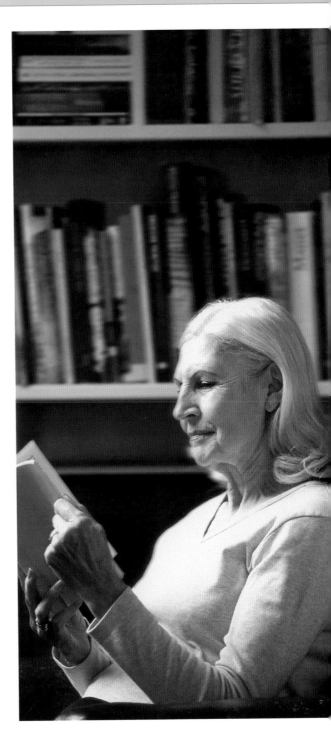

Take a break from stress. Chronic stress raises levels of the hormone cortisol, which is toxic to the memory centre of the brain. Cortisol decreases the brain's ability to use glucose, blocks the effects of neurotransmitters, and actually injures and kills brain cells. He advises people to manage stress by meditating, doing stretches or simply sitting quietly for a few minutes before they begin their day.

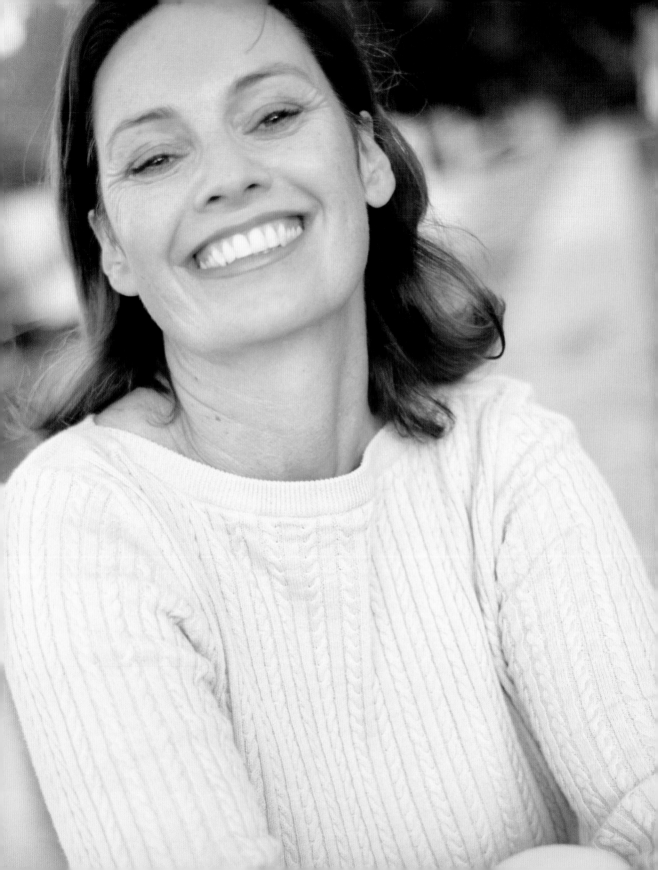

PART 5

An A–Z of Women's Health

abdominal fat

'If a woman takes in more calories than she's expending, she will put on weight and store fat in certain areas of her body, such as the abdomen,' explains Dr Ellen Glickman, a professor of exercise physiology. 'Women are genetically predisposed to store fat in the abdominal area because it's nature's way of protecting the childbearing area of our bodies,' she explains. 'Extra calories get stored as fat around the abdomen and hips to protect a baby against trauma.'

When it comes to abdominal fat, genetics may dictate that women have an uphill climb, but that doesn't mean it's not worth the effort. A firm tummy looks great in everything from swimsuits to jeans. In addition, research continues to demonstrate that having a trim middle can protect against life-threatening diseases, such as breast cancer, heart disease and diabetes. Fat inside the abdomen is more likely to release fatty acids into the liver than fat elsewhere on the body. As a result, excessive amounts of cholesterol and insulin seep into the bloodstream, contributing to the development of disease.

'Women with large bellies also complain of back pain,' says Dr Glickman. 'Back pain is often caused by weak abdominal muscles, so strengthening these muscles helps your back support your body and takes pressure off the back. Where there's less pressure, there's less pain and discomfort.' Here are some strategies to make your belly bulge less noticeably or lose it entirely.

Immediate Solutions
HOME REMEDIES

Drink up. For premenstrual bloating, drink lots of water. This will actually help flush away excess fluid, not increase it. And avoid carbonated drinks and those with lots of sugar, which can blow your belly up like a balloon.

Skip the crisps. Salt makes you retain water, especially before your period. Processed and tinned foods tend to be high in sodium.

Ditch the chewing gum. Chewing gum can cause you to swallow excess air, which may 'inflate' your stomach.

Stand up straight. Imagine a string with one end attached to the top of your head and the other tied to the ceiling. Pretend it's tugging you upright, and your belly will instantly look flatter.

Don't slump. Sitting in a slump accentuates your stomach. To improve your posture, check your chair. If the seat is too high to let your feet touch the floor without making you slump, use a footstool about 10 centimetres (4 inches) high, or place a pillow at the small of your back to help move you forwards in your chair.

Shape up underneath. Body shapers – high-waisted Lycra waist slimmers – can take off an inch or more. The more Lycra they contain, the more control you'll get.

Wear black. Wearing black makes women of all shapes and sizes look thinner and taller.

Long-term Solutions
HOME REMEDIES

🏠 **Aim for at least 30 minutes of exercise most days of the week.** To do that, set a specific time to work out and stick to it. 'Women are increasingly taking on more roles, and they tend to put themselves last,' notes Dr Glickman. 'We put our jobs, children and house before our own health. We claim to have less and less time to be physically active and do daily exercise.

'Most women expend a lot of time and effort counting fat grams and calories,' she points out. 'But what they need to realize is that exercise combined with a reduction in calorie intake is the best way to a flat tummy because you reduce your overall body fat while maintaining lean muscle tissue.'

Start at the top. 'When you do upper-body weight lifting or resistance exercises, your lower body, especially the abdomen, will work to stabilize the body,' says Dr Glickman.

Another bonus: building upper-body muscles, such as those in your arms and shoulders, can make your waistline *look* smaller. Dr Glickman recommends starting out slowly, then working your way up to at least three sets of 12 repetitions.

Sign up for a few Pilates classes. Dancers have used this series of stretching-type exercises done on the floor and on special equipment for decades. Now hundreds of others, including many celebrities, attribute their tight abs to this low-impact form of exercise. For a list of teachers in the UK, visit www.pilates-foundation.org.uk. In Australia and New Zealand, look at www.pilates.net.

Do a clean sweep. Does the pavement need sweeping? Grab a broom and get to it. The back-and-forth motion is a great ab toner. And don't forget the dustpan: bending over works the abs, too.

Get out and garden. Gardening involves bending, lifting, pulling, pushing and digging. The spinal twisting and abdominal contractions you do while digging are a particularly good ab workout.

Go for a walk. According to a study, women who walked regularly were 16 per cent less likely to gain inches at the waist than those who didn't. 'Walking is an outstanding exercise for overall weight reduction for women of all body shapes, all ages and all weight ranges,' says Dr Glickman. 'Research shows that it helps to maintain the integrity of bone, which will reduce the chances of developing osteoporosis.'

Try tennis. As you play, you'll feel it around your middle. Each time you turn to make a stroke, you strengthen the oblique muscles on either side of your abdomen.

Go for a swim. A vigorous crawl stroke can tighten abs. Since you must breathe in and out forcefully as you swim, your abdominal muscles contract constantly. The reaching forwards and pulling back in the butterfly stroke also tones the abs.

Aim for strength. For specific exercises to tighten and tone the abdominals, turn to pages 346–8.

anaemia

Every time you take a breath, oxygen is picked up by haemoglobin, an iron-rich protein in red blood cells, and carried to tissues throughout the body. Women who have insufficient levels of haemoglobin or red blood cells can't get all the oxygen they need. This condition, called anaemia, can result in weakness, fatigue, headaches, heart palpitations, difficulty concentrating and other symptoms.

Anaemia rarely causes serious health problems for women, but doctors take it seriously because something is causing haemoglobin or red blood cells to decline. Heavy menstrual bleeding or insufficient iron in the diet is often to blame. There could also be internal bleeding – due to ulcers, for example, or some forms of cancer, says Dr Barbara Goff, an associate professor of obstetrics and gynaecology. Even haemorrhoids can result in anaemia if they bleed profusely.

Women who are vegetarians sometimes become anaemic because the iron in plant foods isn't as easy for the body to absorb as the iron found in meats. Pregnancy also affects iron levels, which is why women are often advised to take iron-containing prenatal supplements when they're expecting.

Most cases of anaemia are caused by insufficient iron in the diet, but there are other forms of this condition as well. A deficiency of vitamin B_{12} can result in a decrease in red blood cells that may lead to anaemia. This nutrient is found only in animal foods, so strict vegetarians may not get enough. Pernicious anaemia, which often affects elderly adults, is caused by the lack of a stomach protein that's needed to transport vitamin B_{12} from the stomach to the small intestine – the inability to produce the stomach protein leads to inadequate absorption of vitamin B_{12}.

Anaemia always needs to be checked out by a doctor – but once you have the OK from your doctor, there are a variety of home care options that can offer effective treatment.

when to see a doctor

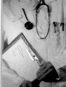

If you have heavy menstrual periods and you're also suffering from constant fatigue: see your doctor right away. The odds are very good that you have iron deficiency anaemia. You'll probably need to get extra iron in your diet, and your doctor will want to ensure that the bleeding is normal and that there isn't an underlying problem.

If your energy is low and you're a strict vegetarian: you could have low levels of vitamin B_{12}, which is found only in animal foods. If you avoid eggs and dairy foods as well as meats, you may need to take B_{12} supplements. The RNI or recommended daily amount is 1.5 micrograms.

If your stools appear black or tarry: bleeding from the gastrointestinal tract is a common cause of anaemia, and it always needs to be investigated by a doctor.

For Immediate Relief
HOME REMEDIES

Increase your iron intake. Women between the ages of 18 and 50 are advised to get 14.8 milligrams of iron daily. Women 51 years and older need only 8.7 milligrams of iron daily.

Eat lean red meats. They help prevent – or reverse – anaemia in two ways: they're rich in dietary iron; and the form of iron that they contain, called haem iron, is easy for the body to absorb.

Enjoy iron-rich greens. Spinach, chard, parsley and spirulina (seaweed) are good sources of iron. The one problem with these foods is that they contain a type of iron called non-haem iron, which is somewhat harder for the body to absorb than the haem iron found in meats.

Put beans on the menu. All kinds of beans, including the humble baked bean, and lentils are good sources of iron. A small can of baked beans provide 3.2 grams of iron, for example.

Drink orange juice with meals. Or finish off your meals with a few slices of orange or grapefruit. Citrus fruits are very high in vitamin C, which enhances iron absorption.

This is especially important when you're eating plant foods that contain difficult-to-absorb non-haem iron.

Save the coffee for later. Along with tea, coffee reduces the body's absorption of iron. It's

THREE THINGS I TELL EVERY FEMALE PATIENT

DR SCOTT A. FIELDS *is a specialist in family medicine. He sees a lot of women who suffer from anaemia, and he always offers this advice.*

1

DON'T TREAT IT ENTIRELY ON YOUR OWN. Many women know the signs of anaemia – such as fatigue around their menstrual periods – and they assume that getting extra iron is all that they need to do. Iron will certainly improve your levels of red blood cells, but it won't correct the underlying problem, says Dr Fields. It's essential that you see your doctor, who will send you for tests to determine what's causing your symptoms.

2

TELL YOUR DOCTOR IF IRON SUPPLEMENTS ARE CAUSING SIDE EFFECTS. Many women with anaemia stop taking iron supplements because they can't cope with the diarrhoea, nausea or other digestive symptoms that sometimes occur when taking them. 'We may try different types of supplements that you'll be able to digest more easily,' says Dr Fields. 'Or we might be able to manage your symptoms with dietary management.'

3

BE PATIENT. 'It usually takes weeks or months for supplemental iron – either from foods or supplements – to correct anaemia,' says Dr Fields. 'In the mean time, rest when you feel tired – and take comfort in the fact that we've found an explanation for your symptoms.'

fine to enjoy these beverages as long as you have them a few hours after meals.

Take advantage of breakfast cereals. If you find that you're eating less meat in order to reduce the amount of fat in your diet, you'll have to make an effort to find other sources of iron in the diet.

Fortified breakfast cereals, which contain added iron, are good choices. A bowl of simple porridge oats, for example, provides only about 1.6 milligrams of iron. A bowl of fortified porridge, on the other hand, may provide more than 8 milligrams.

Take multi supplements. Multi supplements will help your body keep pace with the normal iron losses that take place during menstruation. Premenopausal women should take a multi containing 100 per cent of the RNI or recommended daily amount of iron. Postmenopausal women should take a multi supplement with 9 milligrams of iron.

Don't take iron supplements without checking with your doctor first.

MEDICAL OPTIONS

Ask your doctor about the Pill. Some women lose so much blood during menstruation that they're almost always anaemic. Your doctor may recommend that you go on the Pill: it will normalize your periods and help prevent excessive blood loss, says Dr Goff.

Report strange cravings. It doesn't happen very often, but women will sometimes develop powerful, nearly overwhelming cravings for unsavoury substances, such as dirt, clay or even cigarette ash. This condition, known as pica, is often a sign of iron deficiency anaemia. Doctors aren't sure if iron deficiency causes pica or if it's the other way around – that pica causes iron deficiency anaemia because women eat so much of the non-nutritious substances that they don't get enough healthy foods in their diet. In either case, be sure to report unusual cravings to your doctor. If you're suffering from pica, taking supplemental iron will often cause the cravings to disappear, sometimes in as little as 24 hours.

arthritis

To many women, the word *arthritis* brings to mind an image of a snowy-haired grandmother leaning on a cane or an elderly aunt struggling to open a jar with stiff fingers. Actually, although the incidence increases with the years, arthritis can affect women at any age, including during childhood. Nearly three out of every five people with arthritis are under 65.

Arthritis is the number-one cause of disability in the West, affecting millions of men and women. Predictions are that the numbers affected will rise sharply.

The term *arthritis* (literally, 'joint inflammation') actually refers to a group of more than 100 diseases and conditions that can cause pain, stiffness and swelling in the joints. If not diagnosed and treated, arthritis can cause irreversible joint damage. With treatment, however, women with arthritis can minimize the discomfort and avoid permanent damage.

The two most prevalent forms of arthritis are osteoarthritis, which is the focus of this chapter, and rheumatoid arthritis, which is beyond the scope of this book.

The pressure of gravity and the wear and tear of everyday life cause some kinds of osteoarthritis, which was once called degenerative joint disease. Genetic predisposition also plays a role in developing osteoarthritis. The resulting damage to the joints and surrounding tissues leads to pain, tenderness, swelling and decreased function.

Osteoarthritis primarily affects the cartilage, the slippery tissue that covers the ends of both bones in a joint. Healthy cartilage is thick enough to let the bones glide smoothly over each other and absorb energy from the shock of physical movement.

In osteoarthritis, the cartilage breaks down, wears away and becomes thin, so the bones rub together and cause pain, swelling and stiffness. Over time, the joint can lose its normal shape. Small, bony growths called bone spurs can form on the edges of the joint, and bits of cartilage can break off and float inside the joint space, causing more pain and damage.

In its early stages, osteoarthritis may cause swelling, but its onset is subtle and gradual, usually involving only one or two joints, such as the knee, hip and hand. Pain is the earliest symptom.

For Women, Osteoarthritis Is the Most Common Type

Osteoarthritis affects more than 8 million people in the UK. It is the most common type of arthritis that affects women, mostly after the age of 45. The risk increases with age, especially if there's a family history of the disease.

'Often a woman's mother, grandmother or aunt had osteoarthritis,' says Dr Jeffrey R. Lisse, a clinical researcher in osteoporosis. 'We now know that there's a genetic component to it. It tends to run in families.'

A woman in her fifties, for example, can begin to feel pain and stiffness in her knee, then recall a sports injury or accident when she was a young adult. Being overweight can also cause damage. Obese adults tend to wear out their joints more quickly than do those at a healthy weight.

Fortunately, having arthritis doesn't have to mean the beginning of the end of playing golf, cooking gourmet meals from scratch or doing anything else that you love.

Here's how you can ease the pain if you already have arthritis, and possibly lower your risk of developing it if you don't.

when to see a doctor

If you have severe pain or disability that interferes with normal activities: contact your doctor straight away. Many remedies take at least 8 weeks to start working, so it's best to get an early, accurate diagnosis.

For Immediate Relief
HOME REMEDIES

Grill some wild salmon for dinner. The omega-3 fatty acids in fish oil may ease arthritis pain by providing anti-inflammatory building blocks. 'Fish oil has a mild anti-inflammatory effect by decreasing prostaglandins, which cause inflammation,' says Dr Lisse. Good food sources of omega-3s include salmon, tuna, sardines and mackerel. Experts suggest eating them two or three times a week. Fish oil is also available in supplements. Three grams, or 3,000 milligrams, a day of EPA and DHA (omega-3 fatty acids found in fish oil) is the suggested dose.

Eat your other vegetables. Research has shown that people with high intakes of vitamin C and beta-carotene had a reduced risk of knee pain and disease progression. To be sure that you get enough of these nutrients (as well as other plant-based protective compounds, such as lutein and lycopene), eat lots of carrots, sweet potatoes, broccoli, spinach, fresh tomato sauce and tomato juice, oranges, kiwi fruit and strawberries.

Take some E and D. In studies, vitamin E eased arthritis pain better than a placebo (inactive substance) or a non-steroidal anti-inflammatory drug (NSAID) such as aspirin or ibuprofen. To get the amount of vitamin E that most experts recommend, you'll need a supplement containing up to 3 milligrams. The research also showed that osteoarthritis progression was three times higher in people with low levels of vitamin D, so taking a multivitamin/mineral supplement that supplies 100 per cent of the RNI is a good idea.

Walk away pain. 'Walking is great exercise for women with arthritis because it helps keep muscles warm and flexible, which eases pain,' says Dr Lisse. 'Start slowly, then build up to walking for at least 30 minutes 3 to 5 days a week.'

Concerned that you might do more harm than good? In several studies involving people with osteoarthritis of the knee, none has shown any harm from 30 to 45 minutes of moderately brisk walking on a good walking surface while wearing well-designed shoes.

If walking does cause pain, try walking more slowly, or use some type of special shoe insert or orthotic. And take a good look at your walking shoes: it may be time for a new pair. If the pain continues, stop the brisk walking and contact your doctor.

Long-term Solutions
HOME REMEDIES

Apply heat. For chronic arthritis pain, place a heating pad on the painful site for 10 to 15 minutes three times a day. Heat can be very soothing for sore, stiff muscles and joints. It relaxes them so they move more freely.

Warm up to water walking. Stiff joints and tight muscles can be loosened up by water walking, where the water supports you. For specific water-walking exercises, see pages 349–52.

Go for glucosamine. Glucosamine is a natural substance that furnishes the building blocks needed to make and repair cartilage. In a Belgian study that followed two groups of people over 50 who had mild to moderate osteoarthritis, one group received 1,500 milligrams of glucosamine daily, while the other was given a placebo. After 3 years, the group taking the glucosamine showed little or no joint deterioration. That group also reported improvement in their symptoms, such as pain, and in joint function. The placebo group's joint deterioration worsened, and they did not feel that their symptoms improved.

Though the study focused on arthritis of the knee, Dr Nancy Lane, a rheumatologist, says, 'If it's going to work on the knee to reduce pain, it may work for other joints.' The experts aren't sure exactly how glucosamine works. Made from extracts from crab, lobster and shrimp shells, it contains the chemical building blocks the body needs to make and repair cartilage.

In addition, some research shows that glucosamine soothes knee pain as well as ibuprofen does, but without the stomach upset, bleeding or ulcers that long-term use of high doses of NSAIDs can cause. Studies also show that it can slow cartilage loss, although it may work only for mild to moderate arthritis.

'Glucosamine may prevent further wear and tear on the joints by maintaining the integrity of cartilage,' says Dr Lisse. We recommend 1,500 milligrams a day in two or three doses. You should take it for at least 8 weeks before deciding whether it works for you.

Try SAM-e. Some experts believe that this supplement may improve joint mobility and relieve the pain of osteoarthritis by boosting levels of an amino acid, adenosine triphosphate (ATP) and

THREE THINGS I TELL EVERY FEMALE PATIENT

DR JEFFREY R. LISSE, *clinical researcher on osteoporosis, offers this special advice.*

1

USE A CREAM. 'I have some luck with capsaicin cream with my patients,' says Dr Lisse. Capsaicin is a substance found in hot peppers, and in this topical analgesic cream, it acts on nerve endings to ease arthritis pain. The cream doesn't work instantly, so repeated applications are key. Also, it produces a burning feeling when you first apply it, but this side effect diminishes over time. Follow label directions carefully, and thoroughly wash hands after each application to avoid stinging if you accidentally contact your eyes or other sensitive areas later. Capsaicin cream is available on prescription.

2

EXERCISE. 'It's important to exercise daily to keep the joints and muscles flexible and moving. If you stay physically active, you'll see an improvement in symptoms,' says Dr Lisse.

3

KEEP YOUR WEIGHT DOWN. 'Obese women have more problems with arthritis because extra weight puts pressure on the joints. Keeping weight within the normal range may lower the risk of developing osteoarthritis,' says Dr Lisse. 'For the woman who already has arthritis, keeping her weight in check will reduce the pressure, which eases pain. If you're overweight and can't lose it on your own, talk to your doctor. He can put you in touch with a dietitian who can design a weight-loss programme tailored to your tastes and needs.'

supporting cartilage production. Some studies have shown that SAM-e may help relieve mild osteoarthritis pain almost as well as NSAIDs, but without digestive discomfort.

We recommend a dose of 200 to 400 milligrams three times a day. Sam-e is available on the internet.

MEDICAL OPTIONS

 Ask about new medicines. If taking NSAIDs causes gastrointestinal problems, ask your doctor to prescribe a different drug.

COX-2 inhibitors such as celecoxib (Celebrex) and rofecoxib (Vioxx), for example, are prescription drugs that block pain and inflammation but cause less stomach irritation than NSAIDs do.

For more information: Contact Arthritis Care (www.arthritiscare.org.uk, telephone 020 7380 6500) or the Arthritis Research Campaign (www.arc.org.uk, telephone 0870 850 5000), Arthritis Foundation of Australia (www.arthritisfoundation.com.au, telephone 02 9552 6085), Arthritis New Zealand www.arthritis.org.nz, telephone 04 472 1427).

back problems

The next time you're walking down the street or shopping at the supermarket, take a look around you – eight out of 10 people that you see will experience back troubles at some time in their lives.

'Back pain can come on suddenly and drop you to your knees, or it can be a chronic, long-term condition,' says Dr Stephen Hochschuler, a back specialist.

It's not surprising that back problems are as common as they are. The back is subjected to enormous amounts of stress. Whether you're sitting, standing, bending over, lifting bags and boxes or simply turning to look behind you, the muscles, ligaments and bones in the spine feel the strain. The lower back, called the lumbar region, is especially vulnerable because it supports a

when to see a doctor

If you've hurt your back and the pain hasn't improved after 3 days: you should definitely make an appointment to see your doctor. You may have suffered nerve or tissue damage that won't improve unless you seek medical treatment.

If the pain is excruciating and nothing you do seems to help: you may need to take prescription drugs to reduce the pain, muscle spasms or inflammation.

If you've lost bowel or bladder function, or if you're having numbness, tingling or a loss of muscle strength: you could have suffered nerve damage that may require surgery or other medical treatment.

tremendous amount of weight. That's why it's the most injury-prone area of the entire spine, says Dr Hochschuler.

Men and women suffer from back pain equally, but women have some special risks. After menopause, when a woman's oestrogen levels decline, the bones begin to lose calcium at an accelerated rate. This makes them thinner and weaker than they should be. This condition, called osteoporosis, increases the risk of spinal fractures. Osteoporosis affects both men and women, but women with osteoporosis greatly outnumber men.

Another problem is the design of the spine itself. The bones of the spine, called vertebrae, are separated by shock-absorbing discs that are somewhat similar in structure to iced doughnuts: they have a tough outer coating that surrounds a soft centre. Over the years, the discs lose moisture and flexibility. They literally shrink and lose some of their ability to absorb shocks or impacts. In some cases, the discs actually rupture, or herniate: the soft material in the centre leaks out and puts pressure on tissues in the spine, including the spinal nerves.

'As women start getting into their thirties and forties, the early signs of degenerative disc disease can begin,' says Dr Deborah Saint-Phard, an expert in sports medicine. As women get older, their risk of developing osteoporosis rises – and the bones themselves become increasingly susceptible to damage. 'Even if there's very little stress put on the back, compression fractures are common in women with osteoporosis,' she says.

For men and women, extra weight is among the main risk factors for back problems. Even if you're only a little over your ideal weight, those extra pounds are supported by the back. Year

THREE THINGS I TELL EVERY FEMALE PATIENT

DR DEBORAH SAINT-PHARD, an expert in sports medicine, advises her back patients to do the following:

1

BE CONSCIOUS OF HOW YOU MOVE. 'Little stresses accumulate to cause back problems,' says Dr Saint-Phard. 'Bend your knees when lifting objects – even if you're just picking up a feather. Just because you don't feel pain doesn't mean that you're not creating abnormal stress on the back.'

2

CHANGE POSITIONS OFTEN. Whether you've recently hurt your back or simply want to avoid problems later, don't spend too much time in any one position. Sitting for extended periods can increase pressure on the spine.

FIND EXERCISES THAT WORK FOR YOU. Regular exercise is among the best ways to manage – and prevent – serious back problems, but there isn't a one-size-fits-all exercise plan. 'What works to relieve back pain for one woman may cause it in another,' says Dr Saint-Phard. 'If you try a new exercise and have backache the next day, move on to something else.'

3

after year, they put unnecessary stress on the spine. Even if your discs hold up and your bones remain strong, the muscles and ligaments in the back will feel the strain.

Keeping your back strong requires a combination of strategies, including getting enough calcium in your diet, watching your weight and keeping the muscles and ligaments strong and flexible.

Even if you do everything right, there's a good chance that you'll eventually suffer a bout of back pain. Most back problems are 'self-limiting', which means they'll get better on their own. In the meantime, of course, the pain can be excruciating. Here are a few ways to quickly ease the discomfort of minor backaches and strains – and some long-term strategies for keeping your back strong and healthy.

For Immediate Relief
HOME REMEDIES

Ice the pain. 'Right after you hurt your back, the first thing you should do is apply ice to the area,' says Dr Hochschuler. 'Ice will constrict the blood vessels, which reduces blood flow and decreases swelling.'

Ice works best within the first 48 hours after an injury, Dr Hochschuler adds. If you don't have an ice pack at home, you can wrap a flannel or dishcloth around some ice cubes. Apply the pack for only 5 to 10 minutes at a time. Or fill a few paper cups with water and freeze them. Peel back the paper and apply the ice directly to the sore spots, in a circular motion, for no more than 5 to 10 minutes at a time.

Follow ice with heat. When you've hurt your back, most of the swelling occurs within the first 2 days – which is why applying ice is the best initial treatment. After 2 days, however, you want to *increase* blood flow to the area, which will help the damaged tissues heal.

'Put a heating pad on the area for 20 minutes at a time, using a lower setting in order to avoid a burn,' says Dr Hochschuler. Another option is to lounge in a hot bath several times a day. 'Standing in a hot shower will also help relieve the pain,' says Dr Saint-Phard.

Take anti-inflammatory drugs. Over-the-counter pain relievers are among the best treatments for back injuries because they inhibit the body's production of prostaglandins, chemicals that excite nerve endings and cause pain. Aspirin, ibuprofen, naproxen and acetaminophen all can be helpful, says Dr Hochschuler.

Get some rest – immediately. Back pain is your body's way of telling you that you've done something wrong. Don't ignore the message: stop whatever you've been doing, and give your back a chance to recover.

If you hurt your back playing golf, stop playing and take a break in the clubhouse. If you've been working in the garden, put down the rake and take the rest of the day off. Staying active when the muscles and ligaments are irritated will only increase the damage – and increase the risk of long-term damage.

Even if the pain is severe enough to warrant bed rest, limit it to 2 days. Staying inactive for longer than 2 days will cause the back muscles to weaken and become stiff and inflexible.

Walk it off. 'If you can tolerate it, go for a short walk,' says Dr Hochschuler. Walking is a gentle aerobic activity that gets the blood moving and stretches out stiff muscles. 'It can also relieve some of the tension that could be contributing to your back pain,' Dr Hochschuler adds.

Try water walking. 'If walking on hard surfaces is too painful, try walking in a pool (if you have access),' says Dr Hochschuler. 'It's less painful because the water creates an environment of near weightlessness. Start out slowly, and as it becomes easier, walk faster.'

Long-term Solutions
HOME REMEDIES

Change positions often. It's not unusual for back problems to persist for weeks or even months. One of the best ways to relieve stiffness and also prevent future problems is to change positions frequently. This is especially important if you spend a lot of time sitting, which puts a tremendous amount of stress on the lower spine, says Dr Saint-Phard.

'Every 20 minutes, take a break and change your position,' she advises. If you tend to get so focused on your work that you lose track of time, set an alarm or the beeper on your watch. When you hear the alarm, get up and walk around. Do some stretching exercises. Or simply stand up for a while. The change in position will prevent muscles and ligaments in the spine from 'locking' into position.

Lift with your knees, not your back. 'It's of paramount importance that women use their knees and hips to bend down and pick up children or groceries,' says Dr Saint-Phard. Whether you're picking up something light, like a piece of paper, or something heavy, like a large box, bend your knees and get in a squatting position. 'The back should remain fairly erect while the knees bend, as opposed to bending forwards at the waist,' she explains.

Bend your knees when you sleep. One reason that people often wake up with stiff backs is that they sleep on their stomachs. This causes the back to arch, which puts a lot of pressure on the muscles and ligaments.

'If you have back pain at night or in the morning, it's a good idea to sleep with the knees bent,' says Dr Saint-Phard. 'Lie on your side, and put a pillow between your legs. If you're lying on your back, place the pillow beneath the legs.'

Try not to twist. 'The spine does not like to be bent or twisted, especially when you're lifting things,' says Dr Saint-Phard. 'Remind yourself to keep your spine straight whenever possible,' she advises.

Plan before you move. A lot of back injuries occur when people are doing simple, everyday activities – but doing them the wrong way. When you're vacuuming or making the bed, for example, do you bend forwards at the waist? If so, you're putting a lot of unnecessary pressure on the back. 'Use your leg, hip and buttock muscles to help you when you move the vacuum cleaner,' Dr Saint-Phard advises. When you're making the bed or unloading the dishwasher, bend your knees or even kneel down. Your goal should be to keep your back as straight as possible.

Try to relax. Anxiety and stress cause your muscles to tighten, and tight muscles often lead to back pain.

If you already have back problems, emotional stress invariably makes the pain worse. That's why back specialists advise their patients to do everything they can to reduce the tension in their lives.

One technique that often helps is progressive relaxation, says Dr Hochschuler. It's very easy to do. While you're sitting or lying down, focus on your muscles one at a time. Start with the muscles in your toes; tighten them for a few seconds, then relax. When you've finished with your feet, move upwards to your legs, hips, back and chest. It takes 10 to 20 minutes to tense and relax all the muscle groups. When you're finished, you'll find that a lot of the tension and stress in your body – and your mind – will have melted away.

Strengthen your back muscles. It's a good idea to keep your back muscles in good shape, as this can help you recover from injury quicker. For specific exercises to strengthen the back, turn to pages 353–57.

ALTERNATIVE THERAPIES

Give willow bark a try. Aspirin is among the most effective remedies for back pain, but it may cause stomach irritation or other side effects. An alternative is to use the herb willow bark, which contains a compound called salicin – the same active ingredient that's found in aspirin.

For long-term back pain, willow bark may be superior to aspirin because it's less likely to cause side effects. Health food shops sell a variety of willow bark remedies and it is available online. Look for products containing 250 milligrams of white willow bark, along with 200 milligrams of white willow bark extract that's been standardized to contain 15 per cent salicin. The recommended dose is two to four capsules daily. Willow bark is safe for most people, but those who are allergic to aspirin or other over-the-counter pain relievers may be allergic to willow bark as well. Do not take if you are on blood-thinning medication.

MEDICAL OPTIONS

Ask your doctor about TENS. If you've had long-term back pain, your doctor may recommend a procedure called TENS, short for transcutaneous electrical nerve stimulator. Acupuncture-like needles are inserted into the soft tissues and muscles surrounding the bones. A small electrical current passes through the needles, which interrupts pain signals.

Researchers found that back patients treated with TENS required smaller amounts of painkillers. They also slept better and reported feeling better overall.

For more information: Visit the website of the charity Back Care, at www.backcare.org.uk. Or, in Australia, see www.badback.com.au.

blemishes, pimples and spots

The teenage years are the prime time for acne, but even women in their thirties, forties and beyond can suffer from occasional spots. The only difference is that teenage acne is mainly guided by heredity; adult women can often blame hormonal fluctuations. Even women who never had acne when they were young may have flare-ups in later years – either in conjunction with the menstrual cycle or with the onset of menopause, says Dr Leslie Baumann, a specialist in cosmetic dermatology. Treatments for acne have become increasingly sophisticated in the past few decades. You can't prevent the occasional pimple from popping up, but with a combination of medication and home remedies, it's usually easy to keep acne flare-ups under control.

when to see a doctor

If your acne is accompanied by menstrual irregularities, thinning hair, weight gain or visible facial hair: call your doctor. You might need blood tests to check for excess androgens, 'male' hormones that can cause acne outbreaks.

If you have acne-like bumps on your face, especially on the mid-face (forehead, nose, cheeks and chin) and facial redness and you can also see broken blood vessels, which resemble threads, through the skin: you could have a condition known as rosacea, sometimes called 'adult acne'. Rosacea may require treatment with antibiotics or other medication.

If the acne doesn't get better with home care: your doctor may recommend medications, including birth control pills, oral antibiotics and other drugs to get the outbreaks under control.

For Immediate Relief

HOME REMEDIES

Use benzoyl peroxide. A topical antiseptic, it kills the bacteria that cause the inflammation, swelling and discomfort of acne. Available over the counter in cream, gel or lotion form, benzoyl peroxide (such as Clearasil) may be the only treatment that you need.

After washing your face, spread a thin layer of benzoyl peroxide over the affected areas. Individual dosages and product formulations vary, so follow your doctor's advice.

Generally, benzoyl peroxide should be used once a day at first; as your skin gets used to it, gradually increase to six or eight times daily or as needed during outbreaks.

Try salicylic acid. Another over-the-counter remedy, salicylic acid (which is similar to the active ingredient in aspirin), reduces inflammation and loosens the bonds between dead cells, allowing them to shed more easily.

Clean your skin thoroughly, then apply a thin

layer of salicylic acid (such as Neutrogena Clear Pore Wash or Acnisal) to the acne pimple areas. This medication may cause drying of your skin. Dosage varies for each individual and product, so it's best to follow your doctor's instructions. Usually, you start with one application per day and gradually increase to three applications per day as needed.

ALTERNATIVE THERAPIES

Apply a clay paste. Clay has been used for centuries for deep-cleaning oily complexions and removing impurities from the skin. To prepare a poultice for blemishes, combine ½ teaspoon of cosmetic clay (available at health food shops and some cosmetics counters and from online suppliers) with ½ teaspoon of water. You may need to prepare more of the mixture if you have a larger area to treat or if you want to use it as a facial mask.

Mix well, then apply a thin layer of the clay mixture over the entire face for deep cleaning, or just on the blemishes, and let the clay dry. If the area you're treating is small, you can leave the poultice on for several hours or overnight, then wash it off. Facial masks for the whole face need to be rinsed off thoroughly immediately after the clay dries. Repeat the poultice treatments as needed once daily. You should use the clay mask only once a week to avoid overdrying your skin.

Use essential oil of lavender. It makes pimples less painful, and because it has antibacterial and anti-inflammatory properties, it may help eliminate them as well. Apply 1 or 2 drops of lavender oil to pimples as needed.

MEDICAL OPTIONS

Ask a dermatologist or your doctor about facial peels. Unlike the mild salicylic acid that's used in home preparations, your doctor may recommend treating acne with a highly concentrated form containing 20 to 30 per cent salicylic acid. It removes the surface layer of skin and can improve acne rapidly.

Try tretinoin. Available by prescription, it's a derivative of vitamin A. It reduces oil production in the skin, taking away the 'fuel' that triggers acne. Applied once daily, tretinoin (Retin-A) will help eliminate pimples that are already present, and it may help others from forming.

Ask about isotretinoin. This is among the most powerful acne remedies, and it's used only for severe inflammatory acne and when simpler (and safer) treatments don't work. Isotretinoin (Roaccutane) is very effective, but it may cause adverse effects such as itching, headaches, photosensitivity or hair loss.

More serious possible side effects include elevations of blood fats, abnormal liver enzymes, inflammatory bowel disease and hearing impairment. The most significant potential adverse effect is that it can cause birth defects if taken during pregnancy. Your doctor will prescribe this medication only if you're absolutely sure that you won't get pregnant while using it.

For Long-term Relief
MIND-BODY TECHNIQUES

 Keep stress under control. Emotional stress doesn't cause acne, but it can trigger outbreaks of spots and pimples in some women by changing hormone levels and increasing oil gland secretion.

If you notice that your complexion tends to get worse during emotionally difficult times, take it as a sign that it's time to unwind and take things a little easier. Try to stay calm by exercising more, working less and practising relaxation techniques such as meditation, deep breathing or yoga, and try to avoid stressful situations.

breast pain and tenderness

Cramps, minor mood changes and food cravings are just a few of the signs that a menstrual period is pending. Many women also experience breast pain. The pain usually starts midway though the menstrual cycle, may get progressively worse until the onset of the period, then dissipates. For some women, it can be severe enough to interfere with normal activities.

'Cyclic breast changes occur in response to fluctuating levels of the hormones oestrogen and progesterone during the menstrual cycle,' says Dr Eric Whitacre, a surgeon. 'The breasts may swell and become tender or painful, which may be due to hormonal changes.'

Breast pain, called mastalgia, can have many other causes and affects women of all ages. But because breast tenderness is generally linked to the menstrual cycle, it's much more common in younger women than in those who are post-menopausal. However, any woman may experience pain due to breast tissue changes.

These changes, referred to as fibrocystic conditions, may cause occasional fluid retention in the breasts. The fluid exerts pressure on breast tissues, which in turn may cause pain, says Dr Whitacre. In addition, some women develop tiny fluid-filled sacs, called cysts, in the milk glands. These cysts are harmless, but they can make the breasts tender for a few days.

when to see a doctor

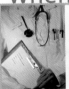

If you've just started experiencing breast pain, regardless of the time of month: make an appointment to see your doctor. It might be due to normal menstrual changes, or it could be related to medication you're taking, such as birth control or supplemental oestrogen or other hormones.

If there's a lump in or near the breast or in the underarm area; a spontaneous nipple discharge, especially if it's bloody; persistent changes in the breast skin, such as puckering or indentations (called dimpling), redness, or scaliness of the breast skin or nipple; pain in the nipple or the nipple turning inwards; or a 'funny' feeling, such as itching or tingling in the skin of the breast or the nipple: these are potential symptoms of breast cancer, and your doctor will probably advise you to have a mammogram or sonogram.

Any type of lump or discomfort in the breasts should be brought to the attention of your doctor right away. In most cases, however, you won't have anything to worry about – and it may be possible to relieve the discomfort with a few simple strategies.

For Immediate Relief
HOME REMEDIES

Wear an exercise bra. It will give the breasts extra support. This is one of the best ways to reduce tenderness and pain. You can wear the bra any time it helps you with the discomfort – even while you sleep.

Take an analgesic. Aspirin and ibuprofen can provide fast-acting relief from monthly breast pain. They inhibit the body's production of prostaglandins, chemicals that cause pain and swelling.

For Long-term Prevention
HOME REMEDIES

Consume less caffeine. Found in coffee, tea, caffeinated soft drinks, chocolate and some over-the-counter medications, caffeine stimulates breast tissue, which may cause an increase in monthly pain, says Dr Whitacre.

Take vitamin E. There's some evidence that vitamin E may reduce breast pain associated with the menstrual cycle as well as the discomforts of fibrocystic breast conditions. 'We're not really sure why it works, but it's worth trying,' says Dr Whitacre.

He advises women with monthly breast pain to take 400 to 800 IU vitamin E daily. Try it for 3 months to see if it helps, he advises.

Try evening primrose oil. Found in over-the-counter supplements, it's rich in gamma linolenic acid, which can inhibit the action of prostaglandins. Evening primrose oil can also reduce painful inflammation. The research is inconclusive about its effectiveness in treating the discomforts of fibrocystic breast conditions. Although doctors aren't sure how it works, evening primrose oil supplements have been shown beneficial as a treatment for mastalgia associated with the menstrual cycle.

'At our clinic, we advise women to start with a minimum of 1,500 milligrams of evening primrose oil per day,' says Dr Whitacre. If that dose doesn't help, you can increase the amount to 3,000 milligrams daily. 'Sometimes you have to start out high, then gradually taper off,' Dr Whitacre adds. 'We've found that you have to take it for 2 or 3 months to see if it will be beneficial.' It's advisable to take 1,000 to 2,000 milligrams of fish oil daily along with the evening primrose oil in order to provide a balance of omega-6s and omega-3s.

Keep a food diary. Breast pain is sometimes caused by foods or beverages in the diet. If you keep track of what you're eating and drinking, you may find that pain occurs, or gets worse, only when you eat certain foods.

'One of my patients was consuming large amounts of soya,' says Dr Whitacre. 'Soya contains plant oestrogens, and oestrogen is implicated in breast pain,' he explains.

constipation

Grandma got many things right, but when it came to bowel habits, the family matriarch missed some vital information.

All that castor oil she made you swallow on the days you missed a bowel movement definitely wasn't what the doctor ordered.

'A generation ago, people were in the habit of giving children laxatives or enemas if they didn't go every day. But now we know that having a bowel movement anywhere from three times a week to three times a day can be normal,' says Dr John W. Popp, a clinical professor of medicine.

Another common fallacy is that our bodies absorb waste, and our health is threatened as a result of not having a daily bowel movement.

Constipation generally refers to stools that are infrequent, dry and hard, or difficult to pass. As a general rule you're constipated if you have fewer than three bowel movements a week. There is, however, no 'right' number of daily or weekly bowel movements. If you're constipated, the bowel movements may be painful. Some patients also complain of feeling sluggish, bloated and uncomfortable.

The hormonal changes of pregnancy are one common culprit of constipation. Also, when the growing uterus compresses the intestines, sluggish bowel movements can result.

Multiple sclerosis, lupus, Parkinson's disease, scleroderma and stroke all can cause constipation. So can diabetes, an underactive or overactive thyroid and spinal cord injuries. Some medicines

THREE THINGS I TELL EVERY FEMALE PATIENT

DR JOHN W. POPP, a clinical professor of medicine, says that patients with bowel problems take their bowel movements very, very seriously. 'I've had patients come in with photographs of their stool,' Dr Popp says with a chuckle. Yet going to the toilet doesn't have to trigger anxiety. Here's some advice he gives his patients.

ESTABLISH A TOILET ROUTINE. Set aside a regular time each day – after breakfast or when you've finished dinner – for a visit to the toilet. Make sure you're not disturbed. 'Every morning after breakfast, sit down, but don't become upset if you don't produce the perfect-10 BM,' Dr Popp says.

1

DON'T THINK OF HAVING A BOWEL MOVEMENT AS A COMPETITION. 'The key is what's normal for you,' Dr Popp says.

2

ADD FIBRE GRADUALLY. If you're currently eating 5 to 7 grams of fibre each day and set a goal of 25 grams, don't adjust your diet overnight. 'It's a huge mistake to take too much too soon,' Dr Popp advises. 'Always start with a very low dose. And make simple substitutions. Replacing a serving of white rice with brown rice will give you triple the amount of fibre.'

3

trigger constipation, too. The most common medications that may produce constipation are antidepressants, antihistamines for allergies, drugs for Parkinson's disease, diuretics (often called 'water pills') and antacids containing calcium or aluminium. Pain medication, antispasmodic drugs, iron supplements and anticonvulsants used for epilepsy can also slow your bowel movements.

Older adults are more likely to report problems with constipation than young people. That's because they're more likely to take constipating drugs, and they're less likely to exercise, eat adequate amounts of fibre and drink enough fluids.

Constipation in older women may also be linked to pelvic muscles weakened as a result of pregnancy and childbirth.

Yet too little fibre is often the main cause of constipation. The average woman eats about 12 grams of fibre each day, well under the 25 to 35 grams experts recommend.

You don't have to eat a regular diet of sawdust to ease your discomfort from constipation. Try these tips from doctors who specialize in the treatment of bowel disorders.

For Immediate Relief
HOME REMEDIES

Answer nature's call. Yes, the kids are clamouring for breakfast – *now*. That doesn't mean it's prudent to ignore your urge to have a bowel movement. People who ignore the need to go to the toilet may eventually stop feeling the urge – and that can lead to constipation. If you're already constipated, don't sit and strain. It's better to wait until you feel the urge to go, and then try.

Try a home remedy. Dr Craig Rubin, a professor of internal medicine, suggests mixing 8

when to see a doctor

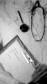

If you've had any change in your usual bowel habits, or if you notice blood in the stool: call your doctor right away. It's probably nothing serious, but these and other changes could be a sign of cancer or other grave illnesses.

'Blood in the stool, a change in bowel habits, a thinning of the stools – all are red flags to call your doctor, especially if they occurred out of nowhere,' says Dr William J. Snape, a specialist in bowel disease.

Yet some patients procrastinate, fearing the truth – and the medical tests, says Dr John W. Popp, a clinical professor of medicine. 'Patients will say, "The doctor is putting a lighted tube *where*? No way." The biggest fear is the fear of the unknown.'

Several other symptoms should send you to a doctor, too: they include weight loss, severe abdominal pain and a change in your bowel pattern, in either the frequency or the consistency of your bowel movements.

Sometimes straining to have a bowel movement causes a small amount of the intestinal lining to protrude from the rectal opening in a condition known as a rectal prolapse. Mucus staining on the undergarments is a symptom.

Abdominal pain and bloating, combined with constipation, could signal that you have an intestinal obstruction.

tablespoons of unprocessed bran, available in most supermarkets, and 8 tablespoons of stewed apples with 80 millilitres (3 fluid ounces) of prune juice. Refrigerate. Take 2 to 3 tablespoons of the mixture after dinner, and then drink a tall glass of water. If needed, increase your dosage to 3 to 4 tablespoons. The mixture will keep for about 2 weeks in the refrigerator.

Find flax (linseed). Two tablespoons of nutty-tasting flax each day may offer enough insoluble fibre to keep you regular. To make a flax-rich breakfast smoothie, combine 240 millilitres (8 fluid ounces) of orange juice, one banana and 2 rounded tablespoons of ground flaxseed. Always refrigerate ground flaxseed.

Consider a little extra help. Fybogel and other over-the-counter fibre supplements may help ease symptoms. Movicol, a laxative that doctors prescribe, has been found to be effective.

Analyse your routine. Have you changed your diet, workouts or work schedule? Any deviation from your routine can trigger a change in your bowel habits. Are you taking any medication that might be constipating? Ask yourself these questions to determine if you are truly constipated: Do I have a hard time passing stools? Am I having fewer bowel movements than normal. Do I have pain during bowel movements? Do I have other problems, such as bleeding? If the answers are yes, you're probably constipated.

MIND-BODY TECHNIQUES

Consider biofeedback for serious cases. Some patients suffer from abnormalities in the structure of the rectum and anus, conditions doctors call anorectal dysfunction or anismus. Women with anismus cannot relax the anal and rectal muscles used during bowel movements. Some people with these disorders may get relief by using biofeedback to retrain their muscles after they receive instructions on the procedure from their doctors.

For Long-term Relief

HOME REMEDIES

Drink when you're dry – and then some more. Juices and other liquids such as water may help make bowel movements softer and easier to pass. Aim for eight 240-millilitre (8-fluid ounce) glasses each day.

Fill up on fibre. 'Fibre is very important, and a lot of people will say, "But I eat bran cereal," and mistakenly think they're getting a whole day's worth,' says Dr Popp. 'I tell my patients a good minimum number to aim for is 20 grams,' adds Dr William J. Snape, a specialist in bowel disease.

If you replace your bowl of Rice Krispies (zero grams) with just 100 grams of Shreddies, say, you start the day with over 11 grams of fibre. Add a couple of apples after lunch and dinner (4 grams apiece), snack on 30 grams (1 ounce) of dried whole almonds in the late afternoon (3 grams) and eat a serving of chopped, cooked broccoli at dinner (5 grams), and you'll easily exceed your daily goal.

Don't forget to eat your vegetables. Brussels sprouts, carrots, potatoes and sweet potatoes with their skins are especially helpful to people with constipation.

Get physical. Doctors aren't sure why, but regular exercise might help your system stay, well, regular. If you have heart disease, emphysema or any chronic illness, ask your doctor before you start exercising or change your routine. Even if you are healthy, don't think you have to be a marathon runner. A 20- to 30-minute walk, every day, should be adequate.

Use laxatives prudently. The key words are *temporarily* and *occasionally*.

'If you're taking a constipating drug like an antihistamine or have an acute illness that causes constipation, it's perfectly acceptable to take a laxative,' Dr Popp says. When you finish the drug or recover from your illness, you should drop the laxative or else you could risk becoming dependent.

'The more you use laxatives, the more your bowel depends on them, and eventually the bowel may stop working,' Dr Popp says.

depression

We all feel sad or discouraged from time to time, and usually we know why. It might be a troubled relationship, problems at work or simply the winter blues. As time passes, we work through the problems, and our moods begin to brighten.

Depression is an entirely different matter. 'It's more than just a down mood,' says Dr Jack G. Modell, a professor of psychiatry. 'With depression, your feelings are controlling you, and you feel as though you just can't get past them.'

It's not clear why, but women are twice as likely as men to suffer from depression. Signs of depression include losing pleasure in daily activities, diminished appetite, difficulty concentrating, changes in your usual sleep patterns and feelings of guilt or worthlessness.

'If you start having three, four or five symptoms every day for most of the day, and the feelings persist for more than 2 weeks, it's time for concern,' says Dr Kelly Conforti, a clinical psychologist.

when to see a doctor

If you're feeling 'blue' and are also experiencing physical problems, such as fatigue or unexplained changes in your weight: see your family doctor. Many symptoms of depression mimic those caused by underlying medical problems.

If your depressive feelings last longer than 2 weeks, or if you're thinking about suicide or death: these are symptoms of clinical depression, and you'll need professional help right away.

If you've had depression in the past, and you suspect that it's coming back: it is estimated that 50 to 60 per cent of people who have had one episode of major depression will have another episode during their lives.

The treatments for depression – everything from medication and 'talk therapy' to changes in lifestyle – are surprisingly effective: up to 80 per cent of those who seek treatment will notice rapid improvement, usually within a few weeks.

For Immediate Relief
HOME REMEDIES

Put pleasure on your schedule. Every day, jot down a few enjoyable activities – going for a walk, enjoying a long bath or simply perusing a magazine that you haven't had time to read – that you're going to do. Give them the same priority that you would a serious business appointment.

'We have too many *should*s in our lives and not enough things that are enjoyable. That can lead to depression,' says Dr Conforti.

Limit coffee to a cup or two a day. Caffeine boosts mood temporarily, but some women feel a letdown when the caffeine wears off, says Dr Neil

Benowitz, professor of medicine at the University of California.

Get enough calcium. Research suggests that women who experience premenstrual depression may feel better when they consume calcium. One study found that women who took 1,200 milligrams of elemental calcium daily in the form of calcium carbonate experienced more than a 50 per cent reduction in their premenstrual syndrome symptoms.

The best sources of calcium are skimmed milk and cheese. Also, many juices and breakfast cereals are fortified with calcium.

ALTERNATIVE THERAPIES

Try St John's wort. This herb appears to help maintain healthy levels of mood-regulating brain chemicals. Dr Varro Tyler, dean emeritus of the Purdue University School of Pharmacy, advises taking 300 milligrams of St John's wort extract three times daily.

It may interact with other medications,

THREE THINGS I TELL EVERY FEMALE PATIENT

DR JACK G. MODELL, a professor of psychiatry, offers the following advice for coping with depression.

1

EXERCISE DAILY. It boosts levels of chemicals in the brain that regulate mood. 'If all you can do at first is 5 minutes, that's fine,' he says. Research has shown that people who exercise regularly are less likely to stay depressed. They'll also recover more quickly when their moods head south.

2

GET SOME SUN. Exposure to sunlight triggers the release of melatonin in the brain. Melatonin regulates your sleep and wake cycles, and it can have a powerful effect on energy and mood.

3

SHARE YOUR PROBLEMS WITH FAMILY AND FRIENDS. Chances are, others have experienced the same feelings. Their understanding and emotional support will go a long way towards helping you feel better.

including some antidepressants. Don't combine St John's wort with other drugs without checking with your doctor first.

For Long-term Relief
HOME REMEDIES

Stay in touch with your friends. It might be the best medicine for depression. A UK study found that 65 per cent of women with depression who met for 1 hour weekly with a volunteer 'befriender' experienced a remission, compared with 39 per cent of those who didn't get the extra support. That's about the same success rate that's seen in conventional therapy or from taking drugs, says study author Dr Tirril Harris, a researcher with the Socio-Medical Research Centre in London.

MIND-BODY TECHNIQUES

Manage negative thoughts. You have a surprising amount of control over the ideas and beliefs that flit through your mind. People are more likely to suffer from depression when they embrace negative thoughts, such as 'I've wasted my life' or 'This is the worst thing that's ever happened'. Turn the thoughts around. When you say to yourself things like 'Things are getting better' or 'I've made mistakes, but I think I can improve things', you'll decrease your feelings of sadness or depression.

Stay in touch with your spirituality. 'Studies have shown that people who are active in their churches or places of worship and feel a connection with God or some higher power have less depression.

MEDICAL OPTIONS

See a professional. Fully fledged depression is unlikely to disappear on its own. If your symptoms are mild, regular visits to a therapist are probably all you need. For more severe depression, antidepressant medications may be added.

'The best treatment is often a combination of therapy and medication,' says Dr Modell. 'Therapy will help you understand why you were having problems in the first place, and the medication will give you the energy and strength to make the most of the therapy.'

Ask your doctor about hormone replacement. Postmenopausal fluctuations in oestrogen and other hormones often contribute to insomnia and fatigue, which can increase the risk of depression.

'Trying oestrogen replacement for a month or two will often solve the problem of sleep deprivation and restore a sense of well-being,' says Dr Neill Epperson, assistant professor of psychiatry at Yale University School of Medicine.

For more information on depression: Visit the website of the charity Depression Alliance at www.depressionalliance.org; the depressioNet is an online resource for Australians who suffer from depression: www.depressioNet.com.au.

fatigue

It's early afternoon, and lunch is followed by one big yawn after another. Ready for a snooze? Join the club: millions of us barely have enough energy to get through the day, and the problem is getting worse all the time.

Westerners are spending more time working and less time sleeping or simply having fun. According to one survey, 60 per cent of women don't get the 8 hours of sleep that they need to feel refreshed and energized.

'Most women need about 8 hours of sleep in order to wake up feeling rested and to have energy throughout the day,' says Dr Lynn Mack-Shipman, an endocrinologist and assistant professor of internal medicine. 'Sleep deprivation is a common cause of fatigue.'

It's not the only one, however. Many women are low in iron. That's the mineral essential for creating haemoglobin, the iron-based protein in blood that ferries the oxygen that the body needs for energy. Thyroid conditions can also lead to fatigue. So can stress, which is almost at epidemic proportions these days.

'The average woman today has many responsibilities, such as a full-time job, child care, housework and taking care of ageing parents,' says Dr

THREE THINGS I TELL EVERY FEMALE PATIENT

DR LYNN MACK-SHIPMAN, an endocrinologist and assistant professor of internal medicine, sees a lot of women whose main symptom is fatigue. Here's what she advises.

1

DO EVERYTHING YOU CAN TO RELAX. 'Stress can zap anyone of their energy,' says Dr Mack-Shipman. 'Practise relaxation techniques. I've actually written a prescription for one of my patients to enroll in a yoga class.'

Yoga isn't the only way to relax, of course. Some women cut back on their work hours. Others practise relaxation techniques such as meditation or visualization. Exercise is a great stress-reducing technique because it stimulates the release of 'calming' chemicals in the brain.

2

FOCUS ON COMPLEX CARBOHYDRATES. Whole grains, pulses and other plant foods are rich in complex carbohydrates, which are broken down slowly during digestion. This allows glucose (blood sugar) to be produced at a steady pace, which helps maintain energy.

3

AVOID SIMPLE CARBOHYDRATES. There's nothing wrong with having a sweet snack on occasion, but the sugars in snacks and soft drinks, known as simple carbohydrates, cause blood sugar levels to rise. The body responds by releasing large amounts of insulin, which can make you feel tired.

Mack-Shipman. The stress from personal and professional responsibilities, along with the physical burden of trying to do too much, leaves many women feeling exhausted all the time.

Because fatigue is a common symptom of medical problems, it's essential to see your doctor as soon as you notice that your energy isn't what it should be. In most cases, however, it's possible to recharge your batteries with a variety of at-home techniques.

when to see a doctor

If you feel as though you sleep well at night, but you're still exhausted during the day: make an appointment to see your doctor. You could have a sleep problem that's preventing you from getting all the rest you need.

Insomnia is probably the most common sleep disorder, but it's not the only one. Your doctor might advise you to have a sleep test, which will measure brain waves, respiration and other factors that can affect the quality of your sleep.

If you've been fatigued for months, and nothing you try seems to help: you should ask your doctor about getting tested for iron deficiency anaemia. If you are anaemic, getting adequate amounts of iron will reverse the symptoms within weeks or even days.

If the fatigue is accompanied by weight gain, intolerance to cold and constipation: these are classic symptoms of an underactive thyroid.

If you have increased thirst and you're also urinating frequently: you could have diabetes, which is often accompanied by severe fatigue.

For Immediate Relief
HOME REMEDIES

Adjust your sleep schedule. Many women get into the habit of keeping late hours – but the alarm clock still goes off at the same time every morning. If you aren't getting enough sleep at night, there's no way you're going to feel energetic during the day. The solution is simple: try to go to bed a little earlier. You can't shift your body's internal clock all at once, so you have to work in increments. Go to bed about 15 minutes earlier than usual. Do this for a few weeks until it feels like the 'right' time. Then move your bedtime back another 15 minutes. Keep doing this until you're getting a full 8 hours' sleep.

Most women can make the transition easily, and you'll find that your energy levels will be higher throughout the day.

Get your body moving. Exercise doesn't produce energy directly; as a matter of fact, it consumes energy. But women who walk, jog, work in the garden or are otherwise physically active generally notice that fatigue is much less of a problem.

'Physical activity stimulates the release of beta-endorphins, hormones that make you feel alive, refreshed and energized,' explains Dr Mack-Shipman.

Exercise is also beneficial because it tires the muscles, which in turn will make it easier for you to sleep at night.

Vary your routine. Women who are new to exercise often complain that doing the same things every day is too boring to stay motivated. That's why many people who start exercise plans drop out within a few weeks or months. The solution is to identify a dozen or more physical activities that you enjoy – it could be swimming, working in the garden, bicycling or even walking round the shops – and swap them around so that you never get bored.

'Try running one day and lifting weights the next. Or do something entirely different, like t'ai chi or ballroom dancing,' Dr Mack-Shipman suggests.

ALTERNATIVE THERAPIES

Energize with essential oils. 'Smelling certain scents can invigorate your body and mind and help you feel more energetic,' says Dr Alan Hirsch, neurological director of the Smell and Taste Treatment and Research Foundation in Chicago. The scents of peppermint and jasmine essential oils are especially energizing, he says.

The easiest way to use 'scent therapy' is to put a few drops of essential oil on a handkerchief, then take a few minutes to enjoy the aroma. Another option is to use an aromatherapy diffuser, available from mail-order catalogues and some health food shops. It will fill the air with the special scents.

For Long-term Prevention
HOME REMEDIES

Get enough iron. Millions of women don't get enough iron in the diet. This is especially common during the childbearing years because women lose a little blood each month

A 'HIDDEN' CAUSE OF FATIGUE

The thyroid is a small gland at the base of the front of the neck. It uses iodine from the blood to produce and store thyroid hormone, which plays a major role in the body's metabolism. Women who produce too little thyroid hormone, a condition called hypothyroidism, will feel tired, weak or depressed.

Doctors estimate that 17 per cent of women will have thyroid problems by the time they reach their 60th birthdays. 'The condition often comes on gradually, over months or years, so it's not always diagnosed right away,' says Dr Gay Canaris, an assistant professor of internal medicine.

As a result, the symptoms often go unnoticed by either the patient or her doctor and are easily attributed to other medical problems, overwork or stress, Dr Canaris adds. Hypothyroidism is diagnosed by a blood test that measures thyroid gland function.

Women with a family history of thyroid disorders, or those with autoimmune conditions such as lupus, have a higher risk of developing hypothyroidism. Women who have recently given birth are also at risk, Dr Canaris says.

Hypothyroidism is easy to treat with medication. Once your hormone levels are back to normal, most thyroid symptoms will improve. 'You just have to take one small pill a day of synthetic thyroid hormone,' says Dr Canaris. 'It's really very simple.'

during menstruation. Even when a woman doesn't have full-fledged iron deficiency anaemia, low levels of this mineral can result in fatigue.

'Some women don't consume enough iron-rich foods, such as red meats, because they are concerned about putting on weight,' says Dr Mack-Shipman. Without sufficient amounts of iron, the red blood cells can't carry as much oxygen, which results in fatigue.

The best sources of iron are lean red meats, poultry, eggs and fish, says Dr Mack-Shipman. Other options include fortified breakfast cereals, potatoes and beans.

The RNI or recommended daily amount for iron is 14.8 milligrams, for women aged between 19 and 50.

Drink plenty of water. 'Dehydration, even in its earliest stages, can make you feel tired and weak,' says Dr Mack-Shipman. Try to drink eight full glasses of water daily, she advises.

Lose weight sensibly. Women who are trying to lose weight often depend upon restrictive diets such as those high in protein and low in carbohydrates, and others that are very low in calories.

These diets aren't very effective for weight loss, and they're even worse for maintaining healthy energy levels, says Dr Cindy Polich, a medical nutritionist.

'Following one of these "starvation" diets can lead to fatigue and weakness,' she says. 'When you don't get enough carbohydrates, you deplete your short-term energy supplies.'

Whether or not you're trying to lose weight, you should choose a variety of foods, focusing on carbohydrates such as whole grains, pulses, and fruit and vegetables. 'The body converts carbohydrates into glucose, which is used for energy,' Polich explains.

Maintain a healthy weight. Women who are above a healthy weight are more likely to experience fatigue.

Extra weight can also increase your risk for a sleep disorder, called apnoea, in which breathing is reduced at night. Your body responds by waking up briefly in order to take a deep breath. You might not be aware of the disturbance in your sleep, but your energy levels are sure to suffer the next day.

fibromyalgia (fibrositis)

Women who develop fibromyalgia (or fibrositis as it is sometimes known) often confuse it with flu, at least at first. It typically causes muscle stiffness, headaches, poor sleep and an overwhelming sense of fatigue. People with fibromyalgia hurt all over, and they are often too tired to perform even

the simplest daily activities. Unlike flu, however, fibromyalgia doesn't go away in a week or two. It's a chronic condition, which means it can last months, years or even decades.

Estimates show that up to one in ten women suffer from fibromyalgia. It's most common in women of childbearing age, but children, the elderly and men can also be affected.

How can you tell if your symptoms are caused by fibromyalgia? The telltale sign is 'tender points' – extremely sensitive areas that generally appear in the neck, spine, shoulders and hips, says Dr Lenore Buckley, a rheumatologist. Depression is another common symptom. Research has shown that between 18 and 36 per cent of people with fibromyalgia suffer from depression at any given time.

Another characteristic of fibromyalgia is poor sleep. It's not that people with this condition sleep too little; in fact, many people with fibromyalgia sleep 10 (or more) hours a night. The problem is that they fail to achieve the deeper levels of sleep that they need to feel refreshed. The lack of deep sleep can interfere with the ability to focus and concentrate during the day. It can also make people feel groggy and 'out of it' when they wake up in the morning.

Scientists still aren't sure what causes fibromyalgia. One theory is that injuries affecting the central nervous system play a role. Some scientists have linked fibromyalgia to changes in muscle metabolism, which may result in diminished blood flow and, in turn, fatigue.

Some evidence indicates that fibromyalgia is triggered by bacterial or viral infections. Research has shown, for example, that 10 to 25 per cent of people with Lyme disease, a bacterial infection transmitted by ticks, will develop fibromyalgia.

Fibromyalgia is a challenge to diagnose because many of the symptoms are similar to those caused by other disorders. If you have tender points and widespread pain that has lasted more than 3 months, and tests show that you don't have lupus, arthritis or Lyme disease, you could have fibromyalgia.

So far, there isn't a cure for fibromyalgia. That doesn't mean you have to live with it for ever. The severity of the symptoms tends to come and go, and it's not uncommon for it to spontaneously disappear.

For Immediate Relief
HOME REMEDIES

Have a massage. 'I have found in my patients with fibromyalgia that a massage stops the pain,' says Dr Denise Borrelli, a massage therapist.

Massage is relaxing, which makes it much easier for people with fibromyalgia to get the sleep they need. 'Some of my patients have been able to cut back on their sleep medication after they started having massages regularly,' says Dr Borrelli.

There are a bewildering variety of massage techniques to choose from. 'I recommend Swedish massage because the long, gentle strokes are very soothing,' Dr Borrelli says. 'I advise against deep muscle tissue massage because it can irritate nerve endings and cause more pain,' she adds.

Depending on where you live, massage can cost anything from £25 per hour. To find a massage therapist in your area, contact the British Massage Therapy Council on 01865 774123 or visit their website at www.bmtc.co.uk. Australian Association of Massage Therapists (AAMT) www.amta.asn.au. Therapeutic Massage Association of New Zealand www.massagecollege.co.nz.

Enjoy pool therapy. Warm-water pool therapy is a great way to relax the muscles and reduce the pain, says Dr Buckley.

Exercise as much as you can. Walking, biking, water exercise and other forms of aerobic exercise have been shown to reduce muscle pain and tenderness. Regular exercise also stimulates the production of endorphins, chemical messengers in the brain that promote feelings of relaxation and well-being.

If you have fibromyalgia, it probably won't be easy to start an exercise programme because your muscles will be sore and achy. But it's worth pushing through the initial discomfort.

'It's very difficult for fibromyalgia patients to get better who are not part of an exercise programme,' says Dr Buckley. 'Regular, gentle exercise, such as walking or warm-water exercises,

when to see a doctor

If you've had widespread pain for 3 months or more: see your doctor right away. It's one of the classic signs of fibromyalgia.

If you feel pain at specific 'tender points': people with fibromyalgia typically have tender areas on the shoulders, elbows, hips or buttocks.

If you're always fatigued, and you can't work out why: fibromyalgia isn't the only condition that can result in low energy or lethargy. If you're exhausted all the time and there doesn't seem to be a good reason for it, see your doctor.

can help loosen up stiff muscles and get the blood flowing again, all of which will help ease pain.' As your muscles get stronger, you'll find you have more energy and endurance, and the intensity and frequency of the pain will gradually diminish.

If you haven't been physically active, start out with stretching exercises before launching into full-fledged workouts, and check with your doctor before commencing a new routine. 'Walking is more of an intermediate exercise for women to work up to,' says Dr Buckley. 'Take a brisk 5-minute walk, then gradually increase the time and intensity until you're walking briskly for 40 minutes three times a week.'

Avoid caffeine. Coffee, tea and other caffeine-containing drinks are Westerners' favourite pick-me-ups, but people often forget just how stimulating they can be. If you have fibromyalgia, consuming caffeine close to bedtime can make it difficult to get the deep, restorative sleep that you need for optimum health.

Your doctor may advise you to limit your consumption of caffeine-containing drinks to one or two servings daily – and to avoid them altogether in the afternoon and evening.

For Long-term Relief
HOME REMEDIES

Take a yoga class. Even though regular exercise is among the best ways to ease the discomfort of fibromyalgia, people are often too tired or sore to get started. One way to get the muscles primed for action is to practise yoga. 'If yoga is the exercise you choose, start with a beginners' class,' says Dr Buckley.

Sign up for aquaerobics. 'Warm-water exercises are very beneficial for fibromyalgia patients because they relax the muscles and decrease pain,' says Dr Buckley. 'The water supports the muscles, so you're not working against gravity,' she adds.

Some people head straight to a local pool, but it's better to sign up for an aquaerobics programme tailored for those with arthritis or other musculo-skeletal problems. 'It's important to make sure that you're doing the moves correctly so you don't hurt yourself,' says Dr Buckley. Your doctor can refer you to a physical therapy programme that includes water exercises.

Try to think positively. It's hard to be upbeat and positive when you're in pain, but it's worth making the effort. Studies have shown that people who dwell on their pain and unhappiness experience a lot more stress – which in turn increases pain.

In one large study, researchers compared drug and non-drug treatments for fibromyalgia. They found that people who exercised or practised cognitive-behavioural therapy – in which they learned to substitute positive thoughts for negative ones – experienced less pain and fatigue. They also performed daily tasks more easily than those who only took drugs. A good place to start is to make an appointment with a psychological therapist. In the mean time, do everything you can to relax. Set aside time each day to meditate, listen to music or simply unwind.

MEDICAL OPTIONS

Consider antidepressants. Even if you aren't suffering from depression, medication such as amitriptyline and fluoxetine (Prozac) can be extremely helpful for fibromyalgia. Apart from reducing muscle pain, these medications also make it easier to sleep, which can significantly boost energy and help you to stay active.

Today's antidepressants are safe and effective, but they may cause side effects, such as a dry mouth or grogginess.

Ask your doctor about drug combinations. In one study, people with fibromyalgia were treated with Elavil, Prozac or a combination of the two drugs. Those who took both drugs experienced twice the improvement of those taking the drugs separately. In fact, 12 of the 19 participants in the study reported improvements of at least 25 per cent.

Researchers suspect that the combination of Elavil and Prozac may change pain perception in people with fibromyalgia. The medications also affect blood flow to pain-receptive regions of the brain, and they enhance the body's production of 'feel-good' chemicals such as serotonin.

Take a sleep aid. 'The main goal in the pharmaceutical treatment of fibromyalgia is to help people get some sleep,' says Dr Buckley. 'The pain often keeps people up at night, and even when they do fall asleep, the pain often wakes them up.'

For more information on fibromyalgia: See the website of the Fibromyalgia Association UK at www.fibromyalgia-associationuk.org.

food allergy

In the past few years, a number of airlines have eliminated the customary practice of handing out bags of peanuts to hungry passengers. The reason: many people – male and female alike – are allergic to peanuts, and for those whose allergy is severe, even the scent molecules that waft from a newly opened bag can trigger life-threatening reactions.

Fortunately, most food allergies aren't this serious. People who eat the 'wrong' foods may break out in hives or welts. Or they may have nausea, diarrhoea or other digestive problems. Once the offending foods clear the system, the symptoms rapidly disappear.

But whether your allergies are minor or severe, there's only one long-term solution: to avoid the foods that make you unwell. This isn't always easy because people with food allergies are rarely allergic to just one food. They usually react to whole groups of foods, such as shellfish or certain grains. Identifying the culprit – and avoiding it – can take some work. As little as $1/5,000$ teaspoon of an offending food can potentially cause a reaction. Women who are allergic to peanuts, for example, could have problems if a cook merely used the same spatula when baking different types of biscuits, one of which contained peanuts. If you're allergic to a certain food or foods, you have to avoid them entirely – probably for the rest of your life. Food allergies occur when the immune system mistakes an entirely innocent protein for a harmful intruder. It overreacts and launches a full array of immune cells to counteract the 'attack', which is what causes the symptoms, says allergy expert Dr Clifton Furukawa.

While most food allergies cause only minor symptoms, people with extreme sensitivities may experience a life-threatening reaction called anaphylaxis, which can literally shut down the airways and cause blood pressure to plummet. Anaphylaxis is more common in people with food allergies than in those who are allergic to insect stings or medications.

Food allergies often begin in childhood, although adults, too, can develop them. Children with food allergies tend to be sensitive to eggs and milk, while adults are more likely to be allergic to shellfish or nuts. Children sometimes outgrow food allergies, but if you developed the problem as an adult woman, it's unlikely to go away.

Researchers are investigating ways to reverse the body's sensitivity to potential allergens in foods, but for now there isn't a cure for food allergies. All you can do is make sure to avoid the 'wrong' foods, and know what to do should an emergency strike.

For Immediate Relief
HOME REMEDIES

Act quickly. If you have a minor food allergy and you accidentally eat what you shouldn't, most reactions can be treated with an antihistamine, and you can simply wait for the symptoms to pass. But for those with severe allergies, waiting can cost them their lives. You have to be prepared to take immediate action – by giving yourself an anti-anaphylaxis injection and getting to a casualty department immediately.

Always carry a self-injector. Women with severe food allergies are advised to keep a self-injector handy. Products such as the EpiPen or AnaPen contain a medication called epinephrine. It helps reverse anaphylaxis by stimulating the heart, opening the airways and reducing swelling of the throat.

If you have a history of food allergies but haven't had a serious reaction for years, it's easy to get complacent and leave the injector at home – either because you forgot it at the last minute or because you thought you wouldn't need it. Don't take that chance. When researchers looked at 32 people who had died from food allergy reactions, they found that only three of them were carrying their injectors.

'I tell patients they should always carry three doses of epinephrine,' says Sandra M. Gawchick, a specialist in allergy and clinical immunology. 'They have one spare in case they drop one, and another spare to buy them time until they get medical help.'

Use the medicine at the first sign of symptoms. Even if you're not completely sure if you're having an allergic reaction, give yourself the injection anyway. 'I advise patients to inject the epinephrine first and ask questions later,' says Dr Furukawa. The sooner you get the injection, the better your chances of making a full recovery.

The advantage of the EpiPen is that it's fully automatic: just remove the safety cap, push the tip against the outer thigh to release the medicine and hold it in place for several seconds. Then get to a casualty department right away.

Practise. It takes time to learn to use self-injectors properly, so it's important to practise ahead of time. 'You need about 30 pounds of pressure to trigger the EpiPen, so if you just tap it lightly, it won't work,' says Dr Ira M. Finegold, an expert in allergy and clinical immunology. 'That's why it's important to practise using it.'

If you experience an allergic reaction and need to give yourself a jab, it's fine to lift your skirt slightly and put the jab into your thigh through tights, Dr Finegold adds. If at all possible, avoid injecting yourself through thick fabric because you could get an infection when the needle goes through dirty clothing.

Avoid alcohol when eating out. Alcoholic beverages can increase the body's absorption of allergy-causing proteins, says Dr Marianne Frieri, a specialist in allergy and immunology.

At home, where it's easier to control your exposure to potential allergens, it's fine to enjoy a beer or a glass of wine. But when you're eating away from home, avoiding alcohol will give you an extra measure of protection.

Never take chances. Many people with food allergies don't take their condition seriously. They may assume that 'just a tiny taste' won't hurt. Or they may depend on medication to get them out of a tight spot. This is a dangerous mindset, says Dr Frieri. 'Food allergies can be life threatening. People need to take their symptoms seriously.'

For Long-term Prevention
HOME REMEDIES

🏠 **Keep a food diary.** It can be tricky to know what food or foods you're allergic to. The only way to find out which foods are friends and which are foes is to keep a comprehensive food diary. Every day, jot down everything you eat. Be specific: don't write 'salad' when you really ate lettuce, onions, tomatoes and grated cheese. At the same time, note any physical symptoms that occur. If you keep the diary for several months, you'll start to narrow down the possible suspects.

Talk to your doctor about an elimination diet. This involves giving up, one at a time, the foods that you suspect are causing symptoms. If you felt that you had a reaction after eating prawns, for example, you would give up prawns for a few weeks. If you don't have additional symptoms, you may have discovered the culprit.

Of course, you might be allergic to more than one food, so you might have to repeat the process several times. Once you have a good idea what's causing the problems, the solution is obvious: you'll have to give up the problem foods completely. Because there are so many ingredients in packaged foods, and because people with food allergies may react to similar proteins that are found in different foods, you'll need to work with your doctor to ensure that you're eliminating the proper foods – and to make sure that you are

STAY ON GUARD FOR HIDDEN ALLERGENS

Women with life-threatening food allergies need to look for harmful ingredients in some unexpected places.

Food is the main offender, of course, but food allergens can also be found in cosmetics, shampoos and other items that you'd never think of eating.

It's possible, for example, for a woman who's allergic to nuts to develop a severe reaction if she uses a shampoo made with almond oil, says Dr Hugh A. Sampson, director of the Elliot and Roslyn Jaffe Food Allergy Institute.

'One of my patients was allergic to nuts – and he developed wheezing and hives when the shampoo, which contained nut oils, got near the lips and eyes,' he says.

Shaving creams, moisturizers and lipsticks are often made with oils made from peanuts, almonds or soyabeans, adds Dr Clifford W. Bassett, an assistant clinical professor of medicine and an expert on allergies.

Even chewing gum is a potential problem for some people because it may contain cow's milk proteins, Dr Bassett says.

Reading the labels may not always help because non-food items rarely list all the ingredients – and those that are listed may be in scientific terms that are difficult to interpret. While nothing is completely foolproof, in some cases it may be helpful to ring the manufacturer – use the Internet to find the number – to inquire about ingredients before using any product that can potentially get into the nose, mouth or eyes.

getting adequate nutrition while the elimination diet is under way.

Read food labels carefully. Packaged foods can contain dozens of ingredients – and sometimes you'll find ingredients where you least expect them. Surprising numbers of packaged foods contain soyabeans, for example. Milk proteins are commonly used in packaged foods, even some that you wouldn't suspect of containing dairy. The terms on food labels can be confusing, so you'll need to work with your doctor to identify possible offenders. For example, many products contain 'casein' or 'caseinates'. These include milk protein, and foods that contain them can cause allergic reactions.

Check labels frequently. Food manufacturers often change the ingredients in their recipes. A food that was 'safe' in the past might contain allergy-causing ingredients in the future. The only way to be safe is to read the labels every time you shop.

Keep foods and utensils separate. Some people with food allergies are so sensitive that the merest brush with an offending food can trigger anaphylaxis. If you are at risk, you have to be careful that you don't inadvertently breathe, taste or touch the foods that you're allergic to. If you're allergic to peanuts, for example, make sure that family members don't use 'your' cutting board when making peanut butter sandwiches. If you're allergic to prawns, eating foods that were fried in the same oil could be just as harmful as eating the prawns themselves.

Telephone restaurants in advance. Eating away from home can be risky for people with food allergies. Asian restaurants, for example, typically use the same woks to cook all the dishes. Even if the chef assures you that your dish doesn't contain a certain ingredient, traces of it might remain on the utensils. Doctors refer to this as cross-contamination. It's worth phoning the restaurant in advance to express your concerns – and to find out if they're willing to accommodate you. If you're allergic to shellfish, for example, let the restaurant know that the steak you've ordered can't be cooked in the same pan or section of the grill that's used to prepare shellfish.

Order simple foods. When you're eating out, it's a good idea to order foods that undergo minimal preparation. A baked potato, for example, is unlikely to be cross-contaminated with other foods, whereas french fries are prepared in oil that may be used to fry other foods.

Wear a medical alert bracelet or necklace. Anaphylaxis and other food allergy symptoms can come on very quickly – too quickly, in some cases, for people to care for themselves. Teach your friends and family about your self-injector so that they can help you during a time of crisis.

It's also helpful to carry a personalized card that lists your name, your doctor's name and phone number, and a list of foods that you're allergic to.

For more information about food allergies: Visit the website of the organization Allergy UK at www.allergyfoundation.com. Allergy New Zealand is at www.allergy.org.nz.

haemorrhoids

Haemorrhoids are one of those intimate conditions that no woman feels comfortable talking about. But there's nothing really that mysterious about them.

Haemorrhoids occur when veins in the rectum become stretched, swollen and inflamed. Basically, they're like the varicose veins that you see on people's legs, except they are in a much more sensitive area.

Most haemorrhoids occur inside the anus, where there aren't many nerve endings. These internal haemorrhoids aren't painful, but if they protrude outside the anus, they can become sensitive and sometimes cause bleeding. Haemorrhoids that start on the outside of the anus, on the other hand, can swell or form a hard lump caused by a blood clot. This type of haemorrhoid, called a external thrombosed haemorrhoid, causes acute pain. Constipation is the main cause of haemorrhoids. When you strain to have a bowel movement, the increase in internal pressure damages the walls of the veins. If you're pregnant, you're especially vulnerable because the growing uterus also causes an increase in vein-damaging pressure.

Haemorrhoids usually go away in a few days to a week, but they can make your life miserable in the mean time. Here are some quick ways to reduce the discomfort and prevent haemorrhoids from coming back.

when to see a doctor

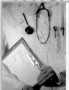

If you're having rectal bleeding, even if it's just a few drops on the toilet paper: see your doctor straight away. Most bleeding is caused by haemorrhoids, but it can also be caused by colon cancer.

If the discomfort is accompanied by changes in bowel habits or unusually thin stools: these are other common symptoms of colon cancer.

If a haemorrhoid is causing excruciating (not just annoying) pain: the haemorrhoid could have a blood clot inside that may need to be removed by your doctor.

For Immediate Relief
HOME REMEDIES

Use baby wipes for a few days. Toilet paper can feel like sandpaper when you have haemorrhoids. 'The best thing people can use is alcohol-free baby wipes,' says Dr Bruce A. Orkin, a specialist in colon and rectal cancer.

Take baths instead of showers. Soaking the area in warm water two or three times a day will shrink swollen tissues and reduce the discomfort.

Soften the stools. When you have haemorrhoids, having a hard bowel movement can be agony. To soften stools in a hurry, use an over-the-counter stool softener or a fibre supplement that contains methylcellulose (like Fybogel), following the directions on the label. Stool softeners may be taken twice a day.

For Long-term Prevention
HOME REMEDIES

Increase the fibre in your diet. Found in fruit, vegetables, whole grains and other plant foods, fibre helps prevent haemorrhoids – and reduces discomfort if you already have them. Gradually increase your fibre intake to avoid bloating.

'Fibre acts like a sponge and soaks up water,' Dr Orkin says. The water makes stools softer, which reduces straining during bowel movements.

According to the experts, everyone should eat 25 to 35 grams of fibre daily. 'I tell patients to choose cereals with 5 to 7 grams of fibre per serving,' Dr Orkin says. Add to that a few servings of fresh fruit, raw or lightly steamed vegetables, and fibre-rich foods such as whole grains and pulses, and you'll automatically get all the fibre that you need.

Drink a lot of water. It's absorbed by stools in the intestine, which makes them softer. Plan on drinking eight full glasses of water daily. If you drink coffee, tea or a caffeinated soft drink, only count that as two-thirds of a serving towards your fluid intake for the day. These drinks can pull water out of your stool.

Go to the toilet straight after breakfast. That's when the body's urge to go is strongest. If you wait until later in the day, you'll probably have to strain more, which increases the risk of haemorrhoids.

Don't dawdle. The more time you spend on the toilet, the more likely you are to suffer from haemorrhoids. You shouldn't need to sit for more than a few minutes to have a bowel movement.

headaches

Millions of people suffer from headaches, with pain that ranges from a mild twinge to the skull-pounding agony of migraines. For reasons that still aren't clear, women are more likely to suffer from headaches than men, with two out of three migraine sufferers being female.

The two most common types of headaches are tension headaches and migraines. Even though they share the name 'headache', they're as different as night and day.

With tension headaches, the pain is felt all over the head, including in the small muscles around the eyes and behind the ears. As the name suggests, tension headaches are often but not always associated with muscle tightness in the back of the neck or on the scalp. The pain is usually mild or moderate, and it tends to be triggered by emotional factors, such as stress, anxiety, fear or anger.

Migraines are much more disabling. They cause moderate to severe throbbing or pulsing pain, usually on one side of the head. The pain of migraines, which can last as long as 3 days, is often accompanied by nausea and sensitivity to light or sound. About 20 per cent of migraines are preceded (or accompanied) by visual disturbances that include wavy lines, dots, flashing lights or blind spots. Some people experience changes in their usual sense of touch, taste or smell prior to the attacks.

Doctors still aren't sure what causes migraines. They have discovered that people who get migraines have overactive areas in the brain stem. It's thought that changing levels of hormones affect this part of the brain, which may be why women get migraines more frequently than men.

'Some women get migraines due to the falling oestrogen levels that are associated with their menstrual cycles,' says Dr Stephen D. Silberstein, who specializes in the treatment of headaches.

Another hormonal factor that contributes to migraines is pregnancy. 'Some women find that they get more migraines during the first trimester, when their levels of oestrogen and progesterone change,' Dr Silberstein explains. 'The migraines usually go away during the second and third trimesters, when hormones level off. Then, after women give birth, they often return within the first week because of falling oestrogen levels.'

Hormonal fluctuations are just one explanation for migraines. Doctors have identified dozens of things that can set them off, including stress, bright lights, food preservatives (such as nitrites and nitrates) or even changes in the weather. Migraines also tend to run in families. If your parents got these head bangers, there's a higher risk that you'll get them, too.

THREE THINGS I TELL EVERY FEMALE PATIENT

DR STEPHEN D. SILBERSTEIN, a doctor who specializes in the treatment of headaches, offers the following advice for women coping with headaches.

DON'T WAIT TO GET HELP. Women often assume that headaches are 'normal' – and they suffer for years or decades without getting help. 'Most women with tension or migraine headaches can get successful treatment that will keep them under control,' Dr Silberstein says. Before your doctor's appointment, keep a journal noting the dates, severity and duration of the headaches; any possible triggers; and the headaches' impact on your life, such as missed workdays, suggests Dr Silberstein.

THEY'RE NOT 'ALL IN YOUR HEAD'. In the past, doctors sometimes dismissed headaches as being a sign of emotional problems. Nothing could be further from the truth. 'Headaches are a biological disorder of the brain, and we can usually control them,' says Dr Silberstein.

TAKE TIME FOR YOURSELF. 'Write a prescription for yourself to relax,' Dr Silberstein advises. 'Schedule time to do anything you want, whether it's listening to relaxing music, meditating or reading a book. Everyone needs this special time to relax – and it may prevent headaches.'

1

2

3

Tension headaches are easier to treat than migraines, but nearly all headaches, regardless of the type, can be managed with a combination of medication and self-care strategies.

For Immediate Relief
HOME REMEDIES

Use over-the-counter painkillers. They're very effective at stopping tension headaches, says Dr Silberstein. Aspirin, ibuprofen, naproxen and paracetamol are all equally effective.

Products such as Migraine Relief and Migraleve contain codeine and paracetamol. Other migraine medications contain ibuprofen. All of the products work for a non-disabling migraine, so you can take these if your pain is not so severe that you are unable to function. Everyone responds differently, so you may have to try several medications to find the one that works best.

Take a hot shower. 'It may relieve tension headaches because the warm water loosens and relaxes muscles in the back of the neck and head,' says Dr Silberstein.

Ice it down. Cold compresses are helpful for all types of headaches because they numb the area and also constrict blood vessels, which can reduce the painful pounding. Apply either an ice pack or a plastic bag filled with ice cubes and wrapped in a towel to the painful area for about 10 to 15 minutes. Or wrap a bag of frozen peas in a towel and place it on your forehead, Dr Silberstein suggests.

ALTERNATIVE THERAPIES

Try feverfew. It's been used for thousands of years to treat headaches, and there's some evidence that it's effective. A common herb, feverfew contains compounds called sesquiterpene lactones, which reduce spasms in blood vessels in the brain. The research isn't conclusive, but feverfew appears to be more effective at preventing migraines than at stopping them once they begin. The recommended doses vary, depending on the form. If you're using fresh feverfew, take one leaf once daily; for freeze-dried feverfew tablets or capsules, take 300 milligrams

when to see a doctor

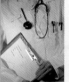

If you're experiencing headaches more than usual, or if the pain seems to be getting worse: see your doctor straight away. Headaches can be caused by a variety of potentially serious neurological problems, including tumours.

If the pain mainly occurs on one side of the head: you're probably suffering from migraines, which are a lot more serious (and painful) than common-or-garden tension headaches.

If the headaches that you experience are accompanied by nausea or vomiting or if you're experiencing auras — visual disturbances that may include waving lines, flashing lights or blind spots in your vision that precede or accompany (or both) the headache: you may be experiencing the classic form of migraines, and you'll probably need medication to get them under control.

daily; for fresh plant tinctures, take 40 drops daily; and for standardized extracts in tablet form, take a daily dose that provides the equivalent of 0.25 to 0.50 milligrams of parthenolide.

One more point about feverfew: many herbs are dried with traditional methods, but this destroys the active compounds in feverfew. It's best to use tinctures made from fresh leaf, or tablets or capsules that contain freeze-dried herb.

Reach for rosemary. This fragrant kitchen spice does more than perk up roasts and poultry – it also appears to prevent some stress-related headaches by keeping the blood vessels dilated. The easiest way to use rosemary is to enjoy it in a tea. Pour 1 cup of boiling water over 1 teaspoon of dried rosemary leaves. Cover and let it steep for 10 minutes, strain the leaves and drink.

For Long-term Prevention
HOME REMEDIES

Drink more fluids if you're active. Some people get migraines mainly when they exercise, possibly because they allow themselves to get dehydrated, says Dr Silberstein. 'To prevent dehydration, make sure you drink eight 240-millilitre (8-fluid-ounce) glasses of water each day,' he advises. 'If you're working out and perspiring, you're losing water, and it needs to be replaced.'

Take riboflavin. Researchers have found that brain cells in some people with migraines produce insufficient amounts of energy. One way to boost energy production and prevent headaches might be to flood the cells with vitamin B_2, also known as riboflavin.

In a study in Belgium, 55 migraine sufferers were given either 400 milligrams of riboflavin or a placebo. At the end of the 3-month study, 56 per cent of the riboflavin group reported a decrease in the frequency of their migraine attacks. In the placebo group, only 19 per cent had a similar benefit.

The amount of riboflavin used in the study was much higher than the amounts that most people get – hundreds of times the recommended daily amount of 1.1 milligrams for women. 'It's difficult to get that much riboflavin from foods, and the study wasn't recommending that all migraine sufferers take the study amount in supplement form,' Dr Silberstein says.

'But women with migraines might consider asking their doctors for advice on whether to try a supplement and the dosage that's right for them,' he adds.

Keep a food journal. There's little scientific evidence that eating certain foods causes migraines, but many people believe that when they stop eating the 'wrong' foods, their migraines disappear. For some migraine sufferers, the desire to eat particular foods, however, can be a warning sign of an impending migraine attack, adds Dr Silberstein.

The next time you get a migraine, take a few minutes to jot down everything you ate in the past 48 hours, Dr Silberstein suggests. If you keep the journal consistently, you may discover that the headaches are consistently preceded by a craving for certain foods.

Some of the foods that are commonly associated with migraines include:

■ Ripened cheeses such as Cheddar, Stilton, Brie and Camembert

■ Fermented, marinated or pickled foods

■ Chocolate

■ Sour cream

■ Nuts or peanut butter

■ Sourdough breads

■ Broad beans or mangetouts

■ Foods with monosodium glutamate (MSG), such as soy sauce, seasoned salt or meat tenderizer

■ Papayas, figs, raisins or avocados

■ Citrus fruit

■ Processed meats, such as salami

■ Alcoholic beverages

Cut back on caffeine. 'Some people get "Saturday migraines" because they drink a few cups of coffee every day during the week, then don't drink any on the weekends,' says Dr Silberstein. 'Caffeine withdrawal is what causes their migraines.'

The solution isn't to drink coffee or tea 7 days a week but to cut back on caffeine overall – or to switch to decaf. This gives the brain a chance to become less sensitive, which in turn can reduce the frequency of headaches.

Keep a regular sleep schedule. Women who keep irregular hours – by staying up late at weekends, for example, then sleeping until noon the next day – are more likely to suffer from headaches than those who keep regular hours. 'Make sure that the bedroom is dark, peaceful and quiet,' Dr Silberstein adds. 'When your body is resting, your brain is resting.'

MIND-BODY TECHNIQUES

Take up yoga or meditation. Stress probably doesn't cause headaches, but it does act as a trigger in those who are susceptible to migraines or tension headaches. Some of the best ways to relax and reduce stress include yoga, deep breathing and meditation, says Dr Silberstein.

Try progressive relaxation. This relaxation technique calls for tensing and then relaxing every muscle in your body, starting with your toes and working upwards to your skull. It can take 20 minutes or more to complete a session, but it's worth it. People who practise progressive relaxation say it helps them feel rested and relaxed – and less likely to suffer from headaches.

MEDICAL OPTIONS

Ask about prescription relief. Medications for migraines are divided into two main groups: those that prevent migraines and those that can quickly reduce the pain of attacks.

Doctors have found that medications – such as sodium valproate (Epilim), also used to control seizures, and amytryptiline, also used as an antidepressant, can prevent migraines. To stop migraines that are already under way, doctors usually prescribe a class of drugs known as 'triptans', which include sumatriptan (Imigran), rizatriptan

(Maxalt), naratriptan (Naramig) and zolmitriptan (Zomig). The medications work by attaching to a receptor for serotonin, a neurotransmitter in the brain.

For the fastest relief possible, doctors often advise people with migraines to use sumatriptan in an injectable form, Dr Silberstein adds.

Consider biofeedback. It's a technique that teaches people to control muscle tension, lower blood pressure and even divert blood away from the head at the first signs of headaches. Biofeedback is simple to learn, but it requires the use of sophisticated equipment that allows patients to monitor changes in their physical signs. Ask your doctor if a referral to a biofeedback specialist would be helpful.

For more information about headaches: Visit the website for the US National Headache Foundation at www.headaches.org. Note that this is an American site and therefore drug names may be different. Or go to the website for the British Migraine Action Association at www.migraine.org.uk; Headache Australia at www.headacheaustralia.org.au; the Neurological Foundation of New Zealand at www.neurological.org.nz.

irritable bowel syndrome

Women who live with irritable bowel syndrome (IBS) soon develop a sixth sense about the locations of public toilets. They have to because the symptoms of IBS – usually abdominal pain, cramping and diarrhoea – can come on with very little warning.

Before leaving the house, women with IBS invariably ask themselves, 'Is my bowel going to act up today?' IBS is very unpredictable. Some women will have sudden attacks of diarrhoea, sometimes several times a day. For others, diarrhoea may alternate with constipation, painful flatulence buildups or other digestive upsets.

There's still a lot of mystery surrounding IBS. Normally, the muscular walls of the intestine contract and relax in a predictable and rhythmic way. Research has shown that in people with IBS, the contractions are stronger and last longer –

although it's not yet clear if this is the underlying cause of the condition. Since doctors haven't discovered what causes IBS, there still isn't a cure. However, there are a number of medications that can control the symptoms. In addition, there are a number of home care strategies that will go a long way towards reducing the discomfort.

For Immediate Relief
HOME REMEDIES

Cut back on coffee and tea. Caffeine may irritate the digestive tract, so it's a good idea to avoid anything containing caffeine.

Take fatty foods off the menu. They're difficult for the body to digest, which can result in more flatulence and indigestion.

Choose soluble fibre supplements instead of bran. Some IBS sufferers find that bran and other foods rich in insoluble fibre worsen their condition. If you're one of them, switch to a soluble fibre supplement.

Be prepared. There will be times when you simply can't afford to be incapacitated with intestinal woes – when you're overwhelmed at work, for example, or you're planning an overseas flight.

For short-term control of diarrhoea, it's fine to take over-the-counter diarrhoea remedies such as loperamide (Imodium).

Reduce flatulence. Bloating or distention due to intestinal flatulence is one of the most common symptoms of IBS and can also lead to cramping and abdominal pain.

Over-the-counter products that contain simethicone (such as Maalox Plus) may help relieve intestinal flatulence. Or you could try an over-the-counter product called Beano, available in some pharmacies and health food shops. It contains an enzyme that assists in the digestion of some sugars and may help prevent flatulence from forming.

Eat less dairy. Some people have a condition called lactose intolerance: they don't produce enough of the enzyme (lactase) that's needed to digest a sugar (lactose) found in dairy foods. If you're lactose intolerant and also have IBS, even small amounts of milk, cheese or other dairy foods may cause symptoms.

If you're lactose intolerant, you might be able to enjoy small servings of dairy foods, especially if you have them with other foods. Or you may have to avoid dairy products altogether. You may have to experiment a bit to find out which approach works for you.

ALTERNATIVE THERAPIES

Relax the intestine with herbs. Chamomile and valerian relax intestinal contractions. Valerian may be especially helpful because it also reduces stress, a common trigger of IBS.

Pour 1 cup of boiling water over 1 to 2 teaspoons of dried chamomile flowers. Cover and let it steep for 10 to 15 minutes. For valerian, take two 500-milligram root tablets 30 minutes before you go to bed.

You can buy herbal teas and supplements at pharmacies and health food shops.

Try peppermint. Another herb that relaxes the intestinal muscles, it appears to be very helpful for those with IBS, says Dr Mark Stengler, a naturopathic doctor.

when to see a doctor

If diarrhoea or other common symptoms of IBS are accompanied by weight loss: see a doctor straight away. You could have a more serious digestive condition, called Crohn's disease.

If you notice rectal bleeding or if you've had recent changes in your symptoms: some of the same signs of IBS can also be caused by colon cancer. You'll need to get a checkup straight away.

In one study, out of 52 people with IBS who took one peppermint capsule before meals for one month, most reported having less abdominal pain, bloating and diarrhoea.

If you decide to try peppermint capsules, look for products that are enteric-coated: they dissolve in the intestine instead of in the stomach, thereby reducing stomach upset. Look for capsules with 0.2 to 0.4 millilitres of oil.

Try cognitive therapy. Studies have shown that using a type of 'talk therapy' can help you feel better by changing the way you view your problems.

Cognitive therapy involves keeping a diary of your symptoms and your feelings about them. A therapist can help you reframe your feelings so you gain control over your IBS symptoms.

For Long-term Relief
HOME REMEDIES

Include more fibre in your diet. It's among the best strategies for controlling IBS. Experts recommend getting 25 to 35 grams of fibre daily. If you start the day with a high-fibre cereal, snack on fruit throughout the day and include several servings of vegetables with meals, you'll almost automatically get all the fibre you need.

There are several types of fibre, and they aren't quite interchangeable. If your main symptom is diarrhoea, try to increase your intake of soluble fibre, found in fruit, porridge oats, rice, barley and psyllium. If constipation is the problem, you'll do better focusing on the insoluble fibre found in pulses, whole wheat and vegetables.

THREE THINGS I TELL EVERY FEMALE PATIENT

DR MARK STENGLER, a naturopathic doctor, suffered from IBS for years. Here are his strategies for getting the symptoms under control.

1

TAKE CONTROL OF STRESS. 'When you're under stress, the sympathetic nervous system gets stimulated and the normal contractions of the intestines are altered,' he explains. Some of the best ways to reduce stress include yoga, prayer and meditation. 'You'll have to experiment to find what works best for you,' he says.

2

EXERCISE REGULARLY. There's no scientific evidence that it controls IBS, but many patients report that it helps. 'Choose an exercise that you really like, such as taking walks with a friend,' Dr Stengler advises.

3

TRY PASSIONFLOWER. A herb, it reduces digestive discomfort, Dr Stengler explains. If you're using a 1:1 tincture, take 20 drops three times daily. If you're using capsules, take two 500-milligram tablets three times daily.

Keep to a regular meal schedule. Having breakfast, lunch and dinner at the same times every day will help regulate digestion and prevent 'sneak' attacks of IBS.

Eat cooked vegetables. They're easier to digest than raw vegetables, says Dr Stengler.

Pay attention to your diet. Everyone with IBS reacts to different foods. If you find that you spend 30 minutes in the toilet every time you eat porridge, for example, you should probably try another hot cereal. It will take some trial and error to find out which foods make your symptoms worse – and which make them better.

MEDICAL OPTIONS

✚ **Talk to your doctor about antidepressants.** Patients with more severe symptoms may benefit from antidepressants. They have been shown to relieve some of the symptoms of IBS, especially when people are also suffering from pain and depression.

Your doctor may recommend one of the tricyclic antidepressants, such as imipramine (Tofranil) or amitriptyline (Elavil). Apart from reducing stress and depression, these drugs may decrease stool frequency, which is helpful for some people with IBS.

Other medications that may be helpful to some people include fluoxetine (Prozac) or paroxetine (Seroxat). These drugs tend to be used when people with IBS are suffering from constipation as well as depression.

Look into hypnosis. Performed by doctors or other trained professionals, hypnosis and behaviour modification techniques may be useful in reducing stress and relaxing the intestinal muscles. Studies show that they may be helpful in reducing abdominal pain and bloating associated with IBS.

kidney infections

Even women who get frequent urinary tract infections are surprised – and dismayed – by how ill they feel when the infection moves upwards from the bladder to the kidneys.

The kidneys are the body's main filters. They remove waste products from the blood and ship them to the bladder for disposal. An infection in the kidneys, called pyelonephritis, can result in excruciating pain. There's also a risk that the infection will spread to other parts of the body.

'Women get kidney infections more than men because they tend to ignore bladder infections, instead of getting them treated straight away,' says Dr Larrian Gillespie, president of Healthy Life Publications.

Kidney infections tend to occur when bacteria that have multiplied in the bladder travel upstream through the ureters, the tubes that connect the kidneys to the bladder. It's common, in fact, for women to have infections in the kidneys and bladder at the same time.

Once you have a kidney infection, you're going to need antibiotics. While you're waiting for the drugs to work, there are a number of ways to reduce the discomfort. You can also take steps to prevent future infections.

For Immediate Relief
HOME REMEDIES

Drink as much as you can hold. Water helps flush the infection from the kidneys, and it also dilutes the concentration of bacteria in the bladder, which can prevent kidney infections from getting started, says Dr Gillespie. For long-term protection, drink at least eight 240-millilitre (8-fluid ounce) glasses of water daily.

Use pain relievers as needed. While you're waiting for antibiotics to work, taking aspirin or ibuprofen will help reduce fever and muscle aches. Just follow the directions on the label.

Apply heat. Women with kidney infections often feel better when they apply a hot-water bottle to the abdomen or below the ribs.

when to see a doctor

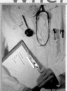

If you have pain in the flank (below the ribs towards the back), fever or nausea and vomiting: see a doctor straight away. These are classic symptoms of kidney infections.

If the urine is cloudy or tinged with blood or if it has an unpleasant smell: you probably have an infection somewhere in the urinary tract — either in the bladder or the kidneys.

MEDICAL OPTIONS

Get a prescription. Kidney infections always require antibiotics and cannot be treated with herbs, says Dr Gillespie. Some women get so ill that they're given the drugs intravenously, but oral medications are usually effective. The antibiotics – such as trimethoprim with sulfamethoxazole, ciprofloxacin or ofloxacin – are usually taken for 7 to 14 days to eliminate every trace of infection.

Reduce bladder irritation. Women with kidney infections often experience intense urges to urinate, even after they've just urinated. An over-the-counter medication called potassium citrate (such as Cystopurin) reduces the 'gotta go' symptoms, says Dr Gillespie.

For Long-term Relief
HOME REMEDIES

Inhibit bacteria with baking soda (sodium bicarbonate). If you have a bladder infection and want to ensure that it doesn't spread to the kidneys, mix ¼ teaspoon baking soda in a glass of water and drink it once a day. It makes the urine more alkaline, which helps prevent bacteria from thriving.

Keep bacteria away from the urethra. Women often get kidney or bladder infections when germs from the anal area get inside the urethra, the tube that carries urine from the body. To avoid kidney infections, when you go to the toilet, always wipe from front to back, which pushes bacteria out of harm's way, says Dr Mary Jane

Minkin, clinical professor of obstetrics and gynae-cology at Yale University.

Wash before sex. Washing the genital area – with soap and water, or simply warm water – removes bacteria that might otherwise slip into the urethra, says Dr Minkin. Urinating after sex is also helpful because it flushes away bacteria that were lucky enough to get inside.

ALTERNATIVE THERAPIES

 Drink cranberry juice daily. Research has shown that cranberry juice contains chemical compounds that make it more difficult for bacteria to stick to cells in the urinary tract. Women who get a lot of infections will often drink one or two glasses of unsweetened cranberry juice daily as a preventive measure.

Dried cranberries, which contain the same infection-fighting chemicals as the juice, are also a good bet.

Eat active, live-culture yoghurt. The 'good' bacteria in live-culture yoghurt help to maintain a healthy balance of bacteria in the body, which translates into fewer bladder infections.

memory problems

Don't be too hard on yourself the next time you lose the car keys. Many women begin experiencing memory lapses around their 50th birthdays, and in adults aged 70 and older, declines in memory are nearly universal. Blanking out occasionally is exasperating, but no big deal.

Occasional forgetfulness isn't a sign of Alzheimer's disease. It doesn't mean that you're destined to spend the rest of your life forgetting names or wondering why you put the post in the freezer. What it probably means is that cells in your brain aren't getting all the nourishment or stimulation that they need to withstand the normal wear and tear of ageing.

'Some people, whether because of their behaviour or their genetic makeup, are able to avoid or slow the usual declines in memory function,' says Dr Stanley Birge, director of the Older Adult Health Center at Washington University School of Medicine. Health problems such as high blood pressure and high cholesterol may contribute to memory lapses and other mental declines, so it's important to talk to your doctor if you find you're forgetting things more than you used to.

But in most cases occasional forgetfulness doesn't mean you're losing your mental faculties. There's a good chance you can significantly improve your memory – and reduce the risk of further declines – with a variety of mental tactics and simple lifestyle changes.

For Immediate Relief
HOME REMEDIES

 Exercise your mind. 'People who remain active socially and are engaged in demanding cognitive activities may be able to reduce the usual ageing of the brain,' says Dr Birge. Crossword puzzles and games of Scrabble will keep the brain challenged. Volunteer work is helpful. So are hobbies, or simply reading magazines and newspapers.

'You shouldn't do just one thing,' Dr Birge adds. 'You need to keep the brain operating at a multitude of activities.'

Review important information. The brain has more trouble taking in new information as you get older. You can overcome this by mentally reviewing information that you want to retain.

The next time you meet someone new, for example, repeat the name in your mind several times. If you tend to lose the car keys, keep them in the same place and mentally visualize where they are.

'The better the preparation, the stronger the memory,' says Dr James McGaugh, director of the Center for the Neurobiology of Learning and Memory at the University of California.

Reinforce your memory with a cup of coffee or tea. Laboratory studies suggest that the caffeine in coffee, tea and fizzy colas may enhance long-term memory when it's consumed shortly after learning new things.

Take a nutritional supplement. As you get older, the small intestine loses some of its ability to absorb vitamin B_{12}, which plays a role in memory and other mental functions. Lean meats, eggs and low-fat dairy foods provide abundant amounts of B_{12}. Vegetarians, however, may need to take a supplement. The RNI or recommended daily amount for vitamin B_{12} is 1.5 micrograms.

Drink more water. People who don't drink enough can get dehydrated, which affects blood flow to the brain, leading to fatigue and making it harder to remember things. Try to drink at least eight 240-millilitre (8-fluid ounce) glasses of water daily.

ALTERNATIVE THERAPIES

Give ginkgo a try. Available in pharmacies and health food shops, this herb improves circulation and helps brain cells get all the nutrients they need to stay healthy. Researchers at the Medical Research Centre at the University of Surrey, found that people aged 50 to 59 who took 120 milligrams of ginkgo three times daily had improvements in memory, concentration and alertness.

'Now we have proof positive that ginkgo can boost memory in healthy young people,' says Douglas Schar, a London herbalist.

Drink sage tea. Folk healers have traditionally recommended sage for improving memory, and new research suggests it could work. Sage contains two chemical compounds – 1,8-cineole and alpha-pinene – which block an enzyme that may be linked to Alzheimer's disease.

The problem with sage is that is also contains a compound called thujone, which may be toxic in large doses. It's fine to enjoy sage tea on occasion, but you shouldn't drink it every day.

Boost cell communication with huperzine A. A supplement based on a Chinese herbal remedy, huperzine A (HupA) is thought to protect the brain's supply of acetylcholine, a chemical messenger that may break down over time.

Studies of people with Alzheimer's disease have shown that 60 per cent of those who took HupA had significant improvements in mental function.

Improve your memory with PS. Short for phosphatidylserine, PS is a component of brain cells that regulates chemical messengers, or neurotransmitters. One study showed that people who took PS found it easier to recall the names of people they'd recently been introduced to.

Long-term Solutions
HOME REMEDIES

Eat brightly coloured fruits and vegetables. They contain chemical compounds called flavonoids, antioxidant compounds that blunt the effects of free radicals, unstable oxygen molecules in the body that may damage blood vessels in the brain and increase the risk of memory declines. In one study, animals that were given flavonoid-rich blueberries or spinach daily were able to reverse memory impairments.

'If you want to slow down the free radical ageing process, blueberries are the leader of the pack,' adds Dr Ronald Prior, head of the USDA Phytochemical Laboratory at Tufts University. 'With 145 grams (5 ounces) of blueberries, you can just about double the amount of antioxidants that most Western people get in one day.'

Take extra vitamin E. Scientists have found that vitamin E reduces levels of memory-clouding free radicals in the brain. Vitamin E is found mainly in nuts, wheat germ and cooking oils, as well as in supplement form. The optimal dose

THREE THINGS I TELL EVERY FEMALE PATIENT

DR STANLEY BIRGE, director of the Older Adult Health Center at Washington University School of Medicine, gives this important advice.

1 TALK TO YOUR DOCTOR ABOUT HORMONE REPLACEMENT THERAPY. The hormone oestrogen protects memory in several ways. It reduces free radical damage, increases blood flow, and stimulates growth factors that are involved in the repair of damaged neurons. Supplemental oestrogen may help after the menopause, when a woman's natural supply of the hormone declines.

2 MAKE SURE YOU EXERCISE REGULARLY. Walking, cycling, and other forms of exercise increase blood flow to the brain. In addition, exercise stimulates different parts of the brain. When people engage in physical activity, their risk of cognitive impairment is dramatically reduced.

3 TAKE CONTROL OF STRESS. Sustained high levels of cortisol and other stress hormones may block the ability to remember important information, such as names or telephone numbers. People who reduce their levels of cortisol – with exercise, meditation or other pleasurable activities – are less likely to experience degenerative damage in the brain.

hasn't been determined, but Dr Birge advises patients to take 800 IU of vitamin E daily.

Enjoy citrus fruits. They're among the best sources of vitamin C, an antioxidant nutrient that promotes healthy blood flow by preventing cholesterol and other fatty substances from accumulating in blood vessels in the brain. Vitamin C also makes vitamin E work more effectively and improves its ability to block cell-damaging free radicals, says Dr Birge.

Add some folic acid (folate). In new research, older people with lower levels of the B vitamin folate in their blood found it harder to hold on to new information that was coming at them quickly.

'Folic acid is one of the most valuable nutrients you can take for healthy memory function throughout life,' says Dr Jay Lombard, director of the Brain Behavior Center in New York. Dr Lombard thinks that folic acid helps memory by 'recycling' chemicals that brain cells need to communicate and fighting artery plaque, which can reduce blood flow to the brain.

Pick the right pain reliever. If you take over-the-counter non-steroidal anti-inflammatory medication, such as ibuprofen, for the treatment of arthritis, it may delay the effects of memory loss. Although these drugs are readily available over the counter, they should not be taken without medical supervision. Older people are particularly sensitive to the drugs' effects on the stomach, which can result in bleeding ulcers.

Battle depression. It can make people feel tired, unfocused and mentally slow. In fact, depression in the elderly is often mistaken for Alzheimer's disease.

'Antidepressant medications do more than relieve the symptoms of depression,' says Dr Birge. They seem to affect the region of the brain (the hippocampus) that plays a key role in memory. 'They also may stimulate the generation of nerve cells,' he adds. By aiding in the repair of nerve cells, antidepressants may help restore memory and other mental functions that have degraded over time.

For more information on memory loss: Visit the website of the British Alzheimer's Society at www.alzheimers.org.uk; Alzheimer's Australia www.Alzheimers.org.au; Alzheimer's New Zealand, www.alzheimers.org.nz

when to see a doctor

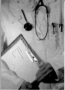

If your memory is progressively getting worse: see your doctor immediately. Memory declines may be caused by potentially serious – and treatable – conditions, such as depression, thyroid disorders or nutritional deficiencies.

If your memory gets worse and you're taking a new medication: many prescription drugs, including those used to control high blood pressure, may cause impairments in memory. Changing to a new drug will often resolve the problem.

phobias and panic attacks

Fear can save your life. When you see a suspicious stranger on the street or when a large, angry dog is coming your way, fear makes your heart beat faster and prepares your mind and muscles for action.

But irrational fear can wreak havoc on your life. Millions of women (and men) suffer from panic attacks – overwhelming sensations of anxiety that come without warning and for no good reason. Others are terrified by things that shouldn't be all that scary, like travelling in lifts or browsing in a busy shopping centre.

Doctors aren't sure what causes panic attacks. They're probably linked to disruptions in a part of the brain called the hippocampus. 'These are people who may be more sensitive than they should be to perceptions of potential danger,' says Dr Jack G. Modell, a professor of psychiatry.

If one or both of your parents suffered from phobias, you're more likely to have them, too.

Women may experience phobias more than men and tend to generally feel more vulnerable.

Don't allow your fears to take control of your life. With a combination of therapy, medication, and a variety of coping strategies, almost everyone can get them under control.

For Immediate Relief
HOME REMEDIES

Hold your breath for 10 seconds. 'It allows carbon dioxide to build up in the body, which reduces hyperventilation and other symptoms of anxiety for some people,' says Dr Kelly Conforti, a clinical psychologist.

Get up and leave. People tend to experience panic attacks at certain times or in certain situations, such as when they're in a crowded place. 'Just leaving the situation and going somewhere else can reduce levels of panic,' says Dr Modell.

THREE THINGS I TELL EVERY FEMALE PATIENT

DR KELLY CONFORTI, a clinical psychologist, gives the following advice for stopping panic attacks.

1

BREATHE SLOWLY AND DEEPLY. 'A lot of panic symptoms are triggered by hyperventilation,' Dr Conforti says. When you force yourself to breathe no more than eight to 12 times a minute, you'll reduce the amount of oxygen in your body, which will help stop you from hyperventilating.

2

BREATHE INTO A PAPER BAG. It increases blood levels of carbon dioxide, thereby reducing feelings of anxiety and panic.

3

DRINK LESS COFFEE. For some people, as little as 200 milligrams of caffeine – about the amount in two cups of coffee – can stimulate the feelings of panic attacks.

In the long run, it's better to get the problem under control than to 'run' when you start feeling anxious, Dr Modell adds. 'But to get relief from a particular attack, getting away is a reasonable thing to do.'

MIND-BODY TECHNIQUES

Play a mind game. Nearly everyone gets anxious when they feel that people around them are judgemental or dominant. 'Try imagining that the person is a turkey, or even the back end of a horse,' Dr Modell advises. 'You'll be less nervous when you take the situation less seriously and see the person in a different light.'

MEDICAL OPTIONS

Sedate your fears. If you need to occasionally get your fears under control – because you're about to take a plane trip, for example – ask your doctor if a sedative would help, Dr Modell suggests. Prescription sedatives won't eliminate fears, but they will temporarily reduce feelings of anxiety and help you cope with the moment. A sedative that is used for severe panic attacks is diazepam (Valium). This may cause drowsiness and driving impairment, so use with care, cautions Dr Modell.

Block panicky feelings. Many people avoid sedatives because they dislike feeling less alert than usual. An alternative is to take a prescription drug called a beta-blocker. 'Beta-blockers don't do much from the neck up, but they block the body's response to fear,' says Dr Modell. They may cause dizziness, he adds.

For Long-term Relief
HOME REMEDIES

Get to know what scares you. People are most frightened by things that seem unfamiliar and alien. Dr Modell advises women to learn everything they can about the things that frighten them most. If you're afraid of flying, read up on how aeroplanes work and what pilots do to control them. If you're afraid of spiders or snakes, learn about their natural habits. 'When you understand that snakes aren't going to run up and chase you, you'll realize that the fears may be excessive and unreasonable,' Dr Modell says.

when to see a doctor

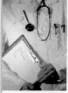

If your heart is racing, you're perspiring and you're having trouble breathing: seek urgent care immediately. The symptoms of panic attacks and heart attacks are very similar.

If you've just started having panic attacks, and you've never had them before: a number of medical problems, including hypoglycaemia (low blood sugar), can trigger symptoms that feel like panic. The side effects from some medications, including decongestants, can also simulate the sensations of panic attacks.

If you're having panic attacks more than a few times a month or if you've avoiding normal activities because you're afraid of attacks: you'll need to see a mental health professional, who will help you find ways to prevent anxiety from interfering with your life.

MEDICAL OPTIONS

✚ **Confront your fears.** One of the best ways to overcome phobias is with a technique called 'exposure and response prevention'. You'll work with a therapist or psychologist, who will expose you, in a slow and controlled way, to the things that scare you most.

Suppose you're afraid of spiders. Your therapist might begin by talking about spiders. Then she'll show you pictures of spiders. Finally, she might ask you to be in the same room with a spider.

'You gradually increase the intensity of the exposure while teaching coping skills,' Dr Conforti explains. About 80 per cent of those who practise this technique will experience partial or even total relief from their fears.

Consider SSRI antidepressants. Even if you don't suffer from depression, this type of medication (selective serotonin reuptake inhibitor) can help reduce the frequency and intensity of panic attacks and phobias. The drugs, usually Seroxat (paroxetine), are usually taken for about 6 months, at which point your doctor may wean you from the medication. In some cases, the panic attacks will stop for good, although many people will continue to take small doses of the medication to prevent recurrences.

For more information on phobias and panic attacks: Visit the website of Pax at www.panicattacks.co.uk or No Panic at www.no-panic.co.uk. Anxiety Treatment Australia www.anxietyaustralia.com.au. The Phobic Trust of New Zealand www.phobic.org.nz.

thinning hair

In some ways, women are luckier than men. Nearly all women will lose some of their hair over time, but they rarely develop bare spots. Even when their hair gets thinner, they can often disguise the changes by styling their hair differently or using shampoos and conditioners that 'bulk' the hair and make it look thicker. Another plus is that when a woman's hair thins, the front hairline isn't lost, as with the telltale receding hairline that many balding men experience.

Despite these benefits, however, thinning hair can be a devastating experience for many women.

'Even though they lose their hair differently, thinning hair may be more of a trauma for women because it is less socially acceptable,' says Dr Diana Bihova, a dermatologist. A number of different factors can contribute to hair loss in women, but fortunately there are options that can help slow, stop or reverse thinning hair, or at least minimize its appearance.

It's normal for a woman to lose anywhere from 50 to 100 hairs daily. The hairs are usually replaced by new ones, which grow at the rate of about $\frac{1}{2}$ inch a month. As women get older and their oestrogen levels fall, the rate of hair loss may slightly exceed the pace of replacement. Known as androgenetic alopecia, this type of hair loss is caused by a combination of genetic factors and high levels of androgens circulating in the blood, which are hormones that affect hair follicles, says Dr Bihova.

Trauma from accidents, divorce and other stressful events – as well as physical problems, such as anaemia, liver or hypothyroid disease – may cause hair to get thinner.

Solving hair loss problems involves addressing the underlying medical problem, as well as caring for your hair to minimize the visual impact of your condition.

For Immediate Relief
HOME REMEDIES

Change your hair colour. The chemicals in hair colours slightly roughen the surface of each hair. This gives hair more body, makes it look fuller, and helps disguise thin spots.

Women who have fine hair to begin with should choose lighter hair colours. Light browns or blondes will blend with the colour of the scalp and make the hair appear thicker.

Add highlights. It is a good idea to highlight your hair because it creates a sense of depth and makes the hair appear fuller.

Or use lowlights. Adding streaks of a colour that is a shade or two darker than your natural hair colour creates the optical illusion that your hair is thicker than it really is.

Wash your hair less often. Every time you shampoo your hair, the cleansing agents remove oils and cause the hair to lie flatter.

If you wash your hair a little less often, perhaps two or three times a week, it will have a little more body and fullness. This is most effective if you have normal or dry hair. If it tends to be oily, wash your hair daily, as usual, and add styling gel before blow-drying to give extra body.

Use protein-based conditioners. Check the label for ingredients called hydrolyzed animal proteins. Known as thickeners, the proteins coat the hair shafts and give the hair more thickness and heft.

Women whose hair is thinning should use a lightweight conditioner. The lighter products don't bring the hair down next to the scalp as much as heavier conditioners.

Finish with a cold rinse. After washing and conditioning your hair, adjust the temperature so that cool water soaks your hair for a few minutes. A cold rinse seals in some of the conditioner, which will give your hair additional body and shine.

Put hair mousse to use. Mousse is a lightweight styling gel that adds a thin, oily coating to the hair shafts and makes them appear fuller.

Wear your hair shorter. One of the best things women can do is wear a shorter cut and perhaps perm it. When the hair is shorter, it's a little more curly and is less likely to lie against the scalp and reveal the thin spots.

Go for a natural look. Consider wearing your hair a little more messy and tousled, rather than always having it smoothly combed. Try a layered look or a shorter blunt cut. That will make it look fuller than before.

Use a blow-dryer. It roughens up the hair shafts and also causes the hair to rise higher off the scalp. To avoid damaging the hair shafts, set the dryer on 'low' and hold it 15 to 25 centimetres (6 to 10 inches) away from your hair.

ALTERNATIVE THERAPIES

Finish with a vinegar rinse. White vinegar makes hair shiny and gives it a thicker appearance. Mix 1 tablespoon of white vinegar and a pint of water in a spray bottle. Spritz it on after you've shampooed and conditioned your hair. Leave it on for about 3 minutes, then rinse.

If you're concerned that the rinse may leave you smelling like a salad, use chamomile tea instead of water. Soaking a chamomile tea bag in warm water before adding the vinegar really reduces the smell significantly and, as a bonus, seems to give more shine to the hair.

Long-term Solutions
HOME REMEDIES

Eat a balanced diet. Women who go on crash diets, or those with eating disorders or other conditions that affect the body's intake of nutrients, may experience hair loss, says Dr Bihova. Protein and iron are especially important for the hair to grow normally.

The best sources of protein include lean meats, low-fat dairy foods, and pulses and whole grains. For iron, enjoy lean meats and fish, and fortified cereal products.

MEDICAL OPTIONS

Use minoxidil. Available over the counter, minoxidil (such as Regaine and generic brands) is an effective treatment for androgenetic alopecia.

'About a third of the people who use it will grow new hair, and another third will maintain the hair they have,' says Dr Bihova.

Available as a liquid, minoxidil is rubbed into the scalp twice daily. It's not an instant cure, Dr Bihova adds. In fact, she recommends seeing a

when to see a doctor

If your hair is thinning and you're premenopausal: see a dermatologist. Younger women who experience hair loss may have medical problems, such as hypothyroid disease or dermatological problems.

If you're taking a new medication and you're losing hair: a number of prescription and over-the-counter drugs – including diuretics, thyroid medication and even ibuprofen – may trigger hair loss in some people.

If the hair loss occurs suddenly and you've developed bare patches: you could have a condition called alopecia areata, which is thought to be linked to family history as well as stress. This condition is often temporary, and your hair may start to grow back within a few months.

If your hair loss is a serious concern to you: it seems that the stress some women experience due to thinning hair problems can create a vicious cycle that only contributes to increased hair loss.

dermatologist for a correct diagnosis of your hair-thinning problem because while minoxidil works for many people, it won't help at all if you don't have androgenetic alopecia. Some women who use minoxidil may start to see results in about 3 months, but for others it may take as long as a year, says Dr Bihova.

When using minoxidil, be careful to keep it off your face, Dr Bihova warns. 'It may cause facial hair growth if you get it on your facial skin.'

MIND-BODY TECHNIQUES

Unload some of the stress in your life. In order to conserve energy during stressful times, your body may slow the rate of hair growth. If you're burning the candle at both ends or dealing with stressful life events, you may want to spend some time unwinding with meditation, regular exercise and other relaxing activities.

urinary incontinence

Women who have gone through pregnancy and childbirth sometimes joke about the frequency of their toilet visits. What they don't laugh about – or in some cases even discuss with their doctors – are the embarrassing 'leaks' that may occur when they sneeze, laugh or bend over to pick up a sock.

'Women might start noticing small stains or dampness on their underwear,' says Dr Gary Lemack, an assistant professor of urology. 'The leaks happen suddenly, usually with strenuous activity, such as lifting heavy objects.'

It is estimated that up to one in three women suffers from urinary incontinence, which is the inability to completely control the flow of urine. Incontinence often occurs after childbirth or menopause because women may lose strength in the muscles (the pelvic floor muscles) that support the bladder. The muscles that surround the urethra, the tube that carries urine from the body, can also weaken over time.

If this is happening to you, don't put up with it. Incontinence is *always* caused by underlying physical problems. Incontinence may clear up on its own, but often it doesn't. The good news is that about 80 per cent of women can reduce or eliminate incontinence with a combination of medical treatments and home care strategies.

For Immediate Relief
HOME REMEDIES

Put your bladder on a schedule. 'Go to the toilet every 2 hours, even if you don't feel like you have to go,' says Dr Lemack. Women who practise 'timed voiding' are less likely to leak urine accidentally.

Drink less coffee. Or at least switch to decaf. The caffeine in coffee and other drinks increases the body's output of urine. Caffeine also stimulates bladder contractions, which can lead to unexpected leaks, says Dr Lily A. Arya, an assistant professor of urogynaecology. She advises limiting caffeine intake to 200 milligrams daily, which is the equivalent of two 180-millilitre (6-fluid-ounce) cups of coffee.

Use a tampon. If you find that you frequently leak urine when you cough, sneeze or exercise, you might want to use a tampon even when you're not having your period. Tampons provide extra support for the bladder, which can prevent urine from escaping, says Dr Mary Jane Minkin, clinical professor of obstetrics and gynaecology at Yale University School of Medicine. Follow the guidelines inside the pack for how long you can safely wear a tampon without increasing your risk of toxic shock syndrome – usually 4 to 8 hours.

Use pads as necessary. You don't want to depend on absorbent pads, such as sanitary towels, because they don't solve the underlying problem. But if you find that you're nervous about having 'accidents', absorbent pads can give you the confidence you need to get out and about. They're also helpful as an interim measure when you're working with your doctor to get your bladder under control.

Control allergies. Women who suffer from hay fever or other allergies may have flare-ups of incontinence due to coughing or sneezing. It's worth trying over-the-counter antihistamines during the allergy season, says Dr Lemack.

MEDICAL OPTIONS

Discuss medication with your doctor. If you're taking diuretics (water pills) for high blood pressure or other conditions, you may have more trouble controlling your bladder. 'Changing to a different drug or changing the timing of taking the drug may be helpful,' says Dr Lemack.

Tighten the urethra. If you've lost strength in

THREE THINGS I TELL EVERY FEMALE PATIENT

DR GARY LEMACK, an assistant professor of urology, gives the following advice for coping with incontinence.

1 KEEP A 'VOIDING' DIARY. For several weeks, record your bladder 'habits'. Write down how often (and how much) you drink, how many times you urinate, and how many 'accidents' you have. The diary will help your doctor determine the best course of treatment.

2 DO KEGEL (PELVIC FLOOR) EXERCISES DAILY. Do Kegels in conjunction with the voiding diary in order to measure progress.

3 CONSIDER YOUR GOALS. For some women, the treatments used to control incontinence are more inconvenient than the symptoms themselves. If your goal is complete dryness, you may need to consider surgery or other medical treatments. On the other hand, if the leaks only happen once or twice a week, you might want to stick with simpler treatments, such as Kegels or the occasional use of pads.

the urethra, your doctor may recommend peri-urethral injections, which add bulk to the tissue and increase urinary control. The injections are effective, but they may have to be repeated over time, says Dr Lemack.

Consider a pessary. Made of rubber, a pessary is a device that slips inside the vagina and helps support the bladder. 'Some are also designed to press the urethra, which can give additional control,' says Dr Morse. 'Pessaries are helpful in some cases, but most women will gain better control with other methods.' You'll need to speak to your doctor about whether a pessary is right for you.

Long-term Solutions
HOME REMEDIES

 Squeeze in some muscle training. One of the most effective strategies both for treating and preventing incontinence is to strengthen the pelvic floor muscles, says Dr Morse. These are the same muscles you use when stopping urine flow in midstream.

All you have to do is clench and relax the muscles about 10 times, and repeat the series three times daily. The great thing about these pelvic floor exercises, called Kegel exercises, is that you can do them any time: when you're lying in bed, watching TV, or standing in a queue at the supermarket.

Tighten at the right time. Kegel exercises are used mainly to prevent incontinence, but you can also use them to stop leaks before they start.

'That means contracting your pelvic floor muscles in anticipation of a cough, laugh or sneeze to prevent urine from leaking out, says Dr Linda Brubaker, a urogynaecologist.

Practise with vaginal weights. The tricky part about Kegels is working out which muscles you need to contract. Your doctor may recommend vaginal weights, which slip inside the vagina, as a training tool. If you aren't clenching the right muscles, the weights will slip out, Dr Minkin explains.

Meet up with a urinary 'coach'. 'For younger women, who are unlikely to have nerve damage or severe incontinence, I encourage going to physical therapy for pelvic floor muscle training,' says Dr Morse. 'In many cases they'll gain enough control to be satisfied with the results.'

Maintain a healthy weight. Women who have too much padding around the middle may have excessive pressure on the bladder. Losing weight – by exercising regularly, reducing the amount of fat in the diet, and eating more fruit and vegetables – may reduce the pressure and improve urinary control, says Dr Lemack.

when to see a doctor

If the leaks are accompanied by sudden, uncontrollable urges to urinate: see your doctor. You could have a urinary tract infection that's irritating the bladder.

If you're leaking urine and you also have pelvic pressure or lower back pain: you could have a condition called cystocele, which occurs when weakened pelvic floor muscles allow the bladder to sag into the vagina.

MEDICAL OPTIONS

✚ **Consider electrical stimulation.** There's some evidence that applying mild doses of electrical stimulation can strengthen muscles and improve the bladder's 'holding' ability. A probe is temporarily placed in the vagina or rectum, and precise amounts of electricity are applied to stimulate the nearby muscles, including those surrounding the urethra, Dr Morse explains. You'll learn how to use the device at a gynaecology clinic, then you'll be able take it home to use on a daily basis.

Supplement your body's oestrogen. The reductions in oestrogen that occur at menopause can result in weakness in the urethra or bladder. 'I will often start patients on an oestrogen suppository or cream if they have evidence of vaginal weakness,' says Dr Lemack.

For more information on urinary incontinence: visit the website of the Continence Foundation at www.continence-foundation.org.uk; the Continence Foundation of Australia at www.contfound.org-au; or the New Zealand Continence Association website at www.continence.org.nz.

urinary tract infections

About the only good thing you can say about urinary tract infections is that they're easy to treat and rarely serious.

The bad news is that they're extremely common. One in five women will get a urinary tract infection (UTI) at some time in her life, and some women get them again and again.

UTIs that occur in the bladder are called cystitis. Those that affect the urethra (the tube through which urine leaves the body) are called urethritis, and infections in the kidneys (the most serious kind) are called pyelonephritis.

UTIs usually occur when bacteria that live around the anus gain entry to the urethra and begin to multiply. Sexual intercourse is a common cause of UTIs, but women who aren't sexually active get them, too. The risk of infections rises after menopause, when declines in the body's oestrogen levels make tissues in the vagina and urethra more vulnerable to bacterial assaults.

If you suspect that you have a UTI, you'll want to call or see your doctor straight away. You can 'diagnose' some UTIs based on symptoms alone; typical symptoms for cystitis, for example, include a burning sensation while urinating and a powerful urge to urinate even after you've urinated. But your doctor may need to perform tests to ensure that the infection hasn't spread to other parts of the body, explains Dr Sanjay Saint, an assistant professor of medicine.

Once you start taking antibiotics, the discomfort will usually disappear within a day or two, Dr Saint adds. After that, you can plan a strategy to prevent infections from coming back.

For Immediate Relief

HOME REMEDIES

Ease discomfort with heat. Placing a hot-water bottle or heating pad on your lower abdomen will relieve uncomfortable cramps or pressure while you're waiting for antibiotics to take effect, says Dr Larrian Gillespie, president of Healthy Life Publications in Beverly Hills.

Avoid coffee or alcohol for a few days. They can irritate the urinary tract when you have an infection. Coffee and other beverages with caffeine also stimulate urination, which can increase discomfort, says Dr Gillespie.

ALTERNATIVE THERAPIES

Avoid acidic foods. Orange juice, strawberries, vinegar and other foods with a high acid content may create a more favourable environment for bacteria in the bladder, says Dr Gillespie.

'Eating these foods when you have an infection can increase the irritation,' she adds.

Put aside the soy sauce. Along with bananas, nuts, cheese and wine, it contains biogenic amines, amino acids that affect sensory nerve fibres in the bladder. Eating these foods when you have an infection may increase urinary 'urgency', says Dr Gillespie.

MEDICAL OPTIONS

Ask your doctor about supplemental hormones. If you're past the menopause and have been getting frequent infections, you may be a good candidate for hormone replacement therapy. Taking low doses of oestradiol, a form of oestrogen, strengthens tissues in the urethra and vagina and helps prevent infections, says Dr Gillespie.

Long-term Solutions

HOME REMEDIES

Wash away bacteria. Removing bacteria from the area around the urethra is among the best strategies for preventing UTIs,

TWO THINGS I TELL EVERY FEMALE PATIENT

DR LARRIAN GILLESPIE, president of Healthy Life Publications, gives the following advice for dealing with urinary tract infections (UTIs).

1 **DON'T WAIT TO TAKE ANTIBIOTICS.** They're extremely effective at stopping UTIs. Most women can be treated with a single 'triple dose', which is more convenient than the older, week-long regimes.

2 **DRINK BAKING SODA (BICARBONATE OF SODA) MIXED WITH WATER.** 'It makes the urine more alkaline for about 24 hours, which takes away the acid environment that bacteria need to multiply,' says Dr Gillespie. When you first notice symptoms, mix 1/4 teaspoon of bicarbonate of soda in a glass of water and drink it once daily until your symptoms have improved, she advises.

says Dr Mary Jane Minkin, clinical professor of obstetrics and gynaecology at Yale University School of Medicine.

Make sure you wash the genital area before having sex – and remember to urinate before and after intercourse. After going to the toilet, wipe from front to back. This helps ensure that anal bacteria don't get moved towards the urethral opening.

Consider alternative forms of birth control. Women who use diaphragms have a higher risk of UTIs. If you use a diaphragm and have recurrent infections, discuss alternative forms of birth control with your doctor.

Drink eight glasses of water daily. Water won't stop an infection in progress, but it dilutes the urine and reduces the concentration of infection-causing bacteria, says Dr Gillespie. Drinking water also promotes urination, which helps remove bacteria from the bladder.

Stay clean naturally. The use of douches, deodorant sprays and other 'feminine' products can irritate the urethra and promote infections. Washing with soap and water is more effective and less irritating.

ALTERNATIVE THERAPIES

Drink a glass of cranberry juice daily. Cranberry juice contains chemical compounds called proanthocyanidins, which help prevent bacteria from sticking to cells in the urinary tract. Blueberries contain the same helpful substances, says Dr Minkin.

when to see a doctor

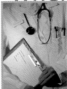

If you have pain in the abdomen and loins, difficulty urinating, a burning sensation when you urinate or frequent urges to urinate: see a doctor straight away. These are classic symptoms of urinary tract infections.

If you have a pain in the loins, fever, chills or nausea that accompanies the typical symptoms of a UTI: you could have a potentially serious kidney infection called pyelonephritis and must see a doctor right away.

If you feel pressure in the lower abdomen, and the urine has a strong smell: the infection could be in the bladder, a condition called cystitis.

MEDICAL OPTIONS

Arrange a plan with your doctor. UTIs respond quickly to antibiotics, but you can get them only with a prescription – which means that you have to put up with symptoms until you can see your doctor. Women who get frequent UTIs sometimes arrange for their doctors to prescribe antibiotics over the telephone when symptoms first appear. This is a reasonable approach if the infections are uncomplicated and your doctor is familiar with your health history, says Dr Saint.

Dr Saint led a study that looked at nearly 4,000 women with uncomplicated UTIs. The researchers found that those who had telephone consultations with their doctors did just as well as those who came into the surgery for an examination.

vaginal dryness

At the menopause, a woman's ovaries stop making oestrogen, the hormone that stimulates the vaginal glands to produce lubricating moisture. The tissues lining the vagina therefore become thinner, and the vagina may become dry enough to make sex uncomfortable.

'In addition to discomfort during intercourse, a woman who's menopausal may have a higher risk of vaginal infections because the natural vaginal environment changes,' adds Dr Debra Papa, an assistant professor of obstetrics and gynaecology. Also, the thinning of vaginal tissues makes women more susceptible to irritation or trauma, which may provide a gateway for an infection.

Women sometimes reach for petroleum jelly (Vaseline) when they're feeling dry, but it's not a good choice: it acts as an irritant in the vagina.

Here are some better ways to enhance moisture and maintain your natural lubrication.

For Immediate Relief
HOME REMEDIES

Use a water-based lubricant. Available over the counter, lubricants such as Astroglide and Replens help prevent dryness by replenishing moisture in the vagina. This reduces irritation and itching and decreases friction during intercourse, says Dr Papa. They're also safe to use with condoms.

Product ingredients vary, so it's best to follow instructions on the package on how to apply.

Switch tampons. Many premenopausal women find that vaginal dryness makes the use of tampons difficult or painful. You may want to try a brand that uses a cardboard or plastic applicator. Or use one that has a slimmer shape or a rounder tip, suggests Dr Mary Jane Minkin, clinical professor of obstetrics and gynaecology at Yale University School of Medicine.

To reduce irritation, it's fine to dab the tampon with a small amount of a water-based lubricant, Dr Minkin adds.

Long-term Solutions
HOME REMEDIES

Stay sexually active. Having sex regularly maintains the elasticity of the vaginal tissues, which get dry at menopause.

Put out the cigarettes. Smoking constricts blood vessels and reduces vaginal circulation, which can cause a decrease in lubrication, says Dr Papa.

MEDICAL OPTIONS

Use an oestrogen cream. Available by prescription, oestrogen creams are applied directly to the vagina. They relieve dryness by strengthening vaginal tissue and promoting the ability of the glands to secrete adequate amounts of moisture, says Dr Papa.

The creams initially need to be applied daily for several weeks, Dr Papa advises. Then they're usually used two or three times a week. Follow your doctor's instructions or those that come in the package for dosage.

Use an oestrogen ring. Oestrogen creams are messy and inconvenient to apply, which is why some women opt for an oestrogen ring. A diaphragm-like device, the ring is kept in the vagina for up to 3 months. It releases steady amounts of oestrogen, keeping the vaginal environment healthy.

Consider oral oestrogen. The medication in vaginal creams and rings mainly stays in the vagina – only small amounts go on to enter the bloodstream.

If you're postmenopausal, your doctor may recommend that you take oral oestrogen. Along with relieving vaginal dryness, supplemental oestrogen helps prevent hot flushes and osteoporosis, a disease in which bones gradually become fragile and more likely to break. It may also help you to guard against heart disease. Women who still have a uterus need to take a

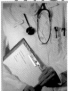

when to see a doctor

If you're getting recurrent infections: visit your doctor. Changes in the vagina's natural acidity can make women more prone to yeast and other infections.

If you're experiencing dryness even though you're premenopausal: vaginal dryness is not a common complaint in younger women. If you're premenopausal and sex is uncomfortable for you, discuss this with your doctor.

progestin, along with oestrogen, to offset the effects oestrogen has on the lining of the uterus, Dr Papa adds.

For more information about vaginal dryness and other conditions associated with menopause: Visit the website of the Amarant Trust in the UK at www.amarantmenopausetrust.org.uk; or the Australian Menopause Society at www.menopause.org.au.

vaginal infections

The tropical rain forests are home to more species of life than any other location on earth. There's something about the warm, moist environments that allow many of nature's creatures to thrive.

Closer to home, quite a few organisms also thrive in a hothouse environment – which is why most women will get a vaginal infection at some time in their lives.

'The vaginal environment usually prevents infections by maintaining a balance between normal organisms and those that can cause infection,' explains Dr Debra Papa, anassistant professor of obstetrics and gynaecology.

A fungus called *Candida albicans*, for example, is often present in the vagina. When the conditions are right, it can multiply out of control and cause a yeast infection. It is estimated that at least 75 per cent of women will get at least one yeast infection in their lifetime.

Infections can also be caused by bacteria, viruses, parasites and species of fungus that are not the *albicans* type. Some infections are transmitted sexually. Others occur when offending germs on the outside of the body manage to get inside. An infection can also be a result of a disturbance in the vaginal environment due to antibiotics, douches, hormones or stress. Regardless of how you get them, vaginal infections often cause a discharge along with intense irritation, itching and odour.

Most vaginal infections can be treated with antifungal creams, antibiotics or other medications. In addition, there are things you can do to reduce the discomfort and prevent the infections from coming back.

For Immediate Relief
HOME REMEDIES

Enjoy an oatmeal bath. Add colloidal oatmeal (such as Aveeno) to a warm bath and soak for a while. 'Yeast infections especially can be pretty severe and intense,' says Dr Papa. 'An oatmeal bath won't stop the infection, but it will relieve the itching and burning.'

Let air circulate. Stay out of tight clothing while the infection is healing, Dr Papa advises. At home, don't wear underwear under your skirt. 'You want to keep the area dry, which will reduce the irritation,' she says.

Sleep in just your nightie. Sleeping without underwear under your nightgown allows the area to 'breathe', which reduces irritation and also makes it more difficult for yeast or other moisture-loving organisms to thrive.

Use a hair dryer. 'When you have an infection, rubbing yourself dry with a towel can be uncomfortable,' Dr Papa says. She advises drying yourself with a hair dryer – set on low, of course.

MEDICAL OPTIONS

Start with a checkup. If you've never had a vaginal infection before, don't assume that your symptoms are caused by yeast. Studies have shown that women often misdiagnose what they believe to be a yeast infection, which means that you could have a more serious infection that requires medical care.

Choose your medication. If you've had yeast infections in the past and you're sure that's what you have, it's fine to use an over-the-counter medication to treat it. Except in rare cases when yeast infections are caused by 'resistant' organisms in the vagina, over-the-counter products work well, says Dr Meg Autry, assistant professor of obstetrics and gynaecology.

There are a number of products to choose from: creams or pessaries. The active ingredient usually will be clotrimazole (such as Canesten). These products are effective for most *Candida albicans* infections. Just make sure you read the label. Different products may require that you use them for different lengths of time.

For most women, the 3-day treatments work just as well as those that are used for 7 days, Dr Autry adds. Although, she continues, 'A woman might have a species of yeast that can't be killed in 3 days.' If your infection doesn't clear up after 3 days, you can try a 7-day product. If that doesn't work, you'll definitely need to see your doctor.

Reduce discomfort with a local steroid cream. The burning and itching sensations of yeast infections sometimes last for a week or more, even after using medication. To ease discomfort in the mean time, you may try an over-the-counter cream containing hydrocortisone (such as Dermacort). Your doctor may also prescribe a combination medicine, such as Dactacort, to treat the infection and relieve symptoms at the same time. These contain both a steroid and an antifungal.

Get a prescription. If your infection is caused by a resistant strain of yeast or other organisms, you'll probably need to take a prescription medication. For trichomoniasis, a sexually transmitted infection caused by a tiny parasite, *Trichomonas vaginalis*, your doctor may advise you to take oral metronidazole (Flagyl). Bacterial infections can also be treated with metronidazole. Resistant strains of yeast usually succumb to a drug called Gyno-Daktarin (miconazole).

For Long-term Relief
HOME REMEDIES

Wash with plain water. Nearly everyone enjoys scented soaps and bath oil, but you should avoid using these products even when you don't have an infection. The chemicals in them can irritate the vulval tissues (the external parts of the genitals) and cause scratching. This may make it easier for infections to establish themselves, says Dr Papa. Douches, too, can be irritating, so if you feel you must douche, use plain vinegar and water, advises Dr Papa.

Change into something dry. After swimming or working out, try to change into dry clothing

THREE THINGS I TELL EVERY FEMALE PATIENT

DR MEG AUTRY, an assistant professor of obstetrics and gynaecology, gives the following advice to women who suffer from vaginal infections.

1

NEVER DOUCHE. 'It's always bad,' says Dr Autry. 'It changes the vaginal environment, and it also increases the risk of upper genital infections. There's some evidence that it may increase the risk of ovarian cancer as well.'

2

BE GENEROUS WITH ANTIFUNGAL CREAMS. It's not uncommon for women with yeast infections to have inflammation outside the vagina. When applying a medicated cream, you may need to put it outside as well as inside the vagina.

3

GET CHECKED FOR DIABETES if you have frequent infections. This is especially true if you have any of the risk factors for diabetes, such as being overweight or having a family history of the disease.

immediately afterwards. It will make the vulval and vaginal areas less hospitable to yeast.

Wear cotton underwear. Unlike nylon and other synthetic fabrics, cotton allows air to get in and moisture to get out, which can reduce your risk of infections. If you wear tights, use the ones with cotton crotches. It's also a good idea to always wear comfortable, not tight-fitting, clothing.

Wipe microbes away. Vaginal infections can occur when bacteria that live around the anus migrate into the vaginal area. One way to prevent this is to wipe from front to back after urinating or having a bowel movement, says Dr Papa.

Keep your blood sugar under control. Women with diabetes have an increased risk of

vaginal yeast infections because they may have higher-than-normal levels of glucose (blood sugar), which can change the vagina's protective balance.

If you have diabetes, keeping your blood sugar levels stable – by eating a healthy diet, controlling your weight and using medication, if necessary – is helpful in preventing infections from getting started, says Dr Papa.

ALTERNATIVE THERAPIES

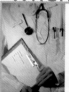 **Prevent infections with yoghurt.** Eating yoghurt won't stop a yeast infection that's already in progress, but there's some evidence that it may reduce the risk of getting them in the future.

'The acidophilus in yoghurt changes the vaginal pH,' says Dr Autry. In addition, when you eat yoghurt that contains live bacterial cultures, the 'good' organisms migrate into the vaginal canal and inhibit the growth of yeast. It may be especially helpful to eat yoghurt when you're taking antibiotics. It replenishes the healthy organisms that are killed by the medication.

One 6-month study found that women who ate 240 millilitres (8 fluid ounces) of live-culture yoghurt daily were much less likely to develop yeast infections than those who didn't eat yoghurt. 'If you have recurrent infections, including yoghurt in your diet is a good approach,' says Dr Autry.

Munch on mushrooms. In a small study, maitake, a delectable Japanese mushroom with scientifically proven immune-enhancing abilities, significantly eased the uncomfortable symptoms of chronic yeast infections in all but one of the 13 women who participated in the study.

when to see a doctor

If you get recurrent infections or have symptoms that don't improve after treatment with over-the-counter products: you may have a strain of yeast that requires treatment with prescription medication. You may also have a type of vaginal infection other than that caused by yeast.

If you develop a greenish or yellow discharge or lower abdominal pain: you could have a vaginal infection, one of which is called trichomoniasis, a sexually transmitted disease.

If you get a vaginal infection after having a new sex partner or if you've had multiple partners prior to the infection: any symptom should be evaluated by your doctor.

'The real culprit in chronic yeast infections is a depressed immune system, which I find to be a common problem for women who undergo constant stress,' says herbalist Douglas Schar, who conducted the study in his London clinic.

'In my experience, raising a woman's immune function makes her less susceptible to chronic yeast infections.'

Maitake is well-known for its ability to increase immune cell count and activity. In addition, it contains compounds that specifically inhibit or destroy *Candida albicans*, the organism that causes vaginal yeast infections. But watch out for some unwanted side effects: mannitol, the natural sugar found in maitake, causes flatulence and intestinal discomfort in some people.

MEDICAL OPTIONS

Take care around your period. 'The risk of almost all vaginal infections increases around the time of a woman's period because blood is an excellent culture medium,' says Dr Autry. 'Sometimes women who get chronic infections may benefit from fluconazole (Diflucan) towards the end of their periods as a preventive measure.'

varicose veins

Women are much more prone to varicose veins than men, possibly because the female hormones oestrogen and progesterone gradually weaken the vein walls, eventually reducing their ability to move blood uphill. No one knows the exact cause of this condition, but several factors may play a role. Women with a family history of varicose veins are much more likely to get them. Other factors that may cause or aggravate varicose veins include pregnancy, a lack of exercise, standing or sitting for long periods of time, crossing your legs and obesity. 'By the time they're in their fifties, nearly one in two women will have to contend with varicose veins,' says Dr Luis Navarro, director of the Vein Treatment Center in New York.

The veins in the legs are in a constant struggle with gravity. It's easy for venous blood, the blood that's going back to the heart, to circulate from other parts of the body because the route it follows is usually downhill. But the venous blood that travels from the leg veins has to make an arduous uphill journey in order to reach the heart. Sometimes the trip takes longer. If portions of the leg veins are weaker than they should be, or if tiny valves in the veins malfunction, blood tends to pool in the leg veins, causing them to bulge like little balloons. These areas of 'stagnant' blood are called varicose veins.

Most varicose veins are the small, 'spider' variety. They are blue or red in colour and can resemble a tree branch or spider's web. These veins cover areas that range from very small to very large. Located close to the surface of the skin, they are usually found on the legs or face but may occur anywhere on the body and often coincide with larger varicose veins. Although spider veins may be unattractive, they rarely cause discomfort and you can pretty much ignore them.

Larger varicose veins, however, make the legs feel tired and sore. These blue, dark purple or green veins may be raised above the skin's surface and are found most often on the backs of the calves or on the insides of the legs, anywhere from the groin to the ankle. They may be quite ropy, or bulging. In some cases the veins cause swelling in the legs or feet or around the ankles. Excess fluid leaks from the blood vessels into the tissues around the veins. The tissues become fragile, and the skin appears thin and may be inflamed. Open ulcers or sores may form and heal slowly.

Once varicose veins have formed, the only way to get rid of them is with surgery or other medical treatments. Most women don't need to do this because the discomfort of varicose veins, assuming there is any, can easily be managed with home remedies.

For Immediate Relief
HOME REMEDIES

Change positions often. Varicose veins tend to cause the most discomfort when women have been standing or sitting for a long time, which allows the blood to pool. 'Get up from your chair, or just get moving if you're standing, and walk around for a few minutes every 1 to 2 hours,' Dr Navarro suggests. 'When you move, the calf muscles flex against the veins, which gets the venous circulation moving again.'

Elevate your legs. When you raise your legs above the heart, blood that's pooled in the veins flows back into circulation, says Dr Navarro. 'You can put a couple of bricks or books under the legs at the foot of the bed, which will give some elevation. You can also sleep with a pillow or two under your feet. This will take the pressure off the veins and prevent the blood from pooling in the lower extremities.' Putting your legs up while you're reading or watching TV is a good idea, too.

Wear compression or support stockings. Available from doctors and in pharmacies, shops that carry medical supplies and department stores, compression stockings put precise amounts of pressure against the leg veins, which can reduce painful swelling. Compression stockings also help prevent varicose veins from getting worse.

'They essentially add an extra layer of muscle to your leg, which helps the calf and foot muscles move blood upwards to the heart,' says Dr Navarro. Two good brands of compression stockings are Scholl and Activa.

When buying compression stockings, here are a few things to keep in mind.

- Different stockings provide different amounts of compression, which is measured in millimetres of mercury (mmHg). For spider veins, you'll need stockings with moderate compression (15 to 20 mmHg). If the veins are bulging, use stockings with more compression (20 to 30 mmHg).

- Compression stockings come in different lengths: calf only, which extend to the knee;

mid-thigh, which reach to the upper third of the thigh; full-thigh, which extend to the groin; and full-length tights. Choose a length that covers all of the veins that you want to compress.

ALTERNATIVE THERAPIES

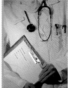 **Take horse chestnut.** Available in health food shops, this herb strengthens veins that have lost their elasticity, which can help ease discomfort. A number of studies have shown that women who take 250 to 312.5 milligrams of the standardized extract of horse chestnut twice daily will have considerable relief from symptoms.

MEDICAL OPTIONS

Consider injections. If your legs keep hurting no matter what you do or if you're simply tired of looking at the unsightly veins, your doctor may recommend a procedure called sclerotherapy, in which a solution is injected into the varicose veins. The solution irritates the inner lining of the blood vessels, making the veins swell, close and eventually disappear. This treatment can be used to eliminate both varicose and spider veins, as long as the main leg vein is not involved.

Apart from the tiny prick of the needle, sclerotherapy is almost painless, although you may have some cramping for a day or two afterwards. Since new veins may form, sclerotherapy is usually repeated every 2 to 4 years.

Talk to your doctor about other options. Doctors have recently developed a technique called the endolaser procedure, which uses lasers

when to see a doctor

If leg pain wakes you up at night or if the area around the varicose veins is swelling, itching or scaling: make an appointment to see your doctor. It's possible that the tissues around the veins aren't getting enough blood and oxygen, or you may have circulatory or arterial problems. You may need medical treatment to remove or seal the veins.

to seal and shrink the varicose veins, says Dr Navarro. 'It's done using a local anaesthetic,' he explains, 'and is used, when the main vein of the leg is affected, as a way to avoid surgery.' At present, this can only be done privately.

Varicose veins involving the main vein of the leg can also be shut down with the use of radio waves. Again, this procedure is only done privately at present.

In some cases, doctors advise removing the veins surgically. This is a more extensive procedure than simply sealing the veins, and it's usually recommended for large varicose veins that can't be controlled with other treatments.

For Long-term Prevention
HOME REMEDIES

Exercise often. 'It's my number-one tip for preventing varicose veins,' says Dr Navarro. 'Try to exercise for 30 minutes at least three times a week. I recommend walking, running, swimming, cycling, yoga, dancing and t'ai chi. They are all great for circulation and building up the calf muscles.'

Do toe raises. It's a good exercise for strengthening muscles in the feet and calves and also for removing pooled blood from the veins. Put your hand on a wall for support, and rise on your toes, as far as you can go. Hold the stretch for a moment, then lower yourself back down. 'Do this for 5 to 10 minutes every day,' suggests Dr Navarro.

Get plenty of fibre in your diet. Women who eat a lot of whole grains, pulses and other fibre-rich foods are much less likely to get constipated. This is important because constipation causes straining, which puts extra pressure on the leg veins.

While some studies have not found a consistent relationship between fibre, constipation and the presence or severity of varicose veins, other research suggests that the diet of industrialized countries may be a risk factor.

'Studies have shown that in countries where people eat diets that are rich in fibre, the incidence of varicose veins is low,' says Dr Navarro. 'When the same people come to Western countries and adopt a low-fibre diet, they have the same risk of developing varicose veins as the rest of the population.' The recommended amount of fibre is 12 to 24 grams daily. All plant foods contain fibre. Some of the best include beans, peas, fruit, potatoes (with the skins on), berries and whole grain breakfast cereals, such as Bran Flakes.

Eat less salt. The average Westerner consumes around 3,000 milligrams of sodium daily, a lot more than the recommended daily amount of 2,400 milligrams. 'Consuming a lot of high-sodium foods causes inflammation and swelling, which makes the discomfort of varicose veins worse,' says Dr Navarro.

He advises women to buy low-sodium packaged foods and to avoid high-salt foods, such as salami and fast foods.

MEDICAL OPTIONS

Ask your doctor to check your medication. Women who take supplemental hormones – either in the form of birth control or as hormone replacement therapy – sometimes develop varicose veins. Taking a lower dose will often provide the same benefits, but without the side effects, says Dr Navarro.

For more information about varicose veins: Visit the NHS Direct Online Health Encyclopaedia in the UK at www.nhsdirect.nhs.uk; or the Health Network in Australia at www.healthnetwork.com.au.

Get fit forever with
exercise

Exercise can help you in so many ways. From increasing your feeling of wellbeing to improving your fitness, exercise is the easiest route to optimum health. And it doesn't necessarily mean hitting the gym. The exercises on the pages that follow can be performed in your own home or at the pool and can help to ease and prevent common ailments such as back pain and arthritis. Follow these simple routines to strengthen and tone your whole body.

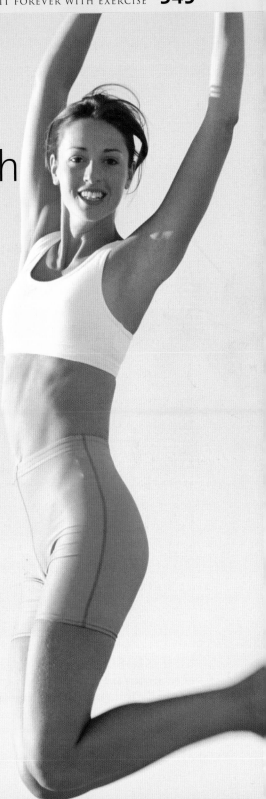

Aim for
strength

Strong, flat abs don't just look great. They also improve your posture and protect your back. Try these exercises recommended to trim and tone your tummy. *(Note:* If you experience back pain while doing any of these exercises, stop and check with your doctor before continuing.)

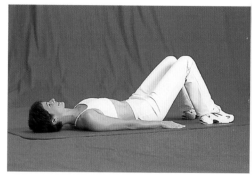

Pelvic Tilt

Lie on the floor with your arms at your sides, knees bent and feet flat on the floor. Press your lower back to the floor so that your pelvis tilts upwards. Straighten your legs by slowly sliding your heels along the floor, and stop when you can no longer hold a full tilt position; hold for a count of six. Next, move one leg at a time back to the starting position, maintaining the pelvic tilt throughout. Hold the starting position for six counts, then relax.

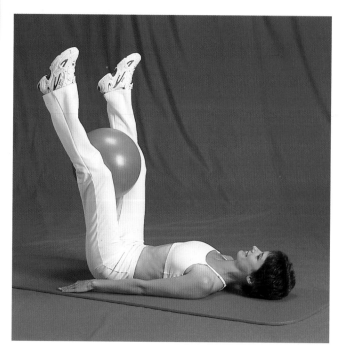

Leg Raise

Lie on the floor and raise your legs straight up. Place an exercise ball between your knees, then do a slight pelvic tilt from the hips. Squeeze the exercise ball for 1 second, then relax.

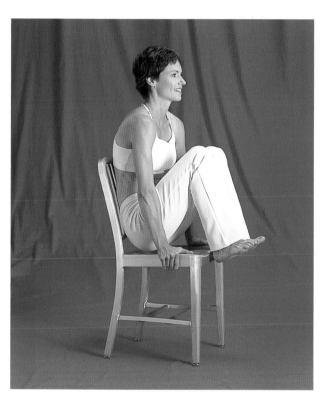

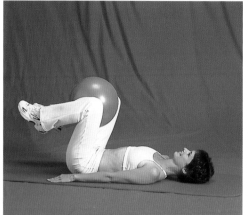

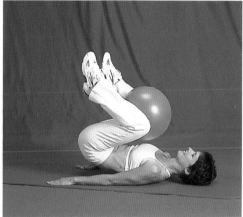

Seated Body Lift

Sit erect in a firm, armless chair and place your
hands on the sides of the chair in front of your hips.
Tighten your abs and support yourself with your
hands as you slowly pull your knees up towards your
chest. Keep your lower back against the chair back.
Hold and then slowly lower. (This move is more
easily performed without shoes.)

Hip Raise

Lie on the floor and place an exercise ball
between your bent knees (top). Lift your hips off
the floor, and bring your knees towards your
chest (bottom). Squeeze the ball for 1 second,
then relax.

Aim for
strength

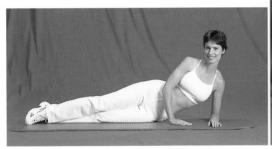

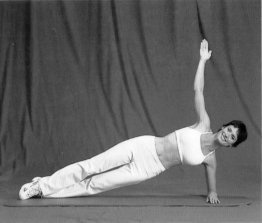

Side Body Lift

Lie on your left side, supporting your upper body on your left elbow, forearm and hand. Your elbow should be directly under your shoulder (left). Slowly lift the rest of your body off the floor so only your forearm and feet are on the floor (right). (Use the other arm for balance. For an advanced move, hold that arm straight up in the air.) For maximum effect, keep your body as straight as possible. Hold for as long as is comfortable or until you can no longer maintain good form, then slowly lower and relax. Repeat on the other side.

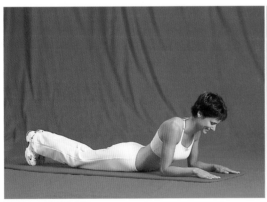

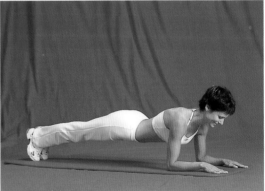

Front Body Lift

Lie face down on the floor, supporting your upper body on your elbows, forearms and hands (left). Slowly lift the rest of your body off the floor until you're balanced on your toes (right). Keep your body straight, and hold for as long as is comfortable, then slowly lower and relax.

Warm up to
water walking

When you have arthritis, warm-water exercise can encourage stiff joints to become more flexible and can relax tight muscles. The buoyancy of the water supports the joints.

A warm-up is essential to prevent pain and injury for all exercisers, but especially for people with arthritis. We recommend starting with the following set of full-body range-of-motion exercises on this and the following spread, done in a pool to increase flexibility. Do these before and after the water walking routine described on page 352.

The warm-up: walk into the water to chest height. (The body part you're working on should be underwater. You'll need to go deeper or crouch down to get your shoulders underwater when doing the first exercise.) Do all of these moves slowly, and never stretch to the point of pain or discomfort. Do at least three repetitions of each, but depending on your individual needs and condition, you can do as many as 10 reps of any move to help loosen a stiff joint. Repeat the entire set of exercises to cool down after your water-walking workout.

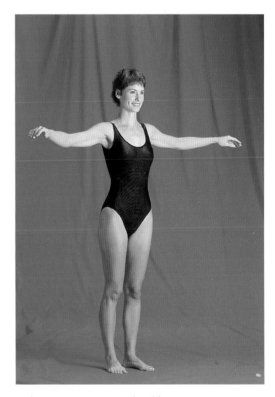

Swing your arms out to the sides.

Warm up to
water
walking

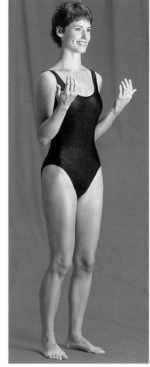

Bend your elbows.

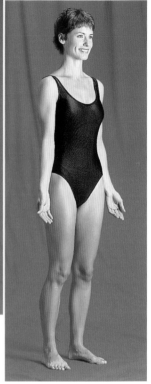

Straighten your elbows.

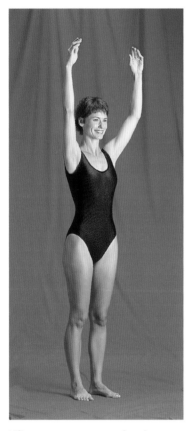

Lift your arms over your head.

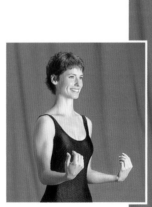

Bend your wrists.

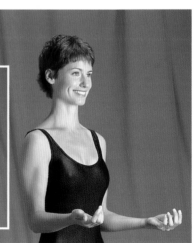

Straighten your wrists.

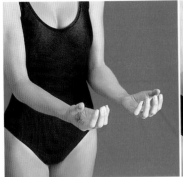 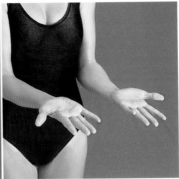

Hold each hand in a loose fist with fingers bent.

Straighten your fingers.

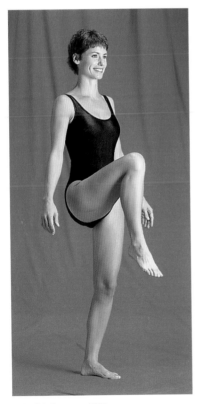

Take high steps, lifting your raised knee towards your chest.

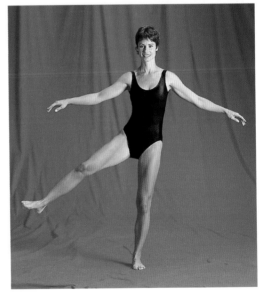

Standing on one leg, swing the other leg out to the side; then switch sides.

Warm up to
water walking

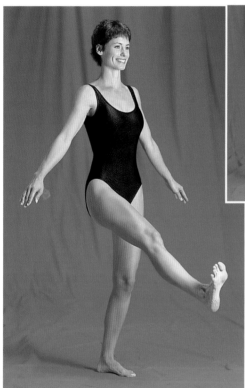

Flex each ankle.

Extend each ankle.

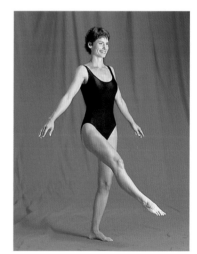

Swing each ankle in a circle.

The exercise: After completing the warm-up routine shown in this photo series, you're ready to exercise. Standing in water that's between hip and waist deep, start walking and swinging your arms. Start slowly, then pick up speed and work up to a comfortable, brisk pace. Start with 5 minutes, then gradually increase the time until you feel it could be rated as moderate, which is described as anywhere from 'still light but starting to work' or 'still comfortable but harder' to 'getting to be somewhat hard'. Do the workout three to five times a week.

strengthen
your back muscles

People who stay in shape don't necessarily have a lower risk for back pain, but they do tend to recover more quickly from back attacks than those who are sedentary and out of shape, says Dr Stephen Hochschuler, a back specialist.

Opposite Arm and Leg Lift

One of the best exercises for your back is also the simplest. It's called opposite arm and leg lift, and it strengthens the abdominal muscles as well as those in the back. It protects the spine and also improves your posture.

When doing the exercise, try to complete 8 to 12 'lifts' with each arm and leg. Rest a moment, then repeat the series again. Doing the exercise two or three times a week will keep your muscles strong and flexible.

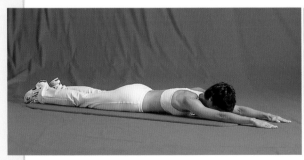

Lie face down with your legs extended straight behind you, toes pointed, and your arms extended straight over your head. Keep your chin up off the floor at a comfortable level.

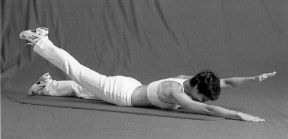

Slowly raise your left arm and your right leg at the same time until they are both a few inches off the floor. Hold, then slowly lower them back to the starting position. Repeat on the other side.

The best exercises for
preventing
back pain

You need to strengthen your abdominal and back muscles in order to support and protect the spine. It's also important to stretch the hamstrings (the muscles in the back of the thighs) and hips. The following exercises will go a long way towards keeping your back strong and pain-free.

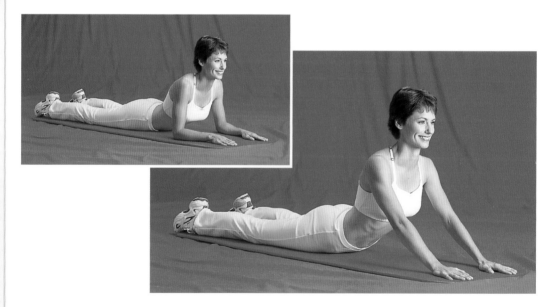

Back Extension

Lie on your stomach. Keeping your hips on the floor, prop yourself up on your forearms and raise your chest (left). Hold the stretch for a few seconds, then raise your upper body by straightening your elbows and arching your back (right). Go as far as you comfortably can, hold the position for 10 seconds, then relax.

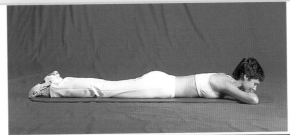

Chest Lift

Lie on your stomach with your hands under your chin (top). Lift your head and feet about 2.5 to 5 centimetres (1 to 2 inches) off the floor; don't arch your back too much (bottom). Hold the position for a few seconds, then lower yourself.

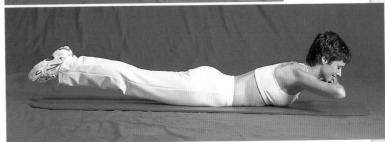

Bridge Lift

Lie on your back with your knees bent and your arms at your sides (top). Slowly lift your pelvis and buttocks off the floor (bottom), hold for about 5 seconds, then lower yourself.

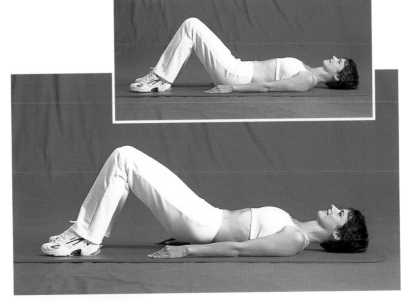

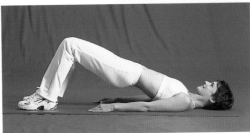

As you get stronger, try to lift your torso until there's a straight line between your knees and shoulders.

The best exercises for
preventing
back pain

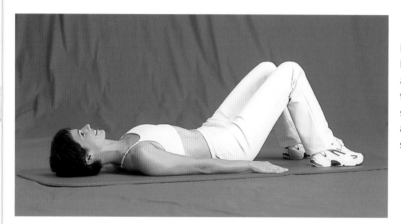

Pelvic Tuck

Lie on your back with your knees bent. Tighten the abdominal muscles and tilt the pelvis upwards until the small of your back presses against the floor. Hold for 5 seconds, then relax.

Mini-crunch

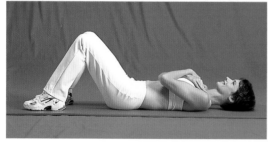 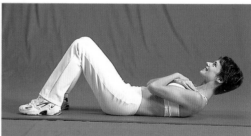

Lie on your back with your knees bent and your arms crossed on your chest (left). Slowly lift your head and shoulders until your shoulder blades come off the floor; don't bend your neck (right). Hold the position for a few seconds, then lower yourself.

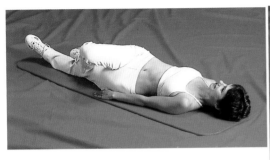 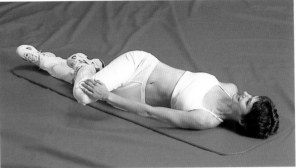

Hip Stretch

Lie on your back with your legs straight. Bend your right leg so it crosses over the left, keeping your foot near your left knee (left). Using your left hand, gently press your right knee towards the floor until you feel a stretch in your right hip and buttocks (right). Hold the stretch for 10 to 30 seconds, then relax. Repeat the exercise with the left leg.

Hamstring Stretch

Lie flat on your back with your legs bent and both feet on the floor. Loop a towel or rope under the arch of your left foot. While keeping a slight bend at the knee, straighten and raise your left leg off the floor and gently pull your leg towards your chest as far as is comfortable. Hold for 10 to 30 seconds, then relax. Repeat on the other leg.

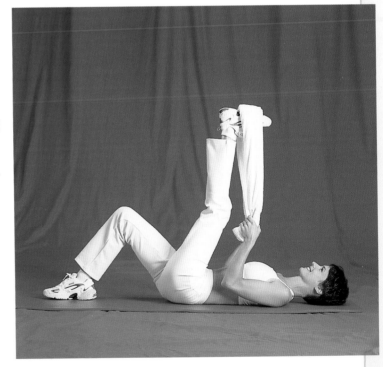

Guidelines for Safe Use of Supplements

Vitamin and Mineral Supplements

Although serious side effects from vitamin and mineral supplements are not common, they can happen. The guidelines presented here are designed to help you use the supplements mentioned in this book safely and wisely.

You should talk to your doctor before using any supplement if you have a chronic illness requiring medical supervision or medication. In fact, if you have any type of health problem, your doctor or pharmacist needs to know about any supplements you're taking before treating you with a prescription or over-the-counter medicine. If you are a woman who is pregnant, breast-feeding or attempting to conceive, do not use supplements unless under the supervision of your doctor.

The vitamin and mineral doses listed below are the Reference Nutrient Intakes (RNI), the UK Department of Health's recommended daily allowance of nutrients sufficient for every individual. Also given below are the safe upper limits for adults, above which harmful side effects can occur. These amounts are the total from both food and supplements. Do not take more than the safe upper limit of any vitamin or mineral without first consulting your doctor. (Note: mg = milligrams; mcg = micrograms; IU = international units.)

Nutrient	Reference Nutrient Intake (RNI)	Safe Upper Limit	Cautions and Other Information
CALCIUM	700 mg	1,500 mg	Taking more than 1,500 mg a day can cause serious side effects such as kidney damage. For best absorption, avoid taking more than 500 mg at one time. If you are over 50, look for a formula that contains vitamin D with calcium since you may need more vitamin D than is supplied by a multivitamin alone. Some natural sources of calcium, such as bonemeal and dolomite, may be contaminated with lead and other dangerous or undesirable metals.
FOLATE	200 mcg for women + 100 mcg for pregnant women	1.5 mg	Folate supplementation before and during pregnancy can help to prevent birth defects.
IRON	14.8 mg for women 19–50 yrs 8.7 mg for women 50+ yrs	17 mg	Iron supplements of 20 mg or more can be toxic in children, with doses of 200–300 mg proving fatal. Adults with haemochromatosis (high iron absorption) should avoid iron supplementation.

Nutrient	Reference Nutrient Intake (RNI)	Safe Upper Limit	Cautions and Other Information
MAGNESIUM	270 mg for women	400 mg	Check with your doctor before beginning supplementation in any amount if you have heart or kidney problems. Doses exceeding 400 mg a day can cause diarrhoea in some people.
PANTOTHENIC ACID	no UK RNI	210 mg	A healthy, balanced diet provides enough of this nutrient to meet your body's needs.
SELENIUM	60 mcg women	0.45 mg	Taking more than 0.45 mg a day can cause dizziness, nausea, hair or nail loss, or a garlic odour on the breath or skin.
VITAMIN A	600 mcg for women	1,500 mcg	Not suitable for pregnant women or those wishing to become pregnant. Excessive intakes in all adults can cause liver and bone damage, hair loss, double vision and vomiting.
VITAMIN B_1 (Thiamin)	0.8 mg for women	100 mg	High intakes can be toxic, giving rise to headaches, irritability, insomnia and rapid pulse.
VITAMIN B_2 (Riboflavin)	1.1 mg for women	43 mg	
VITAMIN B_3 (Niacin)	13 mg for women 19–50 yrs 12 mg for women 50+ yrs	17 mg	High doses may cause flushing and may impede liver function.
VITAMIN B_6 (pyridoxine)	1.2 mg women	10 mg	Taking more than 10 mg a day can cause reversible nerve damage. When selecting a B-complex supplement, check the label for the amount of each ingredient to help you determine its safe use.
VITAMIN B_{12}	1.5 mcg women	2mg	Supplementation is useful for strict vegetarians and vegans who eat few or no animal products.
VITAMIN C	40 mg	1,000 mg	Taking more than 1,000 mg a day can cause diarrhoea in some people. To help maintain levels of vitamin C throughout the day, take half of the recommended dose in the morning and half at night.
VITAMIN D	400 IU (for over 65s, in pregnancy, during lactation, and people with no exposure to sunlight)	1,000 IU (or 0.025 mg)	Taking more than 1,000 IU a day can cause headache, fatigue, nausea, diarrhoea or loss of appetite.
VITAMIN E	Safe intakes are: 3 mg women	800 IU (or 540mg)	Because it acts like a blood thinner, consult your doctor before taking vitamin E if you are already taking aspirin or a blood-thinning medication, such as warfarin.
ZINC	7 mg women	25 mg	Taking more than 25 mg a day can cause nausea, dizziness or vomiting. When levels of zinc are elevated, the absorption of copper can become impaired.

Emerging Supplements

Reports of adverse effects from emerging supplements are rare, especially when compared with prescription drugs, and supplement manufacturers are required by law to provide information on labels about reasonably safe recommended dosages for healthy individuals. Be aware that the potency and dosing strategy can vary significantly among products.

You should note, however, that little scientific research exists to assess the safety or long-term effects of many emerging supplements, and some supplements can complicate existing conditions or cause allergic reactions in some people. For these reasons, you should always check with your doctor before taking any supplements.

We recommend that you take supplements with food for best absorption and to avoid stomach irritation, unless otherwise directed. Never take them as a substitute for a healthy diet since they do not provide all the nutritional benefits of whole foods.

And, if you are pregnant, breast-feeding or attempting to conceive, do not use supplements without the supervision of a doctor.

Supplement	Safe-use Guidelines and Possible Side Effects
COENZYME Q_{10}	Discuss supplementation with your doctor if you are taking the blood thinner warfarin. On rare occasions coenzyme Q_{10} may reduce the effectiveness of warfarin. Side effects are rare but include heartburn, nausea or stomach upset, which can be prevented by consuming the supplement with a meal.
EPA (fish oil)	Do not take if any of the following apply: bleeding disorder, uncontrolled high blood pressure, use of anticoagulants (blood thinners) or aspirin, allergy to any kind of fish. People with diabetes should not take fish oil because of its high fat content. Increases bleeding time, possibly resulting in nosebleeds and easy bruising, and may cause upset stomach. Take fish oil, not fish liver oil, because fish liver oil is high in vitamins A and D – toxic in high amounts.
FIBRE e.g. bran	Do not take if you are allergic to the source of fibre in the supplement, such as wheat or psyllium. Take under the supervision of your doctor if you have diverticulitis, ulcerative colitis, Crohn's disease, bowel obstruction or any serious gastrointestinal disorder, or if you are taking any medication. May cause flatulence or bloating.
FLAXSEED (LINSEED)	If you are on medication, check with your doctor before supplementing with flaxseed because it may negatively affect absorption. Do not take if you have a bowel obstruction.
GLUCOSAMINE	May cause stomach upset, heartburn or diarrhoea.
GLUTAMINE	Available mainly at gyms and online. If you have problems with your kidneys or liver, check with your doctor before supplementing.
QUERCETIN (bioflavonoid)	Available online. In some people, doses above 100 mg may dilate blood vessels and cause blood thinning. Should be avoided by individuals at risk for low blood pressure or problems with blood clotting.

Converting Calories to Kilojoules

CALORIES X 4.186 = KILOJOULES

CALORIES	KILOJOULES (kJ)
1	4.186
10	41.86
25	104.65
50	209.3
75	313.95
100	418.6
200	837.2
300	1255.8
400	1674.4
500	2093.0
600	2511.6
700	2930.2
800	3348.8
900	3767.4
1000	4186.0

Board of Advisors

Dr Rosemary Agostini, primary care sports medicine physician at the Virginia Mason Sports Medicine Center and clinical associate professor of orthopaedics at the University of Washington, both in Seattle

Dr Barbara D. Bartlik, clinical assistant professor in the department of psychiatry at Weill Medical College of Cornell University and assistant attending psychiatrist at the New York–Presbyterian Hospital, both in New York City

Dr Georges C. Benjamin, secretary for the Maryland department of health and mental hygiene in Baltimore

Dr Mary Ruth Buchness, chief of dermatology at St Vincent's Hospital and Medical Center in New York City and associate professor of dermatology and medicine at the New York Medical College

Craig Cisar, Ph.D., professor of exercise physiology at San Jose State University in California, certified exercise test technologist, certified strength and conditioning specialist, and certified personal trainer

Dr Robert DiBianco, director of cardiovascular research at the risk factor reduction and heart failure clinics at Washington Adventist Hospital, and associate clinical professor of medicine at Georgetown University School of Medicine in Washington, D.C.

Dr Leah J. Dickstein, professor and associate chairperson for academic affairs in the department of psychiatry and behavioral sciences and associate dean for faculty and student advocacy at the University of Louisville School of Medicine in Kentucky and past president of the American Medical Women's Association (AMWA)

Dana S. Dunn, Ph.D., associate professor of psychology at Moravian College in Bethlehem, Pennsylvania

Dr David Edelberg, founder of the American WholeHealth Centers in Chicago, Denver and Bethesda, Maryland; section chief of holistic medicine at Illinois Masonic Medical Center and Grant Hospital in Chicago; and assistant professor of medicine at Rush Medical College in Chicago

Dr Jean L. Fourcroy, past president of the American Medical Women's Association (AMWA) and of the National Council on Women's Health

Dr Roger L. Gebhard, professor of medicine in the division of gastroenterology at the University of Minnesota and staff gastroenterologist at Regions Hospital, both in Minneapolis

Dr Gary N. Gross, clinical professor of medicine in the division of allergy and immunology at the University of Texas Southwestern Medical School in Dallas

Dr Scott Haldeman, clinical professor in the department of neurology at the University of California, and adjunct professor at the Los Angeles Chiropractic College

Dr Arthur I. Jacknowitz, professor and chairperson of the department of clinical pharmacy at West Virginia University

William J. Keller, Ph.D., professor and chairperson of the department of pharmaceutical sciences in the School of Pharmacy at Samford University

Robert D. Kerns, Ph.D., chief of the psychology service and director of the comprehensive pain management center at the VA Connecticut Health Care System and associate professor of psychiatry, neurology and psychology at Yale University

Photo Credits

Briony Chappell: Icons pages 151, 152, 154, 157

Nancy R. Cohen/Getty Images: Page 147

John Foxx/ImageState: Page 21

Jules Frazier/Getty Images: Page 102

Michelangelo Gratton/Digital Vision: Pages 99, 105, 106, 107, 111, 116, 122, 136, 137, 139, 141, 148, 155

Vincent Hazat/Photoalto: Page 23

Mitch Mandel/Rodale Images: Pages 67, 68, 69, 70, 72, 73, 74, 75, 76, 266, 267, 268, 269, 346, 347, 348, 349, 350, 351, 352, 353, 354, 355, 356, 357

Ryan McVay/Getty Images: Page 135, 242

Doug Menuez/Getty Images: Page 265

Daisuke Morita/Getty Images: Page 49

Jonelle Weaver/Getty Images: Page 51

BananaStock Ltd: Pages 2, 3, 4, 5, 10, 12, 13, 17, 22, 26, 29, 30, 31, 32, 33, 34, 42, 63, 81, 84, 89, 92, 93, 95, 115,118, 120, 121, 127, 128, 131, 140, 176, 186, 198, 205, 214, 218, 220, 221, 233, 236, 253, 265, 274, 345

Brand X Pictures: Page 18, 52

Comstock: Page 230

Corbis: Pages 8, 79, 129

Digital Vision: Page 165, 240

EyeWire Collection: Page 14

Getty Images: Pages viii, 11, 15, 24, 28, ibid Part 5, 33, 35, 37, 39, 40, 41, 45, 64, 71, 80, 88, 91, 97, 98, 101, 103, 104, 108, 109, 113, 124, 130, 143, 151, 166, 170, 179, 227, 239, 260, 264, 271

Image 100/Royalty Free/Corbis: Page 142

Image Source: Page 78, 86, 273

Rubberball: Page 133

Stockbyte: Page 162

Stock Image/ImageState: Page 43, 83

Websters International Publishers: Page 47

Editorial Credits

Special thanks to Dr Doug Schar, Dr Tom Smith and Dr Michelle Stephenson for the expert advice they kindly provided on this book.

Index

Bold type indicates boxed text; *italics* indicate illustrated exercises

abdominal fat 276
    exercises for reducing *346–8*
ACE inhibitors 230
acne *see* blemishes
acupuncture
    for fibroids **183**
    to stop smoking 113
ageing 22–5, 48, 321
    and constipation 294
    effects of sun 116–17
    and pain relievers 324
    treatment for skin spots 127
    treatment for wrinkles 125–7
    when to go to casualty **25**
Agnus castus (vitex) 61, 156–7, 194, 213
agonists 183
AIDS **143**
alcohol
    and allergies 307
    calories in 86–7
    and cancer 47, 248
    good effects 35, 220
    and high blood pressure 228
    and HRT 206
    and infertility 173
    and osteoporosis 262
    at perimenopause 192
    in pregnancy 166–7
alkaloids 51
allergies
    anaphylaxis 306–9
    food allergies 306–9
    hidden allergens **308**
    nettle remedy 53
    and urinary incontinence 331

aloe 62
alpha lipoic acid 238
alpha/beta hydroxy acids 125–6
alternative therapies for:
    Alzheimer's 273
    back problems 288
    blemishes, pimples and spots 290
    diabetes 240–1
    endometriosis 187
    fatigue 301
    fibroids 182
    high blood pressure 228–9
    PMS 154–7
    thinning hair 329
    urinary tract infections 335
    varicose veins 343
Alzheimer's disease 270–3
    early diagnosis vital **272**
    focusing on fish **271**
    vitamins and 48
anaemia 281–3
    doctor's tips **279**
    when to see a doctor **278**
analgesics 292, 313, 324
androgens 212
angelica 60
angina **217**
anthraquinones 52
antibiotics 189, 191, 334, 335
antidepressants
    for fibromyalgia 305
    for hot flushes 197
    for irritable bowel syndrome 319
    for memory problems 324
    for phobias and panic attacks 327

anti–inflammatory drugs 286
antioxidants 23, 35, 36–8, **218**, 219, **223**, 245
anxiety *see* stress and anxiety
aquaerobics 305
arthritis 280–84
    doctor's tips **290**
    osteoarthritis 46, 281
    water walking exercises *349–52*
    when to see a doctor **281**
aspirin
    for back pain 286
    for breast pain 292
    against colon cancer **21**
    against heart disease 218–19
    for herpes **144**
    side effects **21**, 218
    against stroke 231
atherosclerosis 216

back problems 248–8
    and abdominal fat 276
    bending and lifting **8**
    doctor's tips **285**
    exercises for *353–7*
    in pregnancy 168
    when to see a doctor **284**
baking soda 334
barbecues 252
beans 88–9
beauty treatment 122–9
    anti–wrinkle products 125–7
    bleaches for skin spots 127
    cleansers 124
    doctor's tips **125**
    Retinova **123**
    masks and peels 127–9
    moisturizers 124–5
    puffy eye treatments 129
    use sunscreen with make–up 119–20, 123
benzoyl peroxide 289
beta–blockers 230, 341

bicarbonate of soda **334**
bilberry 60
biofeedback 295, 316
bipolar disorder **138**
birth control *see* contraception
bitters 51
black cohosh 61, 157, 194, 213
bladder irritation 320
    see also urinary...
blemishes, pimples and spots 289–91
    when to see a doctor **289**
blood glucose tests 9, 11, 15–16, 25
blood pressure
    understanding the numbers 225–6
    see also high blood pressure
blueberries 35, 323, 335
bone–density tests 12, 16, 20, 24
brain *see* Alzhiemer's; memory
breast cancer 247–50
    diet to protect from 35, 47, 247–8
    doctor's tips **248**
    HRT and 205, 206
    mammograms 12, 20–1, 25
    self–examination 9, 11–12, 16
    stress and **249**
breast pain and tenderness 291–2
    when to see a doctor **291**
bronchitis and smoking **110**
bupropion 112

caffeine *see* coffee and caffeine
calcium
    and bones/osteoporosis 10–11, 31, 44, 260–1
    and cancer 46, 252
    and depression 297
    and PMS 41, **154**
    in pregnancy **42**
    supplements 18–19, 40–1, 260–1, 358
    when calcium isn't good **19**
calories 14, 18, 29, 85–6, 227

scale of calories worked off by exercise 78
cancer 243–4
    pain **255**
    prevention 45–6, 54, 244–7
    a survivor's story **256**
    see also specific types
carbohydrates 29–30, **299**
cardiovascular disease *see* heart disease
carotenoids 33–4
cervical cancer 256–7
cervical smear (Pap) tests 9, 11–12, 16, 20, 25, 254, 257
chamomile 57, 58
chemo–prevention 250
chewing gum 276
childbirth
    birth plan 169–71
    Caesarian section 169
    episiotomy 170
    medications 169–70
    multiple births **175**
    when to see a doctor **171**
Chinese remedies 182, 337
    acupuncture 113, **183**
chlamydia 189
chocolate **218, 235**
cholesterol
    and free radicals 36
    and heart disease 223–4
    and high blood pressure 228
    lipid profiles 8, 11, 15, 20, 25
    and memory 321
    and reproductive health 111
    and smoking 110
chromium 43, 240
cinnamon 33, 56, 58, 233
clay paste 302
coenzyme Q10 221, 363
coffee and caffeine
    aid for memory 322
    and anaemia 279–80

and breast pain 292
and depression 296
and fibromyalgia 304
and headaches 315
and high blood pressure 228
and infertility 173
and irritable bowel syndrome 316
and osteoporosis 261
and panic attacks 325
and perimenopause 192
and sleep 102
and urinary incontinence 330
and urinary tract infections 334
cognitive therapy 318
colds 44–5
colorectal cancer 21, 25, 251–2
    rye protects against **253**
constipation 252, 293–6
    doctor's tips **293**
    and haemorrhoids 310
    herb for 55
    when to see a doctor **294**
contraception 158–63
    barrier methods 159–60
    condoms (male/female) 145, 158, 159, 160
    emergency 163
    intra–uterine devices 158–9, **161**, 162, **190**
    long–acting hormonal methods 161–2
    oral (the Pill) **146**, 157, 160–1, 179–80, 193, 194, 197–8, 253–4, 280
    symptothermal method 162–3
    tubal sterilization 162
    when to see a doctor **161**
    withdrawal method 162–3
copper 39, 48
cortisol 95, 100
cosmetics *see* beauty treatment
cramp bark 58
cranberry juice 321, 335
cucumber 129

dairy products 31
dang gui 156
dental health 43, **240**
    checkups 6, 11, 15, 20, 24
Depo-Provera 161
depression 296-8
    and diabetes **236**, 241
    doctor's tips **297**
    herbs for **55**
    and infertility 174
    and memory problems 324
    and perimenopause 198
    and PMS 157
    and smoking 111
    and stress 100
    vitamins for 48
    and weight 95-6
    when to see a doctor **296**
DHEA 213
diabetes 232-42
    alternative therapies 240-1
    blood glucose tests 9, 11, 15-16, 25
    cinnamon helps prevent **233**
    and depression **236**
    monitoring **234**
    diet and 237-8, **239**
    and pregnancy 165
    supplements for 238-40
    syndrome X 241-2
    television and **242**
    weight and exercise 235-7
    in young women 43
diet
    antioxidant-rich 23, 36-8
    and cancer prevention **246**
    carbohydrates 29-30, **299**
    DASH diet for hypertension 227, 228
    doctor's tips **38**
    and fertility 174
    fat *see* dietary fat
    forget fad diets **97**

    good-mood foods 5-6
    healthy snacks 91-2, 179
    nutritious 23, 28, **36-7**
    in pregnancy **42**, 167
    protein 31, 152-3
    superfoods 245
    vegan **34**, **239**
    vegetarian and plant based **34**, **156**, 182
    and weight *see* weight
    see also fibre; fruit and vegetables; supplements
dietary fat
    and Alzheimer's 271
    and breast cancer 248
    and colorectal cancer 252
    and heart disease 219
    and irritable bowel syndrome 316
    saturated/unsaturated 31-2
    and weight 89-90
dioxin 186-7
diuretics 151, 230
douches **190**, 339
drinking
    alcohol *see own heading*
    calories in drinks 86
    sugary drinks 238
    water *see own heading*

ectopic pregnancy 189
elderberry 54
electrical stimulation 347
electrocardiograms (ECGs) 8-9, 15
emotional balance 130-41
    anxiety management **140**
    anger management **133**
    bipolar disorder **138**
    doctor's tips **135**
    emotional quiz 131-4
    guilt management **136**
    hidden emotions 228-9
    meditation **139**

pockets of tranquillity 138–9
see also depression
emphysema and smoking **110**
endometrial cancer 252–4
endometriosis 185–8
    doctor's tips **186**
    evening primrose for **55**
    natural treatments **188**
    when to see a doctor **187**
energy, low 59, 198–9
EPA (fish oil) 362
epinephrine 307
essential oils 196, 302
evening primrose 55, 61, 152, **186**, 292
exercise 63–79
    for abdominal fat 277, *346–8*
    aerobic 71
    for Alzheimer's 273
    aquaerobics 305
    for arthritis *349–52*
    for back problems *353–7*
    for brain/mind 273, 321–2
    for endometriosis 186
    for fibromyalgia 316–18
    in forties 13–14
    for general fitness *67–70, 72–6*
    handy hints **65, 79, 93**
    for healthy heart 217–18
    and infertility 172
    for lung cancer 251
    making time 92–3
    for osteoporosis 262, *264–9*
    in pregnancy 166
    for stopping smoking 113
    for stress 106–7
    for urinary incontinence 331, 332
    for varicose veins 343–4
    walking *264*, 277, 287
    water–walking *286–9*, 287
eyes
    cataracts 46–7, 121

examinations 6, 11, 15, 20, 24
macular degeneration 60, 121
puffy eye treatments 129

fall prevention 19
fat *see* abdominal fat; dietary fat; weight
fatigue 311–15
    doctor's tips **299**
    thyroid and **301**
    when to see a doctor **300**
fever 56
feverfew 56, 327–8
fibre
    and cancer 247–8, 252
    and constipation **293**, 295
    and diabetes 238
    general benefits 14, 18, 33, 88–9
    and haemorrhoids 311
    and irritable bowel syndrome 317, 318
    as supplement 360
    and varicose veins 344
fibroids 181–4
    doctor's tips **182**
    when to see a doctor **184**
fibromyalgia (fibrositis) 302–305
    when to see a doctor **304**
fish
    and arthritis 282
    and cancer 245
    EPA (fish oil) 360
    focus on fish for Alzheimer's 271
    general benefits 32–3
    and heart disease 220
    and high blood pressure 228
flatulence 317
flavonoids 51, **218**
flaxseed 33, 55, 61, **186**, 220, 245, 295, 360
flu jabs 15, 21, 23
folate and folic acid 5, 10, 29, 42, 46, 47, 166,
    252, 324, 358
food *see* allergies; diet

free radicals 36–8, **218**, 219
fruit and vegetables
 and arthritis 282
 and cancer 247, 250–1
 general benefits 10–11, 30–1
 and memory problems 323
 superfoods 245
 and weight loss 87–9
furfuryladenine 126

garlic 33, 54, 245
ginger 56 *bis*
ginkgo 60 *bis*, 322
ginseng 53, 59
glucosamine 282–3, 360
glutamine 360
glycolic acid peel 128
goldenrod 62
gonadotropin–releasing hormone (GnRH) 183
gonorrhoea 189
gotu kola 62
grape seed extract 129
guggul 54
gums and resins 51

haemorrhoids 310–11
 when to see a doctor **310**
hair, thinning 327–30
 when to see a dermatologist **329**
hawthorn 55, 228
headaches 311–16
 herbs for 56–7
 when to see a doctor **224**
heart disease 216–24
 angina **217**
 food for **218**, 219–21
 herbs for 54–5
 when to see a doctor **224**
heat treatment 186, 190, 285, 293, 320, 334
height measurement 19–20
hepatitis 57

herbs 49–52
 caution in using 52
 doctor's tips **50**
 herb guide for various conditions 53–62
 for irritable bowel syndrome 317–18
 for PMS 156–7
herpes **144**
high blood pressure 225–31
 checks 7–8, 11, 15, 20, 24, 223, 229–30
 checks: understanding the numbers 225–6
 and memory 322
 and pregnancy 165
 prevention of 54–5
 stress and **229**
 when to see a doctor **231**
HIV/Aids **143**
hives 57
hormone replacement therapy (HRT) 193–4, 200–1
 and alcohol 206
 annual review 202–4
 and bones 207–8
 and cancer 204–6, 249–50, 252
 and depression 298
 and heart 206–7, 224
 progesterone in 253–4
 strategies **203**
 testosterone in 207–8
 types of 209–13
 when to see a doctor **202**
horse chestnut 343
hot flushes 194–7
human papillomavirus (HPV) 9, 257
huperzine 322–3
hydrogenated oils **90**
hypertension *see* high blood pressure
hypnosis 113, 319
hypothyroidism **82**
hysterectomy **182**, **183**, 184, 187–8

ibuprofen 151, 157, 272–3, 292

ice for pain 286
immune system 47
incontinence *see* urinary incontinence
infertility 10, 172–6
    doctor's tips **173**
    in vitro fertilization (IVF) 176
    multiple births **175**
    when to see a doctor **174**
inflammatory bowel disease **57**
insulin resistance 179, 235–6
    see also diabetes
intra–uterine devices 162, 187–8
in vitro fertilization (IVF) 176
ipriflavone 208
iron
    and anaemia 6–7, 279–80
    and fatigue/low energy 199, 299, 301–302
    in pregnancy **42**
    supplements 5, **34**, 39, 199, 358
irritable bowel syndrome **58**, 316–19
    doctor's tips **318**
    when to see a doctor **317**
isoflavones 35, 213
isotretinoin 290

Kegel (pelvic floor) exercises 331, 332
kidney infections 319–21
    when to see a doctor **320**
kidney stones 48

lactose intolerance 317
ladder of fitness 63–79
    exercises 67–70, 72–6
    scale of calories worked off **78**
laryngitis 58
laughter 105
lavender 302
laxatives 296
leptin 81
linseed 33, 55, 61, **186**, 220, 245, 295, 362
lipid profiles *see* cholesterol

lung cancer 250–1

magnesium 37–8, 41, 43, 44, 152, 240, 359
maitake mushrooms 54, 57, 340–41
mammograms 12, 20–1, 25
marriage **221**
massage 114, 303–304
meat 90, 279
meditation **139**, 155–6
melatonin **244**
memory problems 47–8, 321–4
    herb for 60
    when to see a doctor **324**
    see also Alzheimer's disease
menopause 17, 60–1, 200–2
    see also hormone replacement therapy; peri-
    menopause
menstruation
    breast pain and tenderness 303–5
    and endometriosis 185
    heavy periods **279**
    herbs for 60–1
    painful periods **174**
migraines 311–16
    foods associated with 315
    and stroke **231**
    when to see a doctor 312, **313**
milk thistle 241
mind–body techniques
    biofeedback 295
    manage negative thoughts 175, 298
    meditation **139**, 155–6
    mind games 326
    progressive relaxation 155, 241, 288, 315
    spirituality 222, 298
    visualization 174–5, 191
    yoga 304, 315
minerals 4–5, 28–48 *passim*
    see also specific types
minoxidil 329–30
mucilage 51

multivitamins 4–5
mushrooms 245, 340–41
myomectomy 183

nettle 53, 57
nicotine *see* smoking
NSAIDs 282, 284
nutrition *see* diet

obesity *see* weight
oestrogen
    creams and rings 198, 336–7
    guide to types 209–10, 211
    and hot flushes 196
    natural 17–18, 200
    in oral contraceptives 160
    and osteoporosis 207–8, 259, 262–3
    and PMS 152
    and urinary incontinence 334
    and uterine cancer 252–3
    see also hormone replacement therapy
oils, healing 153–4
olive oil 245
osteoarthritis *see* arthritis
osteoporosis 259–63
    bone–density tests 12, 16, 20, 24
    bone–strengthening exercises *264–9*
    bone–strengthening success story **263**
    doctor's tips **261**
    drugs guide 212
    exercise benefits 208
    height measurement 19–20
    and HRT 207–8
    prevention while young 43–4
ovarian cancer 16, 254–6
ovarian cysts 177–80

pain killers 286, 313, 324
panic attacks 325–7
    doctor's tips **325**
    when to see a doctor **326**

pantothenic acid 359
Pap (cervical smear) tests 9, 11–12, 16, 20, 25, 254, 257
passionflower 53, **318**
pelvic examinations 9, 11–12, 16, 20, 25
pelvic inflammatory disease 189–91
    doctor's tips **190**
    when to see a doctor **191**
peppermint 57, 58, 317–18
perimenopause 9–13, 16, 192–9
    doctor's tips **195**
    when to see a doctor **196**
    see also menopause
pessaries 332
pets 107
phobias 325–7
    doctor's tips **325**
    when to see a doctor **326**
phosphatidylserine (PS) 272, 323
phytonutrients 245
pica 283
pneumonia 24, 62
pollutants 186–7
polycystic ovary syndrome 177–80
    and diabetes 242
    doctor's tips **178**
    when to see a doctor **179**
    wrong foods for **180**
posture 202
potassium 34–5, 44
pregnancy 164–8
    and constipation 294
    ectopic 189
    gestational diabetes 233
    herbs should be avoided 52
    high–risk 165–6
    and iron levels 278
    miscarriage 166
    older mums 165–6
    supplements during **42**
premenstrual syndrome (PMS) 41, 150–7

doctor's tips **154**
new life story **153**
when to see a doctor **151**
progesterone 193–4, 196, 199, 211, 213, 253–4
progestogen 160, 206, 210
progressive relaxation 155, 241, 288, 315
prostaglandins 153–4, 285
protein 31, 152–3

qigong 182
quercetin 362

radon 251
reflexology 154–5
retinoids 257
Retinova **123**, 126
riboflavin 314
rosemary 57, 314
rye protects from colon cancer **253**

sage 61, 322
St John's wort 55, 297–8
salicylic acid 289
salt 33
    and high blood pressure 277–8
    and varicose veins 344
    and water retention 276
SAM–e supplement 283–4
saponins 51
saw palmetto 59
schisandra 59
selenium 37, 46, 361
serum ferritin tests 6–7, 11, 15, 20
sex, healthy 142–6
    doctor's tips **145**
    herpes **144**
    HIV/Aids **143**
    low sexual desire 59
    see also contraception; vaginal dryness
sexually transmitted infection (STI) 9, 189–91
    doctor's tips **190**

when to see a doctor **191**
skin
    blemishes, pimples and spots 289–91
    doctor's tips **117**, **119**, **120**, **121**
    cancer 7, 117–8, 257–8
    examinations 7, 11, 15, 20, 24
    herb treatments 62
    psoriasis **119**
    sun protection 116–21
    see also cosmetics
skullcap tea 53
sleep
    and back problems 286
    and fatigue 299
    and fibromyalgia 303, 305
    and headaches 315
    at perimenopause 199
    in pregnancy 168
    and stress **102**
    see also fatigue
smoking 108–15
    and bronchitis and emphysema **110**
    and cancer 250, 257
    and heart disease 218
    and high blood pressure 227
    and infertility 173
    nicotine replacement therapy 112
    and osteoporosis 262
    passive smoking 151–2
    in pregnancy 166–7
    and skin **109**
    and stroke 231
    and vaginal dryness 336
    vitamin C for smokers **32**
sodium see salt
soya foods 213
spinach 19
spirituality 222, 298
statins 206–7, **223**
steroid creams for vaginal infections 339
stress and anxiety 99–107

and acne 291
and Alzheimer's 273
and cancer 247
and diabetes 241
and endometriosis 187
and fatigue 299–300
five minutes tip **100**
and heart disease 222
herbs for 53
and high blood pressure **229**
restoring sleep **102**
and thinning hair 330
and weight 95–6
see also emotional balance
stress–echocardiogram tests 15
stroke 225, 230–1
when to see a doctor **231**
sugar **92,** 153
sugary drinks 238
sun
benefits 105, 216, 261
harmful effects on skin 116–21, 123
harmful effects on vision 121
and psoriasis **119**
and skin cancer 117–18, 123, 257–8
supplements 38–48
for Alzheimer's 271–2
for diabetes 238–40
doctor's tips **45**
for endometriosis **186**
guidelines for safe use 358–60
for healthy heart 221
minerals 4–5
multi 4–5, 245–6, 280
for osteoporosis 260–1
for PMS 152, 156–7
prenatal 173–4
probiotic 190–1
SAM–e 283–4
for vegetarians **34**
syndrome X 241–2

t'ai chi 182
tamoxifen 254
tampons 331, 336
tannins 51–2
tea
benefits of 35, 54
green tea 54, 245, 258
and infertility 173
tea bags for puffy eyes 129
see also coffee and caffeine
television and diabetes **242**
TENS (transcutaneous electrical nerve stimulator) 288
testosterone 177, 179, 180, 207–8, 212
tetanus jabs 7, 11, 15, 21–2, 24
thyme 62
thyroid problems 25, 146, 199
tomatoes 245
transferrin saturation tests 6–7, 11, 15, 20
tretinoin 126–7, 290

urinary incontinence 330–33
doctor's tips **331**
when to see a doctor **332**
urinary tract problems 333–5
doctor's tips **335**
herb for 62
when to see a doctor **334**
uterine artery embolization 184
uterine cancer 252–4

vaginal dryness 336–7
when to see a doctor **337**
vaginal infections 337–41
doctor's tips **339**
when to see a doctor **340**
valerian 53
vanadium 34
varicose veins 341–4
when to see a doctor **343**
vegan diet **34, 239**

vegetables *see* fruit and vegetables
vegetarian diet **34**, **156**
   and anaemia 278
vitamins
   A: 39, **42**, 359
   B complex: 41, **42**, 152, 221, 238
   B1 (thiamin): 359
   B2 (riboflavin): 314, 359
   B3 (niacin): 359
   B6 (pyridoxine): 41, 48, 152, 231, 359
   B12 : 19, **34**, 42, 47–8, 231, 278, 322, 359
   C: **32**, 36, 38, 39–40, 44–5, 46–7, 221, 238, 272, 324, 359
   D: 20, **34**, 40, **42**, 44, 46, 261, 282, 359
   E: 14, 29, 36, 38, 40, 45, 46, 47, 196, 221, 231, 238, 271–2, 282, 292, 323–4, 359
   K: 44
   see also supplements
vitex (Agnus castus) 61, 156–7, 194
volatile oils 51

walking *264*, 277, 282, 287
   water–walking *349–52*
water, drinking
   for bloating 276
   for constipation 295
   as diuretic 151
   for fatigue 302
   general benefits 86
   for haemorrhoids 311
   for headaches 314
   for kidney infections 320
   for memory loss 322
   for skin 123
   for urinary tract infections 335
   use filter 187
weight 80–98
   and arthritis **283**
   body mass index 83, 98, 216–17
   calorie control 14, 18
   and diabetes 235–7

   and dietary fat 89–90
   doctors' tips **84**, **87**
   and fatigue 302
   and fertility 10
   forget fad diets **97**
   and heart disease 216–17
   and high blood pressure 226–7
   if you could change only one thing **85**
   in middle age 13–14
   in pregnancy 166
   sugar and **92**
   thyroid and **82**
   and urinary incontinence 332
   and uterine cancer 253
   also exercise
willow bark 56, 288

yoga 304, 315
yoghurt 321, 340

zinc 37, 39, 359